PUBLIC
HEALTH
IN THE
AMERICAS

conceptual renewal,

performance assessment,

and bases for action

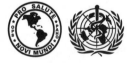

Pan American Health Organization
Pan American Sanitary Bureau,
Regional Office of the
World Health Organization

Pan American Health Organization

Public Health in the Americas.
Conceptual Renewal, Performance Assessment, and Bases for Action.
Washington, D.C.: OPS.

Scientific and Technical Publication No. 589

ISBN: 92 75 11589 3

I. Title   II. Author

1. Public Health
2. Steering Role of the Health Sector
3. Essential Public Health Functions (EPHF)
4. Public Health Workforce
5. Performance evaluation of health services
6. Techniques for evaluation

Book cover illustration: Gustav Klimt, Hygieia. Work/Art "Medicine". Ceiling panel for the Magnum Hall of the University of Vienna, 1900–1907. Oil on canvass 430 X 300 cm., destroyed in 1945 in the Immendorf Castle. Reproduced from the photographic archives by permission of ARTOTHEK. Hermfeldstrasse 8 D-82362 Weilheim, Germany.

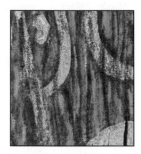

Preface

This book represents the realization of a dream of a work on public health in the Americas that was worthy of being a Centennial publication of the Pan American Health Organization (PAHO). I did not wish this to be a document that analyzed the data on the characteristics of the health of the people of Latin America and the Caribbean. There are other publications that will show in great detail the health situation and the trends that are occurring. Therefore, I am pleased that we have in this book, a work that reflects on the context in which public health is perceived and practiced and sets out the extent to which those functions that are essential to promoting and preserving the public's health are being discharged. No text on the people's health is definitive, it can at best be one of the rivulets that join but enrich the stream of thinking about one of the most important problems of our time-how to improve the health of our people, how to en-

sure that people enjoy that "possession" that is universally valued above all others.

It is proper and natural in considering this as a Centennial publication to revert at least briefly to our origins and the public health of that day. The nature of scientific knowledge of 100 years ago made it inevitable that the major concern would be for infectious diseases, and the appreciation that it was possible to control these through social and sanitary engineering in the widest sense, was a major development. There was no doubt about the role of the government in so modifying the environment that the health of the public would be improved. The data PAHO collected were related to infectious diseases and the possibility of informing decisions about quarantine measures.

But we live in different times. All our countries have undergone health tran-

sitions that have altered their epidemiological profiles. The nature of the burden of public ill health has changed. The data show clearly that it has been the discovery and use of technology that has played a major role in the improvement of the health indicators of populations. We have experienced the power of technology to add years to life, and in the enthusiasm for the magic of the technological imperative for individual benefit we have tended to lose sight of the difference between sick individuals and sick populations. The concern for the health of the public had been consumed by the fervor for individual care as the miracles of scientific research promised ever greater good for individual life and health.

We were witnesses to the growing concern in developed countries about the state of their public health enterprise even in the midst of a veritable cornucopia of scientific advances that augured so well for individual health. The enquiry in the United States showed a public health system in disarray and the situation was little better in the United Kingdom. Attracted as I was to the working definition of public health used in the latter study—"the science and art of preventing disease, prolonging life and promoting health through organized efforts of society," I expressed my disquiet as to whether in our Region we could indeed discern what were these organized efforts of society and how they were made operational. Rudolf Virchow is one of my heroes and many of my concerns of today can be found in his writings. In 1848, as he too agonized over the state of public health, he wrote:

"It is not enough for the government to safeguard the mere means of existence of its citizens, i.e. to assist everyone whose working capacity is not sufficient to make a living. The state must do more. It must help everyone to live a healthy life. This simply follows from the conception of the state as the moral unity of all individuals composing it, and from the obligation of universal solidarity."

We saw the call for solidarity take shape more recently in the call for equity, and this has been a value that has underpinned much of the reform of the health sector that is occupying the attention of almost all our governments. But in the reform movements that sought equity in the delivery of services needed to promote health and prevent illness, the focus was predominantly on the individual and there tended to be neglect of the health of the public. The organized efforts of society were not being focused on the public's health.

But in order to determine how these efforts should be directed, it is intuitively obvious that there must be some measure of the functions that the state must discharge if the public's health is to be promoted and avoidable illness prevented. We have posited repeatedly that the responsibility of the state and that of the government are not coterminous, and this book makes it clear that it is not only the government that has the sole and unique responsibility for discharging all these functions. But let us be clear that there are some that are indeed within the nondelegable responsibility of the government as the principal actor within the state.

The exercise of measuring the extent to which there are essential public health functions and they are being discharged, has been an open and participatory process as indeed any exercise of this nature must be. The selection of the functions is a result of repeated iterations and consultations as a basic premise that in this field there is no absolute truth. It is highly likely that there will be others in different places who will establish different functions as being essential to be discharged in the quest for improved public health. But what will stand is the concept behind the exercise, the methodology that sustains it and the basic and prosaic purpose of providing a measure that is useful for our countries in improving health.

It is especially gratifying to note the emphasis placed here on the acquisition of information, the role of epidemiology in establishing whether the functions are being discharged, and the definition of systems necessary to measure any change that might occur. It is epidemiology that forms the bridge between the concern for the individual and the wider public. PAHO was born out of a necessity for the collection and dissemination of information, and throughout its history there has been steady growth and maturation of the methods and systems for carrying out that pristine mandate. Now in PAHO's 100th year, this Centennial publication shown that provision of information about what is upon the people is the first of the essential public health functions. This certainly speaks to a continuity of focus and purpose.

This work by PAHO is intended mainly for the Americas, but we know that it has informed practice in other agencies and in other parts of the world. The spread of any approach opens one to wider critique, but that is healthy. Perhaps we should say as John Graunt did when he presented the famous Bills of Mortality:

"How far I have succeeded in the Premisses, I now offer to the world's censure. For herein I have like a silly Scholeboy, coming to say my Lesson to the World (that Peevish, and Techie Master) brought a bundle of Rods wherewith to be whipt, for every mistake I have committed."

Any mistakes that there may be are certainly not in the conceptualization of the functions that must be carried out by organized society to ensure the health of the public, nor the methods in applying the tools that have been developed in great part by the public.

I hope you enjoy this Centennial publication of the Pan American Health Organization.

George A.O. Alleyne
Director

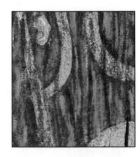

Contents

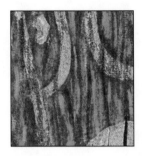

Acknowledgments

The Initiative "Public Health in the Americas" has been one of the main strategic areas of technical cooperation sponsored and guided by the Director of the Pan American Health Organization, Dr. George A.O. Alleyne, during his second term (February 1999–January 2003). The design and general coordination of the Initiative has been responsibility of the Division of Health Systems and Services Development of PAHO, under the direction of Dr. Daniel López-Acuña. Dr. Carlyle Guerra de Macedo, Emeritus Director of the Organization, has counseled and inspired the development of the initiative throughout its different stages. The Coordinators of the Program of Organization and Management of Health Systems and Services, and of Human Resources Development, José María Marín, José Luis Zeballos, and Pedro Brito respectively, have managed at different times the multiple tasks related to implementing the Initiative.

The Division of Development and Research of Public Health Systems at the Centers for Prevention and Disease Control (CDC), of the Department of Health and Human Services of the United States of America, has been actively involved. It was officially designated a PAHO/WHO Collaborating Center during this process. CDC contributed the time of several of its staff members, especially that of Paul Halverson and "Wade" Joseph Hanna, and made available their methodological instruments to measure the performance of Essential Public Health Functions, at the state and county level.

The Latin American Center for Research in Health Services (CLAISS), based in Chile, also participated actively in the implementation of the Initiative, particularly involved were Fernando Muñoz and Soledad Ubilla.

They are many people who in one manner or another contributed to the evaluation of the Initiative tasks summarized in this book. It would be quite a long list to name the over two thousand public health workers in the Americas that had some type of direct involvement in the processes related to the conceptual and methodological development, to the application of the instruments to measure the performance of the Essential Public Health Functions, to evaluate the results of the national exercises, and to prepare the different aspects of this book. Following are the names of those individuals who contributed the most to this task. We hope that in our will to express such recognition we have not unintentionally overlooked some important contributions.

This book, which is the result of collective work, describes the Initiative developments to date. The preparation of its different sections and chapters have been the result of numerous contributions, multiple work sessions, and frequent consultations. The authors shared interest is for the book to reflect, to the highest degree possible, a product resulting from interdisciplinary and participatory consensus.

General Coordination
Daniel López-Acuña

Editorial Committee
Carlyle Guerra de Macedo
Paul K. Halverson
"Wade" Joseph Hanna
Daniel López Acuña
José María Marín
Fernando Muñoz
Soledad Ubilla

Authors
The following persons contributed to the discussion and formulation
of the chapters in its different stages:

Gisele Almeida
Specialist in Health Information
 Systems
Division of Health Systems and
 Services Development
Pan American Health
 Organization/World Health
 Organization
Washington, DC, United States
 of America

Felix Alvarado
Manager
Consultores Asociados
Guatemala City, Guatemala

Natalie Brevard Perry
Health Scientist
Division of Public Health Systems
 Development and Research
Centers for Disease Control and
 Prevention
Atlanta, Georgia, United States
 of America

Pedro Brito
Coordinator
Human Resources Development
 Program

Pan American Health
 Organization/World Health
 Organization
Washington, DC, United States
 of America

Susana De Lena
Researcher
Universidad Nacional de La Plata
Buenos Aires, Argentina

Angel Ginestar
Professor
Instituto Universitario Fundación
 ISALUD
Buenos Aires, Argentina

Carlyle Guerra de Macedo
Emeritus Director
Pan American Health
 Organization/World Health
 Organization
Brasilia, Brasil

Paul K. Halverson
Director
Division of Public Health Systems
 Development and Research
Centers of Disease Control and
 Prevention

Atlanta, Georgia, United States
 of America

"Wade" Joseph Hanna
Deputy Director WHO
 Collaborating Center for Public
 Health Practice
Division of Health Systems
 Development and Research
Centers for Disease Control
 and Prevention
Atlanta, Georgia, United States
 of America

Monica Isabel Larrieu
Consultant
Division of Health Systems and
 Services Development
Pan American Health
 Organization/World Health
 Organization
Washington, D.C., United States
 of America

Daniel López Acuña
Director
Division of Health Systems and
 Services Development

x

Pan American Health
   Organization/World Health
   Organization
Washington, D.C., United States
   of America

Sandra Madrid
Physician Epidemiologist
Primary Health Care Department
Ministry of Health
Santiago, Chile

José María Marín
Coordinator (since January 2002)
Organization and Management
   of Health Systems
   and Services Program
Division of Health Systems and
   Services Development
Pan American Health
   Organization/World Health
   Organization
Washington, D.C., United States
   of America

Graciela Muñiz Saavedra
Consultant
Division of Health Systems and
   Services Development
Pan American Health
   Organization/World Health
   Organization
Washington, D.C., United States
   of America

Fernando Muñoz
Chief
Steering and Sanitary Regulation
   Division
Ministry of Health
Santiago, Chile

Monica Padilla
Regional Advisor in Management
   of Human Resources
Division of Health Systems and
   Services Development
Pan American Health
   Organization/World Health
   Organization
Washington, D.C., United States
   of America

Ana Cristina Pereiro
Chief of Cabinet Advisors
Ministry of Health
Buenos Aires, Argentina

Matilde Pinto
Regional Advisor in Health
   Economics
Division of Health Systems and
   Services Development
Pan American Health
   Organization/World Health
   Organization
Washington, D.C., United States
   of America

Magdalena Rathe
Executive Director
Fundación Plenitud
Santo Domingo, República
   Dominicana

Horacio Rodríguez
Professor
Instituto Universitario Fundación
   ISALUD
Buenos Aires, Argentina

Arturo L.F. Schweiger
Director
Economics and Health Management

Instituto Universitario Fundación
   ISALUD
Buenos Aires, Argentina

Soledad Ubilla
Advisor
Interministerial Coordination
   Division
Office of the Presidency
Santiago, Chile

Manuel Enrique Vázquez Valdés
Consultant
Division of Health Systems and
   Services Development
Pan American Health
   Organization/World Health
   Organization
Washington, D.C., United States
   of America

Guillermo Williams
Director, Health Services Quality
Ministry of Health
Buenos Aires, Argentina

José Luis Zeballos
Coordinator (1999–2001)
Organization and Management
   of Health Systems
   and Services Program
Division of Health Systems and
   Services Development
Pan American Health
   Organization/World Health
   Organization
Washington, D.C., United States
   of America

Curator of the English and Spanish Editions

Manuel Enrique Vázquez Valdés
Consultant
Division of Health Systems and
    Services
Pan American Health
    Organization/World Health
    Organization
Washington, D.C., United States of
    America

Technical Editor for the Spanish Edition

Roger Biosca
United Nations Editor and
    Translator
Barcelona, Spain

Technical Revision of the Translations
María Teresa Gago
Carrie Farmer
Paola Morello
Priscilla Rivas-Loria
Patricia Schroeder
Christiane West
Edwina Yen

Cover Design

Chemi Montes Armenteros
Graphic Designer
Falls Church, Virginia
United States of America

Desktop Publishing

*Barton Matheson Willse &
    Worthington – BMWW*
Leroy Stirewalt and James Taylor
Baltimore, Maryland, United States
    of America

English and Spanish Translation

Translation Services
Pan American Health
    Organization/World Health
    Organization

Text Formatting
Esther Alva
Matilde Cresswell
Carol Lynn Fretwell
Tomás Gómez
Ana Gooch
Maritza Moreno

Division of Health Systems and Services Development
Pan American Health Organization/World Health Organization
Washington, D.C., United States of America

Reference Group

The following network of experts participated in the conceptual and methodological development of the instruments as well as in the performance measurement of EPHFs. The group was consulted, provided their observations and formulated valuable suggestions. It included the following: *Orville Adams, Mohammed Akther, Celia Almeida, Edward Baker, Louis Bernard, Stephen Blount, Charles Boelen, David Brandling-Bennett, Jo Ivey Boufford, Paolo Buss, Xinia Carvajal, Isabella Daniel, Margaret Gilson, Charles Griffin, Rodrigo Guerrero, Knox Hangley, Allen K. Jones, Deborah Jones, Bernardo Kinsberg, Elsie Le-Franc, Setephan Legros, Jorge Lemus, Alejandro Llanos, Christopher Lovelace, Michael Malison, Henry Migala, Daniel Miller, Ray Nicola, Tom Novotny, José Rodríguez Domínguez, Marhuram Santoshan, Steve Sapire, Pomeroy Sinnock, Olive Shisana, Alfredo Solari, Giorgio Solimano, Alan Steckler, Roberto Tapia, Mary Lou Valdez and Barrington Wint.*

The "Public Health in the Americas Initiative" held an experts consultation meeting in september 1999, in PAHO Headquarters, Washington DC to validate the definitions of Essential Public Health Functions and the components it comprises. In addition to the book authors the following experts participated in the meeting: *Anabela Abreu, Mohammed Akhter, Celia Almeida, Cristian Baeza, Louis E. Bernard, Pierre Buekens, Xinia Carvajal, Juan Antonio Casas, Carlos Castillo-Salgado, Pedro Crocco, Rochika Chaudhry, Enrique Fefer, Luiz Gâlvao, Margaret Gilson, Charles Godue, Rodrigo Guerrero, Knox Hangley, Alberto Infante, Allen K. Jones, Sandra Land, Stephane Legros, Jorge Lemus, Alejandro Llanos-Cuenteas, Jay McAuliffe, Michael Malison, Glen Mays, Ray Nicola, Horst Otterstetter, José Romero Teruel, Mirta Roses Periago, William Savedoff, Alfredo Solari, Giorgio Solimano, Gina Tambini, Barrington Wint and Fernando Zacarías.*

Support Group for the Measurement of the EPHF in the Countries

The measurement of the EPHF was preceded by three subregional workshops, which took place in Costa Rica, Argentina and Jamaica and by some national training workshops. Among the participants in the workshops were focal points selected by the national authorities, PAHO staff members from headquarters and from the countries, as well as a group of facilitators that later helped in the application of the instrument in the countries and terrirories that participated in the exercise. The group of facilitators was comprised by:

Isidro Avila Martínez, Charles Godue, Deyanira González de León, Angela Gonzalez-Puche, Jackie Gernay, Marise Guay, Renato Gusmao, Knox Hangley, Margaret Hazelwood, Sandra Land, Monica Larrieu, Fernando Lavadenz, Elsie Le Franc, Marlo Libel, José María Marín, Paola Morello, Graciela Muniz Saavedra, Fernando Munoz, Anne Roca, Ana Gabriela Ross, Luis Ruiz, Patricia Schroeder, Debora Tajer, Clovis Tigre, Soledad Ubilla, Hélène Valentín, Manuel Enrique Vázquez Valdés, Barrington Wint, Edwina Yen and José Luis Zeballos.

In addition to the English and Spanish editions of this book, the instruments to measure the performance of the EPHF are available in portuguese, french and dutch. Special recognition must be given to the Quebec Public Health Institute for their collaboration in the preparation of the French version and its application in the francophone countries, as well as the PAHO Representations in Brazil and Suriname for their work in the elaboration of the portuguese and dutch versions, respectively.

This measurement exercise could not have been carried out without the collaboration of the PAHO country offices and their technical and administrative teams. Similarly, it is an understatement to say that this work, in which 41 countries and territories participated, could not have been completed without the collaboration of the national authorities and the staff members who served as focal points for the project.

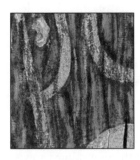

Navigational Chart

The following section is designed to give the reader some hints on how to "navigate" through this book. This is because its modular structure allows for different points of entry. The modules, while complementary, need not be approached in a linear fashion. In fact, each chapter affords an opportunity to begin reading a clearly differentiated unit that can be analyzed separately. These individual analyses combine and connect to form a complete picture of the topic at hand.

Readers from the field of public health, from both academia and the sphere of practice—that is, policy-making, management, and health care—will surely recognize many signposts that will enable them to enter certain sections directly. Readers from different spheres of activity or other disciplines whose link with the work in public health is less direct, on the other hand, will require a more detailed perusal of the chapters.

In any case, the leitmotif of this work is the construction of an approach involving: first, an overview that enables us to view with fresh eyes and sufficient conceptual and analytical problem-solving capacity the responsibilities of state and non-state public entities in contemporary work in public health in the Region of the Americas (Parts I and II); second, the possibility of translating this conceptual framework into highly practical working definitions, which have made it possible to measure the performance of the essential public health functions appropriate to the health authority in all the Latin American and Caribbean countries (Part III); and third, the formulation and discussion of different processes and instruments that permit a shift from measurement to action, from the diagnosis of strengths and weaknesses to improvements in public health practice, focusing efforts on institutional development and strengthen-

ing of the public health infrastructure (Part IV).

Part I presents two gateways or points of entry that are particularly relevant to the understanding of this work. These are discussed in two chapters, one in the Public Health in the Americas Initiative, and the other on strengthening the steering role of the health authority. Both offer complementary dimensions that intersect. That point of intersection is the exercise of the Essential Public Health Functions by the health authority. Either of the two chapters could have been used to open Part I of this book, since they have areas of convergence and offer common inferences, and because there were positions that supported both options. After much discussion, the authors have opted to begin with the arguments that identify the *raison d'être* that they consider fundamental: the need to strengthen public health practice in the Region and, subsequently, to address the concomitant challenge of strengthening the steering role of the different levels of the health authority (national, subnational, and local), whose basic responsibilities include the exercise of the essential public health functions (EPHF).

Part II deals with the conceptual revitalization of public health. Throughout its chapters, it explores the complex, diverse web in which the concept was born, nourished, and in which this sphere of action developed. This is key to promoting an understanding of the historical path of public health, not only among people from other fields and disciplines, but among public health specialists and other health professionals as well. It will enable them to more fully grasp the importance of conceptual revitalization in this field, the relationship between social practices and public health, and the origins and relevance of the concept and categories of the EPHF.

For this reason, in each chapter included in Part II, the concept of public health acquires increasing importance in an effort to move from theory to practice looking relentlessly for the connection among the two. As a result, the essential conceptual issues are presented to increase their understanding within the current global state of affairs, and for their efficient implementation at the same time that reflection and debate on the subject is stimulated opening the area under discussion for future proposals. Thus, in chapter three a selective summary is included on the history of health and public health which identifies the basic factors that have determined its evolution. The basic challenges are identified as well as the need to ponder on the conceptual basis in an effort to reorient its practice. It concludes with a summary of the most important initiatives that have preceded the existent one.

In Chapter four the central areas of public health are revised, as well as its objectives, actors and the distinctive elements for its promotion and practice in the health systems. Public health is conceived as health of the population which is comprised mainly of public goods and is a responsibility of society and the State that is to serve them. Chapter five provides an in-depth look at the concept of social practices and its relationship with public health emphasizing the great potential that exists to utilize it for a comprehensive, inclusive and sustainable public health practice.

Chapter six underscores the importance of its theoretical revision linking it to a practical exercise through the introduction of the operational concept known as the 11 Essential Public Health Functions. This is an explicit and precise formula of the fundamental attributes that should be the responsibility of the State, particularly of the sanitary authorities. Finally, Chapter seven presents the framework for action. The purpose is to identify the necessary elements required to implement the concepts and complete the connection between theory and practice. Thus, in parts III and IV, a link between proposals and actions is sought.

In Part III the basis for the measurement of the performance of the Essential Public Health Functions, and the results of its application in 41 countries and territories of Latin America and the Caribbean are presented. Thus, a valuable self-evaluation tool is presented that allows the National Health Authority to identify the existent strengths and weaknesses to exercise the EPHF as part of its steering role. This tool, moreover, facilitates the use of objective criteria in decision-making, which should lead to an improvement in public health practice. Furthermore, it places the exercise in the broader context of health system performance evaluation, attempting to bring measurement closer to the elements of structure, process, and results, so that it can impact managerial decision-making and the allocation of resources.

Finally, Part IV describes some paths that must be followed, based on the knowledge that this tool provides. It leaves the door open to the possibility of developing new processes and instruments to meet the challenges that emerge from this performance measurement exercise: the need to pay greater attention to the institutional development of the health authority and to upgrading the public health services infrastructure; the importance of improving knowledge about financing, expenditure, cost analysis, and budgeting for the EPHF; the imperative of resolutely promoting the development of the public health workforce and the possibilities offered by international cooperation in all these areas.

The character of this collective work has been inclusive and pluralistic from the outset. The authors have attempted to harmonize the history, institutional direction, experience, and different visions of public health found throughout our Hemisphere. They have engaged in a broad dialogue with experts from the Region throughout the preparation of the work and have made the necessary adjustments to respond to the individual situations of the member countries.

They have sought not only to conduct a systematic performance evaluation of the EPHF and thereby conclude the task entrusted to them by the Governing Bodies of PAHO, but have also left room for us to continue exploring all that remains to research, to learn, to measure, and to transform.

The basic corollary that emerges from this effort is that we must continue navigating the new and the old waters in this exciting and critical area in order to lay a broader, better foundation for the development of health in our societies and consolidation of human security in our countries.

PART I

The Initiative "Public Health in the Americas" and its Rationale

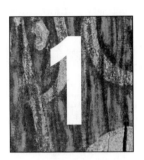

The Initiative Public Health in the Americas and the Need to Improve Public Health Practice in the Region

1. Introduction

The proposed reforms in the public health sector address the need to strengthen the steering role of the health authority. An important part of this role is the exercise of the essential public health functions (EPHF) for which the State is responsible at the national, intermediate, and local levels.[1] For the State to fulfill its responsibilities in this area, it is imperative to create instruments that will facilitate a situation analysis of the health authority's exercise of these functions. Such an analysis will identify the strengths and weaknesses of the health authority and thus lay the foundations for concerted insti-

tutional development efforts to improve public health practice.

Health sector reform processes have focused mainly on structural, financial, and organizational changes in the health systems, as well as modifications in the delivery of health care to the public. Up to now, improvements in health system performance have targeted the following areas: reducing inequalities in health status and access to services; health care financing; reducing gaps in social protection in health; boosting the effectiveness of health interventions; and promoting quality in care. However, changes designed to strengthen the steering role of the health authorities and improve public health practice have received far less attention. Aspects related to public health have largely been neglected, as if they were not a social and institutional responsibility—precisely when state support is most needed to modernize the infrastructure required for the exercise of the essential public health functions.

Reintroducing public health into the program for transforming the sector demands that its scope and function be clearly defined and its basic concepts applied. For this reason, the concepts and methodologies linked with the EPHF must be developed, for they are the wellspring of this instrument's great potential for mustering the will and the resources to strengthen the public health services infrastructure and the steering role of the health authorities.

2. The Concept of EPHF and their Link to Public Health Practice and the Strengthening of the Health Authorities' Steering Role

The concept of public health that supports the definition of the EPHF is that of collective intervention by the State and civil society to protect and improve the health of the people. It is a defini-

---

[1] PAHO/WHO, Essential public health functions. Document CD 42/15. The XLII Directing Council, Meeting of the Pan American Health Organization. The LII Regional Committee, Meeting of the World Health Organization. Washington D.C., September 2000.

tion that goes beyond non-personal health services or community/population-based interventions to include the responsibility for ensuring access to services and quality health care. It also involves activities to promote health and development of the public health workforce. Thus, public health is not referred to as an academic discipline, but rather, as an interdisciplinary social practice. It is a concept that goes beyond the notion of public goods with positive externalities for health, since it encompasses semiprivate or private goods whose dimensions make their impact on public health an important factor.

The concept of public health is frequently confused with that of the State's responsibility in health, when actually the two are not synonymous. Public health goes beyond the responsibilities that are the purview of the State, yet at the same time does not cover all that the State can do in the field of health. Although the State has a series of responsibilities it cannot delegate in executing or guaranteeing fulfillment of the EPHF, they represent but a fraction of its responsibilities in health. It is certainly a very important fraction whose proper exercise is not only fundamental for improving health and the quality of life of the population, but is part of the State's steering role in health—a role characterized by responsibilities in strategic management, regulation, finance modulation, incurance monitoring, and delivery harmonization.

In addition, many non-state public dimensions form part of the universe of action of public health. Thus, there are areas in which civil society promotes changes in the population that result in an improvement in people's health. There are also aspects of social capital

that represent a contribution to culture and health practice as both an individual and a social value and the result of collective intervention that combines with state action in this area.

Likewise, it is important to mention the difficulty of drawing a clear distinction between the scope of public health in the delivery of disease prevention and health promotion services for specific population groups—that is, in collective interventions—and in the delivery of personal health care. The traditional concept of public health is identified basically with the first of these dimensions. However, in the second dimension, there is no doubt that public health has some important responsibilities related to the guarantee of equitable access to services, quality in care, and use of the public health perspective in the reorientation of health services delivery.

In order to restore the concept of public health and place it at the heart of the processes aimed at transforming the system, it is important to typify and measure operational categories such as the EPHF to determine the degree to which they are fulfilled by the State at the national and subnational level.

Thus, the EPHF have been defined as the structural conditions and aspects of institutional development that permit better performance in terms of public health practice. However, as explained in Part I of the book, in order to reach this conclusion, it has been necessary to develop indicators and standards for the EPHF to help characterize the critical elements that will make it possible to identify which aspects of public health practice need to be strengthened. This approach complements the definition of the thematic areas of public health

action, defined by the object of intervention of the action taken. The concepts are actually linked in practice, forming a matrix that yields a set of institutional capacities used in a variety of key interventions. The basic premise is that if the functions are well-defined and encompass all the institutional capacities required for good public health practice, the necessary infrastructure will be created for the good operation of each sphere of activity or key area of the work in public health.

Defining and measuring the EPHF are thus conceived as a contribution to the institutional development of public health practice. They are a first step in developing capacities and competencies. Furthermore, better defining which functions are essential helps to improve the quality of the services and develop a more precise definition of the institutional responsibilities necessary for their exercise.

Moreover, the accountability of public entities to the people for the results of their work begins with the part that is most inherent to them, the part that is exclusively their own—not with responsibilities that they share with other administrative areas involved in general decisions on health policy. The legitimacy and power of the health authorities to bring other actors together to devise intersectoral interventions to promote health therefore increase with the definition of the essence of their operations and the capacity for more accurate performance measurement.

Performance measurement with respect to the EPHF should ultimately permit better identification of the resources needed to guarantee an adequate public health infrastructure and better analysis of financing, expenditures, costs, and the necessary budgets. This information, moreover, is essential for the national and subnational governments, as well as the international organizations that provide technical and financial cooperation.

Finally, the characterization and measurement of EPHF performance are key to improving the training of the personnel that carry out the work in public health. This process provides a better foundation for specifying the competencies required for the exercise of the EPHF and for identifying the pertinent professional and other staff profiles. This goes hand in hand with improvements in training and continuing education in public health and will help inspire training institutions to reorient their efforts in public health toward greater relevance and quality in their work.

3. Nature and Scope of the "Public Health in the Americas" Initiative

As mentioned in the two previous sections of this chapter, in 1999 PAHO decided to implement the "Public Health in the Americas Initiative", with the following main objectives:

- Development of a regional definition of the EPHF, obtained by consensus after an extensive debate among experts from academe, the government, and professionals working in public health.

- Development of instruments to measure their performance as the basis for improving public health practice.

- Development of the methodology and instruments to support the formula-

tion and implementation of some national, subregional, and regional lines of action that will help to strengthen the public health infrastructure and thereby enhance the leadership of the health authority at all levels of the State.

The Initiative, promoted by the Director of PAHO, Dr. George Alleyne, on assuming his second mandate in February 1999, has been coordinated by the Division of Health Systems and Services Development and has enlisted the efforts of all technical units in the Organization, as well as the PAHO delegations in each country. It has also benefited from the participation of PAHO's Director Emeritus, Dr. Carlyle Guerra de Macedo, who served as an advisor and collaborator on the project. The Initiative has developed the performance measurement instruments for the EPHF in collaboration with the U.S. Centers for Disease Control and Prevention (CDC) and the Latin American Center for Health Systems Research (CLAISS).

The project has also involved many examples of interaction with experts from the academic world, scientific associations, health services, and international organizations, forming a network that has been consulted on many occasions, thus enriching the conceptual, methodological, and instrumental development of the Initiative.

The scope of the Public Health in the Americas Initiative can therefore be summarized as follows:

- Promotion of a common concept of public health and of its essential functions in the Americas.

- Development of a framework for measuring the performance of the essential public health functions, applicable to all the countries of the Region.

- Support for self-evaluation of public health practice in each country, based on EPHF performance measurement, within the conceptual and instrumental framework developed by the Initiative.

- Support to the countries in identifying the activities necessary for strengthening the public health services infrastructure and formulating institutional development programs that will lead to an improvement in public health practice—programs whose progress can be evaluated periodically through EPHF performance measurement.

- Laying the foundations for a regional program to strengthen the infrastructure and improve public health practice, based on the conclusions derived from EPHF performance measurement in the Region.

- Publication in September 2002 of the present book, *Public Health in the Americas*, which brings together the different elements and results of the project and provides an overview of the degree to which EPHF are being exercised in the Americas.

After the initial call issued by the Director of PAHO, the member countries enthusiastically welcomed the Initiative and closely collaborated in its different stages. This led to a debate on the EPHF in the 42nd Directing Council of September 2000 and the adoption of Resolution CD 42/18 (see box), which urged the Member States to participate

THE 42nd DIRECTING COUNCIL,

Having considered document CD42/15 on essential public health functions;

Taking into account that the Pan American Health Organization has implemented the *Public Health in the Americas* initiative, aimed at the definition and measurement of the essential public health functions as the basis for improving public health practice and strengthening the steering role of the health authority at all levels of the State;

Considering the need for health sector reforms to pay greater attention to public health and to increase the social and institutional responsibility of the State in this regard; and

Taking note of the recommendation of the 126th Session of the Executive Committee,

RESOLVES:

1. To urge the Member States to:

(a) Participate in a regional exercise to measure performance with regard to the essential public health functions to permit an analysis of the state of public health in the Americas, sponsored by PAHO;

(b) Use performance measurement with regard to the essential public health functions to improve public health practice, develop the necessary infrastructure for this purpose, and strengthen the steering role of the health authority at all levels of the State.

2. To request the Director to:

(a) Disseminate widely in the countries of the Region the conceptual and methodological documentation on the definition and measurement of the essential public health functions;

(b) Carry out, in close coordination with the national authorities of each country, an exercise in performance measurement with respect to the essential public health functions, using the methodology referred to in Document CD42/15;

(c) Conduct a regional analysis of the state of public health in the Americas, based on a performance measurement exercise targeting the essential public health functions in each country;

(d) Promote the reorientation of public health education in the Region in line with the development of the essential public health functions;

(e) Incorporate the line of work on the essential public health functions into cooperation activities linked with sectoral reform and the strengthening of the steering role of the health authority.

in the regional exercise to measure performance with respect to the EPHF and to use the results obtained to carry out interventions develop their infrastructure and improve public health practice. It also requested the Director of PAHO to support these activities in the countries, conduct a regional analysis of the state of public health in the Region, and adopt EPHF performance measurement and institutional development as a line of work for improving public health practice in PAHO's technical cooperation programs at the regional and country level, articulating it with efforts to strengthen the steering role of the health authority within the framework of the new generation of health sector reforms.

The present document outlines the principal conceptual, methodological, and empirical developments stemming from the institutional efforts of PAHO, which have benefited from the broad and committed participation of the member countries. In addition, it provides an overview of the exercise of the EPHF in 41 countries and territories of the Region of the Americas, based on the performance measurement exercises conducted jointly by the participating countries and the Secretariat. The book concludes with a discussion on a number of strategic issues for strengthening the public health infrastructure in the countries of the Region and, with some comments aimed at contributing useful insights to lay the foundation for a regional program to improve public health practice in the Americas.

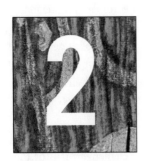

The Steering Function in Health and the Institutional Strengthening of the National and Subnational Health Authorities

1. Regional Scenario

The reform of the State and the decentralization of the political, economic, and social life of the countries have made the redefinition of institutional roles in the health sector a priority in the Region of the Americas to guarantee the full exercise of the health authority and strengthen the steering role of the State in health system performance and the sectoral reform[1] processes.

The essential health responsibilities of the State are undergoing significant changes as a result of a general shift in the balance between the State, the market, and civil society. This is expressed

in the trend toward the separation of functions in the system: steering role, financing, insurance, purchasing and delivery of services, as well as the description of activities, in some countries, to one or more public and/or private actors or agencies. Consequently, these circumstances demand greater institutional capacity on the part of the health authority to manage, regulate, and carry out the EPHF.

The national ministries of health in the countries of the Region are faced today with new realities in sectoral organization, which have been exacerbated by the health sector reform processes currently under way. This has led to the need for a swift and flexible definition of better ways to improve their capacity to exercise their new steering role in the sector.

Progress in State and sectoral decentralization, together with the emergence of new actors in the public and private sec-

tor, are shifting responsibility for service delivery, especially personal health care, away from the national ministries of health. The delivery of public health services and the execution of regulatory activities in health are undergoing similar changes; here, intermediate and sometimes local agencies have assumed responsibility for these functions to one degree or another, consistent with the redistribution of competencies and geographic divisions established by the country.

Many sectoral reform processes in the countries of the Region have been moving in the direction of the separation of sectoral functions, leading to the institutional disaggregation of activities connected with the steering role, financing, insurance, purchasing and provision of services. However, most commonly, all five functions are concentrated in a single institution, or a small group of institutions, a problematic arrangement that segments the population according to

[1] PAHO/WHO. The Steering Role of the Ministries of Health in the Processes of Health Sector Reform. Document CD 40/13. XL Meeting of the Directing Council of the Pan American Health Organization, XLIX Meeting of the Regional Comittee of the World Health Organization, Washington, D.C., September, 1997.

whether or not it belongs to the formal economy and contributes to some form of health insurance, and its ability to pay. As a consequence, striking differences in insurance coverage and service delivery arise.

This is compounded by other important, longstanding factors. Health services have not attained a level of development that can be described as efficient, equitable, harmonious, and of good quality. Lack of coordination is a problem, combined with the simultaneous duplication of efforts and gaps, mainly in personal and non-personal service coverage in rural areas and among the disadvantaged populations of major cities.

Exclusion in health and the other side of the coin, the lack of social protection in health, are characteristic of vast proportions of the Hemisphere's inhabitants. The health sector in many countries of the Region has been unable to provide full and comprehensive coverage to all citizens. Marginal groups with no access to basic health services can be found in virtually every country. At the same time, urban centers have extremely costly, high-quality services to which the majority of the population has only limited access.

Other significant factors compound the situation: the inefficiency of sector institutions; structural weaknesses in managerial capacity, which make institutional development in health management imperative; the high cost of care, often associated with growing numbers of interventions with little or no effectiveness; and poor quality services with low levels of user satisfaction. Emerging problems, such as AIDS, are accompanied by other reemerging problems, such as tuberculosis, cholera, malaria, and dengue. The

rise in chronic pathologies and the growth of the elderly population has heightened the demand and the need for more frequent and complex care, which consumes a considerable volume of resources. Populations are beginning to have greater expectations of the health services, demanding higher quality care and the use of costly innovative technologies. This has given the State regulation, control, and surveillance functions in these areas. However, it does not always have the institutional organization, the critical mass of human resources, and the necessary financial resources to exercise them.

The Region today is witnessing an increase in its population, combined with economic stagnation, rising unemployment, growth of the informal economy, a deepening of absolute and relative poverty, and a widening of the disparities in income distribution. All of this is causing the economic, social, ethnic, and cultural exclusion in the countries to assume increasingly serious proportions. At the same time, the current mechanisms for social protection in health that should guarantee the population a series of benefits through public health measures—either through the ministries of health or the social security systems—are incapable of addressing the new problems in this area.

The current situation in many countries of the Region, especially in Latin America and the Caribbean, is characterized by high economic and social volatility, a breakdown in governance, and the alarming growth of poverty and inequity. Now more than ever, this makes it imperative to ensure that the changes introduced in the social sectors, health among them, contribute to the creation of inclusive societies for all cit-

izens and not to greater exclusion, marginalization, and lack of social protection, including protection in health.

At the dawn of the new millennium, the countries of the Region find themselves faced with an enormous challenge of growing proportions: to guarantee all citizens basic social protection in health that will help to eliminate the inequalities in access to basic quality services for all people and give excluded social groups the opportunity to receive comprehensive care to meet their needs and demands in health, regardless of their ability to pay.

In light of these challenges, it is of the utmost importance to strengthen the steering role of the national ministries of health in the sector, as well as the leadership of the sector as a whole in health advocacy and its negotiations with other sectors. Leadership is needed that will enable governments to stay firmly on track to promote the health of their peoples in the midst of the sectoral reform processes.

In the final analysis, this strengthening of the steering capacity in the health sector should be guided by the goal of reducing inequities in health conditions, within the framework of integrated and sustainable human development and the elimination of unjust inequalities in access to personal and non-personal health services and in the financial burden linked to it.

2. Tasks Comprising the Exercise of the Sectoral Steering Role by the Health Authorities

The phenomena outlined in the preceding section clearly point to the need to reconfigure and adapt the responsibilities and operations of the health authorities—especially the national ministries of health—to strengthen their steering capacity, defining the substantive, nondelegable responsibilities that are proper to them.

This implies building institutional capacity in the following areas: in sectoral management, in the regulating and controlling of goods and services connected with health, in the exercise of essential public health functions, in the modulation of financing, in the monitoring of coverage, in overseeing the purchasing of services and in harmonizing the delivery of health care to bring about the changes necessary to attain universal and equitable access to quality health services.

The changes in the organization of health systems and the nature of the work of the health sector, coupled with a growing awareness of the importance of other sectors in improving the health status of the population, have gradually been defining a series of basic, well-differentiated functions that, taken as a whole, constitute sectoral regulatory action. There is a growing tendency to avoid concentrating all these functions in a single institution, as in the past, creating instead a series of complementary institutional mechanisms to carry out the differentiated functions in a separate and specialized manner.

These tasks can be divided into various categories and will always be subject to different groupings and alternative interpretations. The proposal that follows is one of the many ways of establishing a taxonomy of tasks for exercise of the sectoral steering role. Here, the work is divided into in six major categories (Figure 1).

Figure 1. Sanitary Authority Tasks for the Health Sector Reform

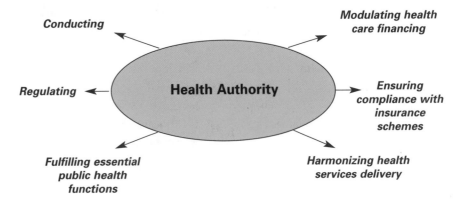

It should be noted that the range of competencies exercised by the national ministry of health will depend on the degree of public responsibility in health, the degree to which sectoral action is decentralized, and the structural separation of functions in the institutional structure of each country.

In some cases, these functions already exist in practice or are set out in codes, laws, or regulations. In others, new competencies are involved that require institutions to strengthen and often modify their operations, their organizational structure, and the professional profile of their managerial, technical, and administrative staff.

2.1 Sectoral Management

Sectoral management is the capacity of the entities that exercise the sectoral steering role to formulate, organize, and direct the execution of the national health policy through the definition of viable objectives and feasible goals, the preparation and implementation of strategic plans that articulate the efforts of public and private institutions in the sector and other social actors, the establishment of participatory mechanisms

and consensus-building, and the mobilization of the necessary resources to carry out the proposed actions.

In order to do this, the national ministries of health need to develop and/or strengthen their institutional capacity to carry out the following activities:

a) Analysis of the health situation and its determinants, with emphasis on identifying inequities in health conditions and access to services, and on the impact on the population's current and future demands and needs;

b) Periodic evaluation of sector operations, institutional operations, and system performance, especially in terms of monitoring and evaluating the impact and dynamics of the sectoral reform processes;

c) Development of methods and procedures for prioritizing health problems, vulnerable populations, programs, and interventions, based on the criteria of effectiveness, cost, and positive externalities;

d) Formulation, analysis, adaptation, and evaluation of the public policies that impact on health and sector policies;

e) Building of national consensus on the strategic development of the sector, leading to the development of State policy in health;

f) The setting of national and subnational health objectives, in terms of health processes and outcomes. These will serve as the basis for coordinating the work of public and private actors in the sector and for developing guidelines for efforts to improve public health practice.

g) Direction, involvement, and/or mobilization of sector resources and actors and those of other sectors that influence the formulation of national health policy and actions to promote health;

h) Health advocacy;

i) Promotion of social participation in health;

j) Coordination of the technical, economic, and policy assistance that multilateral and bilateral agencies devoted to technical and/or financial cooperation in health can provide for the formulation and implementation of national health policies and strategies;

k) Political and technical participation in regional and subregional organizations and agencies for policy coordination and economic integration of relevance to the health sector, to promote greater sensitivity in these entities to the health interests of the population and the health sector.

2.2 Sectoral Regulation

Some of the sectoral regulation tasks involved in the exercise of the steering function are:

a) Development and refinement of national health legislation and its necessary harmonization with the health legislation of countries participating in regional integration processes;

b) Analysis, sanitary regulation, and oversight of basic markets allied with health, such as public and private health insurance, health service inputs (such as drugs, equipment, and medical devices), health technologies, mass communication involving goods and services related to health, and consumer health products, as well as sanitary conditions in public establishments and the environment;

c) Analysis, technical regulation, and oversight of health service delivery, certification, and professional practice in health, as well as training and continuing education programs in the health sciences;

d) Establishment of basic standards and guidelines for health care; development of quality assurance programs; formulation and application of frameworks for the accreditation, certification, and licensing of institutional service providers; and health technology assessment.

Many of these tasks are performed in some extent but must be improved and broadened to fully meet the objective safeguarding health as a public good. Moreover, institutional structures do not always have the capacity or resources to fully execute the types of regulation and control indicated above.

2.3 Exercise of the Essential Public Health Functions pertaining to the Health Authority

If there is one area of action in the sectoral steering role that cannot be ignored it is the exercise of the essential public health functions proper to the health authority, especially those with high positive externalities for the health of the population and/or that constitute public goods in the field of health.

Exercise of the steering role in health involves substantive, nondelegable tasks on the part of the national or subnational health authority. These are fundamental to the work of the ministry of health as the agency responsible for safeguarding public well-being in health. These functions can be delegated to or shared by several levels and institutions within the state apparatus, but the primary mission of the national ministries of health is to ensure that they are exercised as effectively as possible.

This section delves no further into this topic, since the subsequent sections that constitute the bulk of this book are devoted to the conceptual and methodological underpinnings that have produced a regional consensus on 11 essential public health functions considered to be the purview of the national health authority. These sections also measure the performance of these functions in more than 40 countries and territories of the Region and discuss the lessons learned from that exercise in order to take action to improve public health practice and reinforce the infrastructure that makes it possible.

2.4 Sectoral Financing Tasks

The structural separation of sectoral functions characteristic of the sectoral reform processes in the Region shows three major trends in financing.

The first is the creation of autonomous national funds independent of the ministries of health. These funds pool the following resources: the public revenues from general taxes; specific taxes for health purposes, when they exist; and workers' and/or employers' contributions, when steps have been taken to merge the social security health funds with general State appropriations for this purpose. This can involve a single public insurance system or several insurance systems, public or private, that either compete with or complement one another.

The second trend is an increase in the share of public sector financing that comes from the taxes collected by intermediate-level and local State entities and/or from resources of the national fiscal authority, transferred from the central government as block grants earmarked for activities in health.

The third trend is related to the growing share of private health insurance and certain prepaid service modalities in the composition of global sector financing in certain countries of the Region—services that are paid for by the beneficiaries themselves and/or their employers, at least with respect to some types of coverage that supplement the compulsory plans established by the State.

The combination of these three elements in countries that have taken steps to eliminate the segmentation of insurance coverage and health service delivery produced by differentiated financing systems (public services not linked to specific contributions; compulsory social security-type health insurance plans, paid for with subscriber premiums; mutual aid societies or *obras sociales*; and private health insurance or prepaid health plans) imply new challenges and responsibilities for the ministries of health in the organization of sectoral financing.

These developments in sectoral financing give the ministry of health responsibility for: a) establishing the policies needed to ensure that the different financing modalities have the necessary complementarity to ensure equitable access to quality health services for the entire population; b) smoothing out and correcting any deviations that may occur in sectoral financing, and c) developing the capacity to oversee the sectoral financing process.

2.5 Responsibilities in Insurance

The countries of the Region are immersed in intense processes of change in the institutional organization of their health sectors, in the structure of health care delivery, and in the systems for financing it, which together have come to be known as health sector reform. Implementation of these agendas for change has opened up an opportunity to move toward equitable access to health care. However, to accomplish this, it will be necessary to secure effective coverage for excluded groups, particularly those working in the informal sector of the economy and those who are marginalized for cultural, ethnic, and/or geographical reasons.

An important part of these sectoral changes in health are the reforms in the scope and modalities of social security health coverage. This dimension of sectoral change has not always reached the most disadvantaged population groups. Thus, there will be a real opportunity to turn this situation around if progress is made in the design, implementation, and evaluation of innovative mechanisms to expand the coverage of social security in health, targeting groups that do not participate in the formal sector of the economy or have the financial wherewithal to subscribe to the customary social security health plans.

New formulas must be found that rely more heavily on the social capital of excluded groups; that attempt to rationalize the regressiveness of out-of-pocket expenditures in health, which today impose a greater financial burden on households and the most disadvantaged population; that take advantage of community mechanisms for cooperative organization to find responses to complement the social protection in health currently offered through state interventions and the social security health systems, which, regrettably, do not cover all citizens.

The degree to which the social security health system is developed in each country (and not just the number or the coverage of social insurance plans) is what determines the State's responsibility for ensuring a basic package of services or guaranteed health plan that offers coverage to all inhabitants or special population groups (the poor, the elderly, etc.). When this responsibility exists, it generates a role ordinarily reserved for the ministries of health or some of their deconcentrated agencies: that of guarantor of the insurance established. For this, mechanisms are needed that permit the fulfillment of a social mandate often found in the countries' national constitutions.

A second element that has a bearing on this dimension of the sectoral steering role is related to the public, private, or mixed nature of the service providers that participate in the compulsory coverage plans.

Thus, the ministries of health in countries in which this separation of functions is under way or has been consolidated must develop the institutional framework required to perform the task. They must therefore broaden their range of capacities to enable them to:

a) Define the content of the guaranteed basic coverage plans that must be available to all citizens covered by social security health systems that are public in nature;

b) Monitor the administration of these plans by public and private health insurance and/or service delivery institutions (directly or through the supervisory authorities or similar agencies), guaranteeing that no beneficiary of the compulsory social security health plans is denied insurance for reasons of age or preexisting conditions;

c) Enhance the purchasing power of public and/or private health services through group plans, when public insurance is involved, to ensure delivery of the guaranteed packages of services or coverage plans offered by the current social security health systems.

These three aspects of the exercise of the steering role in insurance tend to be poorly developed in the ministries of health of the countries of the Region and their deconcentrated territorial agencies. This implies the particular need to intensify actions to foster progress in this area.

2.6 Tasks in Health Service Delivery

Health service delivery is perhaps the sectoral function that has undergone the most pronounced changes in the countries of the Region over the past two decades. This is the result of two simultaneous phenomena: first, the decentralization and/or deconcentration of sector activities, particularly those related to the delivery of public health services and personal health care; and second, growing private sector participation in health care delivery, either to implement the guaranteed coverage offered by public or social health insurance, or to operate private insurance or direct, out-of-pocket, fee-for-service plans.

With varying degrees of deconcentration, the ministries of health were long accustomed to directly managing the delivery of public health services and personal health care through the hospitals and outpatient clinics of their own service networks. They are now delegating or have already delegated this responsibility, having fully or partially transferred these competencies to intermediate levels of government (states, departments, or provinces) and/or the local level (municipios or cantons), or to decentralized autonomous regional agencies devoted exclusively to health service delivery.

Exercising the steering role thus poses the challenge of properly orchestrating the many public and private service providers to take advantage of their in-stalled capacity in a rational and complementary way and to define basic standards for health services to give users a reasonable guarantee of quality in the services they receive.

3. Institutional Development of National and Subnational Health Authorities for Exercise of the Steering Role

The preceding section's review of the tasks involved reveals numerous challenges. There is a considerable lack of consistency between the new functions of the national ministries and their structures, competencies, and professional profiles. What they *do* have in this area is more appropriate to the functions currently exercised by the intermediate, local, or regional entities, which are responsible for the delivery of personal and non-personal services and for the exercise of certain health authority functions.

Given the decentralizing, deconcentrating, or privatizing trends that currently characterize the organization of the sector, the ministries of health need to assume a series of new tasks, which can be summarized as follows:

a) Define the criteria for allocating the resources to be channeled to the decentralized or deconcentrated public agencies and/or facilities that provide personal and non-personal services. In so doing, it is important to utilize the criteria of need, performance, and impact. Resources can be allocated through direct transfers from the ministry of health or from the ministries of economy, finance, or the treasury, based on well-defined criteria;

b) Harmonize the plans of action and management models of the decentralized or deconcentrated public agencies responsible for health service delivery in the country;

c) Define the content of the basic public health services that are the purview of the State, and, based on the criteria of complementarity, distribute competencies and resources among the different levels of public administration (central, intermediate, and local) that must assume them;

d) Furnish technical cooperation to the decentralized or deconcentrated service providers to guarantee a streamlined process for the transfer of authority and the development of the necessary institutional capacity for the full exercise of their functions;

e) Define mechanisms for the redistribution of current and capital expenditures to compensate for any inequities that may be generated by the decentralization processes;

f) Establish mechanisms for hiring or for service management agreements that will serve as the basis for resource allocation, based on a series of performance measurements expressed in terms of processes and outcomes.

The tasks enumerated above establish the national ministries of health as the harmonizers of the work of the decentralized or deconcentrated public agencies that act as service providers rather than the direct administrators of service delivery—a definition that demands the rapid development of new institutional capacities.

It is also necessary to design and execute a complete and ambitious transformation of the structures and functions of the ministries of health in order to adapt the technical capacity and expertise of their staff at all levels to the new demands and realities. An analysis of outcomes and processes will enable the ministries of health of the countries to initiate and move forward with the transformation of the steering role in health required by sectoral reform.

However, in order to spearhead the actions to improve health and become the full embodiment of all the competencies of the national and subnational health authorities, the ministries of health must consolidate their institutional capacity for the effective exercise of the steering role.

This is not simply an issue of governance in health, although that must be considered to understand the political economy involved in the exercise of the sectoral steering role and, to a certain point, develop it. It is a complex issue that requires a clear will to action, backed by political mandates and government authority.

Exercise of the steering role in health demands an imaginative effort by the State, in an intense dialogue with civil society, that will result in specific measures to guide progress in the sector and correct the imperfections of the health systems; that will make it possible to meet the basic objectives of protecting and improving the health of individuals; and that will guarantee equitable access to health services, regardless of the ability to pay.

All of this requires good organization, which often involves a profound reengineering of the current national ministries of health, coupled with adequate financing of the level of effort required to faithfully execute the basic tasks described in the section above.

It is often assumed that this whole task exists or must exist without realizing that behind it must be the capacity for organization, a critical mass of human resources trained for this purpose, and the financial resources and public health infrastructure that make it possible.

Finally, two thoughts on the exercise of the steering role by the health authorities are worth considering:

First, the modern steering role in health is not simply the development of the ministry of health's leadership in sectoral matters and advocacy to convince other sectors to take part in improving health. Nowadays it is necessary to think in terms of shared leadership among the different levels of government with responsibilities in health, especially in countries with a federal structure or in confederations of autonomous communities. Increasingly, what is involved is state health pacts whose corollary must be territorial management and coordination of the competencies of the local, intermediate, and central health authorities, both de jure and de facto.

Second, a neutral steering role is inconceivable. Behind the act of governing, directing the efforts of the sector, conducting activities in health, building a consensus between the State and civil society, are social values that plot the course. These values are not personal in nature, but public and collective; they have to do with the demands that society places on the legitimate, constituted public authorities. In this regard, especially within the framework of the profound social and economic inequities that characterize our Hemisphere, it is very difficult to conceive of an effective steering role that does not seek to improve social cohesion, that does not make its goal the reduction of inequities—in access to health care, in the financial burdens that people must bear to gain access to health services, and in the health conditions of the population. It is very difficult to conceive of an exercise of the steering role that does not have a redistributive function, anchored in solidarity and aimed at combating poverty and meeting the millennium development targets.

PART II

Public Health's Conceptual Renewal

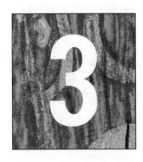

Origins and Current Scenarios

1. Health and Public Health through the Ages

The fear of death and of life-threatening situations can be traced back to the very origins of society. Consequently, a tribe's need to defend and protect its members against multiple threats was what kept it united. In a world without scientific knowledge, disease was explained as the punishment of gods and spirits for the sins of the individual or group, whereas health was regarded as a blessing or reward for virtuous behavior.

Prevention was achieved through virtue and cure was the result of magic. This period of magic and myth gave rise to many health-related beliefs and values that have lasted, with some changes, for generations, centuries, and even millennia. These are still significant today and, at times, fundamental. One of these inherited concepts with major repercussions for society has been the acceptance of the duality and the union

between the spirit, soul, or mind and the body. Another, and no less important one, is the notion of the relationship between the health of the individual and that of the social group to which he/she belongs.

With the dawn of agriculture came new patterns of material and social organization that revolutionized public health: a more reliable food supply and better protection against environmental factors brought with it, no doubt, a spectacular improvement in health status over that of the pre-agriculture era.

As humankind's knowledge of nature increased so did its potential for rational explanations and *scientific* health interventions. Beliefs begin to be supplemented with reason, and philosophy began to transform itself into the cultivation of knowledge.

Natural explanations began to emerge for health and disease, thus increasing

the chances for specific interventions, while medicine became an area of knowledge and a profession. Prevention took on greater relevance, as it became possible to associate disease with impurity or *dirtiness*; thus, the concept of hygiene emerged as the first organized response in health protection. Moreover, there was growing recognition of the environment's role in health and disease. This idea helped give rise to the miasmatic theory of disease, complemented by the humoral theory of body functions. Individual and collective health was improved through a kind of assimilation with beauty, art, and care of the body.

This model of development was already present in prehistoric societies, as evidenced in the historical record of different civilizations.

According to the Etruscan inscriptions, dating back to the beginnings of historical records (5000/6000 B.C.), the practice of curing was already established as a socially significant activity; the Code of Hamurabi (3000 B.C.) mentioned *physicians*, and in ancient Egypt, *medicine* acquired a defined position and its own social status, although linked to and regulated by religion. Imhotep (2980–2900 B.C.) was the first physician to be confirmed by history (18 centuries before Aesculapius) and the Ebers and Smith Papyri were the first known medical texts, the former consisting of a list of remedies and prayers and the latter a surgical textbook. Health was no longer viewed as exclusively magic. The ancient Egyptian society's food systems (silos and distribution) and concerns about the environment and the body can also be viewed as *public health* measures.

Meanwhile in the East, the Chinese figure Fu Nsi (circa 2950 B.C.) was Imhotep's contemporary. The *Nei Ching*, the internal medicine classic of Yellow Emperor Huang Ti (27th century B.C.) was also written around the same time as the Egyptian papyri. The yin and yang, or cosmic theory of complementary opposites, appearing proportionally in the human body and generating balance—health—and imbalance—disease—emerged as the first known attempt at a general and universal explanation that was not strictly religious in nature.

The sacred Vedas of ancient India (circa 2000 B.C.), particularly in the *Ayurveda* system of medicine, include explanations of health and magical cures recorded by Dhanvantari, the god of medicine. However, the Vedas also reflect an awareness of the symptoms and signs of disease and prescribe treatments to cure them (especially herbal remedies). Moreover, religious customs in both China and India prohibited any cutting or mutilation of

corpses, thus precluding the development of knowledge in the areas of anatomy and pathology.

However, in Greece a true revolution in knowledge occurred that also encompassed health. Building on Babylonian and Egyptian foundations, and perhaps also those of China and India, Hellenistic civilization laid the groundwork for the transition from magic to science. In health, this change began with the myth of Aesculapius (circa 1200 B.C.), the god of medicine, who was also a physician. Temples doubled as *therapeutic centers* where, in addition to the role of faith in curing the sick, health was restored through diet, therapeutic baths, and exercises, often preventive in nature. Opportunities for observation began to be pursued, although primitively, as were attempts to make use of accumulated knowledge. However, it was not until the 4th and 5th centuries B.C. that philosophy, drawing on this greater individual and institutional freedom of thought, created the necessary climate for a qualitative leap in knowledge. Empedocles (5th century B.C.) built on the theory of the four basic elements of the universe—fire, air, water and earth—with his hypothesis of the different fluids or *humors* found in the human body. The grand contributions of the different schools of philosophical thought, such as those of Socrates and Plato, culminated in the work of Aristotle (who was also a biologist), and covered almost all areas of knowledge. These contributions established the essential characteristics of scientific knowledge as well as the intellectual and basic instruments for its production and validation (the *Organon*). Moreover, they facilitated an understanding of the natural world and of man (physics and metaphysics), as well as his behavior (ethics).

It is against this marvelous backdrop, this explosion of human creative genius, that Hippocrates (460–380 B.C.) and his collaborators authored the wondrous *Hippocratic Collection* (Corpus Hippocratum) on medicine and health. The importance assigned to observation and logic in diagnosis and treatment was far more than just the basis of semiology and remedy research; it was also the origin of epidemiology and the study of public health. Indeed, the text on *Airs, Waters, and Places* explores human ecology and the relationship between health and living conditions, laying the foundation for the *integral view of the patient in his/her environment*. This text also introduced the term's *epidemion* and *endemeion*, referring to the presence of disease in the community. The reach of Greek culture expanded with the campaigns of Alexander the Great and was incorporated in Greco-Roman civilization. The medical school founded in Alexandria (300 B.C.) was both a product of and participant in that process, which was already emphasizing the importance of the *basic sciences* of medicine. Good examples in this regard include Herophilus in the field of anatomy and Theophrastus in physiology.

Overall, the most specific contribution of ancient Greece to the field of public health is found in the areas of hygiene and the physical culture of the human body. Health and beauty are confused with one another and hygiene becomes associated with well-being and physical prowess.

Rome succeeds Greece. Medicine was expanded and affirmed by proponents such as Aulus Cornelius Celsius (30 A.C.), Asclepiades (120 A.C., an opponent of the humoral theory) and Galen (160 A.C.), the latter of whom became the prototype of the traditional physician. Rome's contribution to public health is even more important. Prior to that time public health had not been distinguished from the field of medicine and only occasionally contemplated, most notably during health calamities, and was practiced by the same actors. Rome moved to differentiate the content of public health from that of medicine. Thus, key measures, such as the development of a common water supply, urban sanitation, hygiene and refuses disposal systems, public baths, hospitals, and public assistance to patients, was established to protect the health of the population. In many instances, such measures became part of the legal framework, specific institutions were created for their development, and they were almost always adopted as social practices.

In each historical experience of the ancient world, health was always associated with the values embraced by society and backed by the institutions responsible for representing them, as well as existing knowledge, in order to explain and intervene in life. The progress resulting from the predominance of positive values and the corresponding social institutions, from their capacity to act (i.e. knowledge and means), and from effective leadership, was accelerated in situations of global change. Thus in the historical context, progress occurred relatively slowly in ancient Egypt and civilizations of the East and faster in the Greek and Greco-Roman civilizations.

In the 1300 years that followed the 2nd century, the prevalence of values aimed at promoting conformity and limiting creativity limited the development of the field of health. In the West, religious dogmatism again exerted control over social forces, filling the voids left by decadence and restricting freedom. Magic once again prevailed over science; Providence over action, salvation of the individual soul over cares of the body and concern about the population. Consequently, public health lost its recently acquired identity and medicine remained stagnant—or even lost ground—as it was relegated to isolated practice in a handful of monasteries or by closely watched practitioners or the lower social classes.

Progress occurred under the relative liberalism of Islam, including Avicenna's work in the field of chemistry and the creation of *modern* public hospitals. Moreover, there was progress in the East: India's Brahman period (800 B.C.–1000 A.C.) evidenced development of the *Caraka Samhita* and the *Susruta Samhita*, which reinterpreted humoral theory by incorporating the spirit and made headway in dietary and medicinal treatments; in China, medical materials, moxibustion, and acupuncture were developed. And by the end of the period (16th century), the Chinese pharmacopeia, the "Ben Cao Gang Mo," was published. However, in the West, advances were also being made with respect to health calamities and other critical situations, including the leper's code of the Third Lateran Council (1179) and introduction of the concept of quarantine during the bubonic plague epidemic of the 14th century, which developed despite the predominance of miasmatic theory.

The Renaissance and mercantilism, which revolutionized creativity in the arts and "globalized" the world, also changed the social order, laying the foundations for a new Cultural Revolution for humankind, and by extension, new scientific and productive transformations. The revival or strengthening of values such as reasoning and freedom, captured by illuminism, positivism, and subsequently, utilitarianism and liberalism, broke down many of the barriers to human creation and led to a new social order that promoted the expansion of knowledge and the urbanization of agrarian societies due to industrialization. The ensuing impact on health was impressive and multifaceted.

The adverse effects of the grinding poverty in urban slums and mining towns during the initial stage of industrialization were widely offset by the associated political advances and progress in the area of knowledge.

With respect to the social sphere, the extremes of the new productive regime provided ample incentives for the emergence of real socialism, social democracy, and the welfare state, and consequently, for reforming capitalism, improving representative democracy, and the rule of law. They also led to an understanding of the relationship between health and living conditions. Moreover, this expansion of productive forces encouraged a scientific revolution that is still under way, fueling the growth of knowledge and technology.

The advent of microbiology reinforced the foundations of hygiene, replaced the *miasma* theory, established a direct causal relationship between disease and its agents—etiology—and at the same time that the discoveries were being made in the physical sciences, paved the way for the control of specific communicable diseases and the development of medicine. Thus, microbiology ushered in a new era of medicine and public health.

However, the most revolutionary changes have occurred only in the past 300 years, as a culmination of the progress begun centuries earlier. The huge toll exacted by the Black Plague of 1348 brought about the acceptance of natural causes for the disease and led to the introduction of *surveillance systems* and quarantine measures. With these steps, public health started down a long road toward reacquiring its identity. During the 17th century, Girolamo Fracastoro demonstrated the contagion principle, thus creating conditions for debate on the idea of prevention. The closing years of the 18th century witnessed the development of the first vaccine (smallpox; Jenner, 1779) and the pioneering brilliance of Johan Peter Frank and his *method for a complete medical policy*, which states that governments should be responsible for the health of their citizens. The exhaustive systematization that ensued laid the groundwork for the reforms carried out by Bismarck in 1884, which then became a model for health services organization. Meanwhile in France, Dr. J.I. Guillotin (1792) successfully lobbied the National Convention to create a health committee. Some decades earlier, in 1748, Sweden enacted the first law providing for the mandatory collection of health data, followed by similar initiatives in other countries. Improvements in health information, the linking of health to a person's social status (Virchow, Villermé, Chadwick, et al) and scientific advances in fields such as microbiology expanded the scope and methods of epidemiological research, allowing even faster progress in the field of public health.

Generally speaking, the French and American Revolutions transformed political thinking around the world, usher in the return of democracy as an idea and a desirable form of government. These "suprastructural" manifestations responded to accelerated transformations in the means of production, through transformations that upheld the principles of the private ownership of the means of production and the bases of the market economy and industrialization, which were complemented by liberal-democratic political regimes. The ideological context and productive basis stimulated creativity, conflict and change.

This transformation continued and expanded during the 19th century, resulting in a true health revolution. *Scientific medicine* was reaffirmed through experimentation (Claude Bernard) and microbiology (Pasteur and Koch). England's Poor Law Commission submitted its report in 1838, amending the Elizabethan Poor Law of 1601. Moreover, England created its own public health institute, with other European countries following suit during the latter half of the century. Health care systems were organized on more solid institutional foundations, and public health acquired definitive status. During this same period, organizational models for health and social security services emerged that have been guiding health care systems since (Bismarck model).

The 19th century ended with an explosion of progress in the knowledge of communicable diseases (i.e. tuberculosis, malaria, and yellow fever). These advances, together with the need to reduce health risks for international trade and the national elite, resulted in interventions targeting specific diseases. In turn, these efforts led to improvements in sanitation and hygiene, and moreover, underscored the need for international cooperation in health. Indeed, the first two international sanitary congresses were held in Paris during 1851 and 1859, followed by others until the Office of Hygiene and Public Health was finally created in 1907. In the Region of the Americas, the first two international sanitary conventions between Argentina, Brazil and Uruguay were held in Montevideo in 1873 and 1884, respectively, while a third took place in Rio de Janeiro in 1887. These meetings were the precursors to the first *Pan American Sanitary Conference (Washington, D.C. 1902), which created the Pan American Sanitary Bureau.*

This process of constant, accelerated change reached its climax during the 20th century. The opposing forces of the capitalism that was dominant at the time gave rise to conflicts in the world of socialism—such as uprisings, the cold war, and fiascos, as well as economic crises and wars that shook the world. The ideas of people and civil society gradually gained acceptance in social areas such as human rights, citizenship, and the democratic rule of law. Liberal representative democracy was acknowledged as the dominant system for legitimizing production based on the market and private initiative. Productivity and production flourished, fueled by technology and new forms of organization. Wealth, however, was concentrated and social inequalities, both between and within countries, became more pronounced.

The end of old-style colonialism brought about a proliferation of the number of *independent* countries at the periphery of the exercise of world power. International mechanisms for debate and conflict resolution, whether through treaties or organizations, succeeded in reducing the chances of war with the potential for world destruction, but by the same token, had the effect of maintaining a large number of *low intensity* conflicts. Scientific and technological output is both a driving force and result of the entire process, providing—sometimes unexpectedly—opportunities to satisfy or create needs, while giving rise to important ethical and social questions. As is the case with wealth and power, knowledge is also concentrated and selective, so the breakdown and *homogenization* of culture clash head on with a multiethnic, multicultural world.

In terms of health and public health, the 20th century witnessed many sensational successes, but also some painful failures. Spurred on by scientific advances, the predominance of positive values, and more effective institutional organization and resources, health care experienced a dramatic expansion, becoming at once more complex and effective. The health of populations around the world improved rapidly, and we are now able to celebrate memorable victories in the struggle against disease, such as those over smallpox and poliomyelitis. However, enormous social inequalities remain with respect to the level of health, exposure to risks, and access to care.

Health care systems are expanding and becoming more complex. Their organization has acquired more diversified reference points such as the state socialism models of Beveridge, and more recently, a number of innovations and combinations. Consequently, a great deal of progress is being made in public health, but there are also failures. While public health has achieved importance and prestige in some cases, in others it has been put aside and shows shameful omissions, such as those observed in the cycle of sectoral reforms based on the principles of the *Washington Agreement*, which have been carried out by numerous countries over the past two decades. Despite the successes, in the overall balance, the distance between what is possible—not the ideal—and what has been achieved has increased. This gap results in the suffering, disability and avoidable deaths that make up the enormous and disgraceful social debt in health that, in the Region of the Americas, is already adding up to approximately 1 million unjustifiable and avoidable deaths annually, as well as millions of years of life lost.

The history of public health in the 20th century has been full of ups and downs, especially in the Region of the Americas, which is the focus of this analysis. The first three decades of that century were a continuation of the movement under way at the close of the 19th century, in which the expansion of trade and the capacity to intervene with the development of the science of etiology stimulated efforts in the areas of sanitation, hygiene and disease control, especially with regard to malaria, cholera and yellow fever, which held serious consequences for trade and immigration. Important successes were achieved in this regard, such as completion of the Panama Canal (1914), rehabilitation of the Region's major ports, and the eradication of yellow fever in Havana and Rio de Janeiro. During the second half of the 20th century, major institutional development occurred in the United States, where, from the time of the Shattuck Report (Massachusetts), public health services were created at the individual state level. This effectively marked a change in responsibility for health, which, up until that time had been almost exclusively the domain of the local level. In 1912, the Federal Public Health Service was created, from the Marine Hospital Service.

World War I did not succeed in interrupting this process, but instead offered opportunities to develop measures and enhance knowledge. In these opening decades of the century, the linkage between the reduction of poverty and sanitary improvements was strengthened, and the first schools of public health were founded in the U.S. (i.e. Johns Hopkins and Harvard), and later in Latin America (i.e. São Paulo, Venezuela, Chile and Mexico). With this, public health completed its institutional development cycle, creating mechanisms for the autonomous reproduction of knowledge, techniques and human resources. Consequently, nongovernmental organizations began to enter the field of public health. Some even entered the international arena, exemplified by the pioneering efforts of the Rockefeller Foundation. The American Public Health Association (APHA) was founded in 1872, followed by a number of other professional and scientific associations with specific concerns, such as tuberculosis and cancer. Meanwhile in Latin America, steps were taken to create the public ministries of health and social security institutions, which continued developing until the 1950s.

The Russian Revolution (1918) and the arrival of bona fide state socialism altered the world's political and ideological landscape, thus introducing an element that would prove to be very important to political development in the remaining years of the 20th century.

The greatest failures of public health in that period were the limitation of its practice to sanitary/hygiene conditions and the control of communicable disease despite knowledge of the social dimensions of health, and its limited coverage, especially in Latin America.

The 1930s witnessed the rise of Nazism and fascism, with their assaults on human rights, intolerance, and colonialist aggression that ultimately led to confrontation with the major powers in World War II. This decade also began with the worldwide recession of the 1930s (the Great Depression in the United States began in 1929), which required new economic thinking to cope with the crisis, including a call for the individual states to take on greater responsibility, and pointed to the need for a new institutional order to improve financial stability. This provided the motivation for creating the institutions of the Bretton Woods system at the end of WWII. *The 1940s were witness to WWII, and afterwards, to the creation of the United Nations and World Health Organization (WHO),* as well as to a renaissance of humanism. During this period, the sciences experienced extreme growth, and economic production accelerated its diversification—in terms of organization and products—which would continue throughout the rest of the century and bring about profound changes in consumer behavior, living conditions, and expectations of the population. Although public health continued to develop, it was increasingly taking a back seat to health care.

The period of the 1950s and 1960s began with a sense of peace and unity after the tragedy and barbarism of WWII, which were subsequently replaced or altered by the *ideologies* of the Cold War. Nevertheless, it was a period of renewed Pan-Americanism and regional cooperation, especially after the critical phase of European reconstruction.

Latin America experienced prolonged growth and expanded its process of industrialization and the State's role in the economy; planning for development came into fashion. At the same time, de facto regimes replaced budding democracies, prompted by the struggle against communism—a trend that intensified with the Cuban Revolution. Meanwhile in the United States, there was a population explosion—the *baby boom*—and a great expansion of public health care programs; public health services were consolidated and strengthened (i.e. NIH, CDC, EPA, and FDA), thus completing the epidemiological transition. In Latin America, a significant expansion in the supply of personal health care services was consolidated, thanks to a major reorganization of health systems. Public health consolidated the expansion of its objectives, although it remained a second-tier priority of governments. Moreover, the most recognized achievements of public health continued to take place in the areas of communicable disease control and basic sanitation, such as the failed effort to eradicate malaria, smallpox eradication, and the expansion of the coverage of the water supply as well as excreta and waste disposal. Latin America's population reached the apex of its natural growth thanks to lower mortality and high fertility rates, thus accelerating the urbanization process. The Region adjusted to the increase in chronic diseases, while coping with high incidences of communicable disease and vitamin deficiency disorders. There was a proliferation of public health schools and institutes, which began to work together in efforts to coordinate and exchange information.

The Pan American Health Organization (PAHO) experienced continuous growth and activity in its sphere of action. By the end of the period, the "Health for All" initiative and its core strategy of primary health care succeeded in increasing public health expectations. However, the strategic vision of transforming these efforts was minimized due to an exaggerated emphasis on the first level of care, thus the transforming potential of these initiatives was not fully realized.

By the end of the 1970s, the dynamic factors that fueled growth in the previous period began to lose steam, leading first to the foreign debt crisis in Latin America and then to "the lost decade" of economic growth, the 1980s. During the 1970s and 1980s, the United States and Canada experienced a turbulent economic period with high rates of inflation, including downturns in investment, production growth and employment, as well as clear signs of unrest among some sectors of the U.S. population with respect to the problems of racial segregation and the Viet Nam War. The failure of communism in the Soviet Union and other countries increasingly led to an easing of Cold War tensions, whose symbolic end was the fall of the Berlin wall. In Latin America, health was hit by the economic crisis, which led to cutbacks in health resources and the negative effects of social injustice (i.e. the concentration of wealth, and the unjust and avoidable disparities that the previous growth period had not significantly addressed). Political violence reached critical proportions in some areas and common violence rose. Then, public health took on a new dimension: *peace.* Accordingly, emphasis centered on the social dimension of health, by demonstrating its relationship to development. A host of other actors become concerned about health, as did international cooperation for health, particularly the international development banks such as the World Bank and the Inter-American Development Bank, as well as NGOs and civil society associations.

The failure of *bona fide socialism* and the economic crisis of the 1980s prompted a return to liberalism—or *neoliberalism*—whose basic principles are reflected in the so-called "Washington consensus." This led to the promotion of a series of health sector reforms, which occurred simultaneously and/or complemented other economic and state reforms. Yet these reforms did not show a great deal of concern for public health; on the contrary, in some cases the already weak institutional infrastructure of public health services was further marginalized. However, progress was made in several areas: the expansion of coverage for some services; polio eradication; greater participation by the health sector in the struggle for peace and social participation in the "redemocratization" of countries operating under totalitarian regimes during the previous period; emphasis on health promotion; and growing recognition of the importance of health for sustainable human development. The last decade of the century played out amid the new process of globalization and a growing consensus on the need to reconsider, review, or improve on the "Washington consensus" and many of its effects, a topic that will be discussed further on in this chapter.

Beyond simply recovering its identity, public health has undergone profound changes in the last three centuries (XVIII XIX and XX) years in terms of its conceptual underpinnings and implementation. In the 18th century, the "century of the Enlightenment," the profusion of ideas from illuminism, utilitarianism, and liberalism, which had such a big impact on politics (i.e. the French Revolution, the nature and organization of the State, the Napoleonic Code, representative democracy and capitalism, and other societal transformations) reached the sphere of public health with considerable delay. The mechanisms responsible for transforming general ideas into public health practice were developed slowly, whether with respect to knowledge, techniques or institutions. Public health remained restricted to the miasmatic theory and, in practice, to limited actions targeting hygiene and the control of epidemics. The Industrial Revolution and the ensuing urbanization process helped to speed up the change. The 19th century arrived with an expanded vision of health and its relationship to social conditions, undermining the dominance of miasmatic theory, which was finally discarded, with the proof of microbial etiologic agents. Throughout the first half of the century, the main public health paradigms targeted the social dimension, especially living and working conditions. By the end of the century, the resulting social reforms and institutional reorganization—the State and insurance systems—were superceded by the practice of specific etiology and its control. In practical terms, the new public health interventions were, as in the past, centered on the definition of regulations and the monitoring of compliance and inspection. The 20th century began under the influence of the same paradigms, emphasizing concern about sanitation and the control of specific diseases. Concern about society, as well as the organization and management of health services, gained momentum in conceptual understandings, with still more progress coming after World War II. Further on in this chapter, the current and future challenges in the field of public health will be examined, while Chapter 4 addresses the new conceptual underpinnings, with a view to achieving more effective practice in public health.

In short, in the past few centuries, the combination of values—although only partially taken from humanism and solidarity—with the expansion of knowledge and public institutional reorganization, has pushed health and public health into a process of even more rapid change, leading to spectacular successes. At the end of the last century and into the present, the control of endemic disease has been pursued, with the additional incentive of commercial interests and the concern of the elite about protection. This led to considerable efforts in environmental sanitation and vector control, following the sanitary model.

The scientific foundations of medicine have been strengthened and made more effective, and health care has expanded rapidly, largely due to performance evaluation, the demands of workers, and the growth of social security systems. This expansion has brought medical care closer to public health, also understood as a process of organizing health care delivery, whose costs and growing complexity demand a collective response. However, the conflicts and injustices persisted, and even increased, during the process. The State created and strengthened its health agencies, yet the assistance it provided varied from country to country and over time. Scientific progress supplied more and better intervention instruments; however, most of these involved personal care. The international organizations have committed themselves increasingly to health. And more recently, global financing and regional institutions have come on board. The concept of health is becoming increasingly comprehensive and expansive, moving beyond the boundaries of medical care and even those of the so-called health sector. Although institutionalized practices do not adequately reflect this knowledge, particularly in the developing world, the necessary conditions are nevertheless in place to evaluate these practices and the concepts implied with respect to the new realities.

Some basic conclusions can be drawn with respect to this overview of the history of health and public health:

1. Health and public health are social and historical constructs.

2. Their nature is cumulative and changing throughout history.

3. Progress in health is made through the combination of values incorporated into social practices, with the expansion of knowledge and its applications and the creation of a public institutional infrastructure that promotes synergy among them.

4. The concurrence of politically significant interests (economics, groups, etc.) during stages of expansion and/or changes in the social production process, together with adequate leadership, increase the power of this combination of factors.

The following sections provide more insight and detail regarding some of the fundamental components of health at present, as well as the current and future challenges facing public health.

2. Present Context

The different components of social life have never been as interconnected as they are today. This interconnectivity is found in all aspects of human life and has increased with the development of national societies and global society. An all-encompassing vision is increasingly necessary in order to understand the parts in that unique space of what is universal or abstract, of what is specific or concrete. Health, which is determined and also explained in this context or contexts, is no exception. Among the several approaches in this regard, we have intentionally narrowed our focus in this document to the following four sets of interrelated yet differentiable phenomena that reflect the immense complexity of the current reality and its implications for health and public health: globalization and its manifestations; political processes; the environment and the population; and necessary development.

2.1 Globalization and Its Manifestations

Globalization stands as a substitute for the geopolitical bipolarity and ideological confrontation of the Cold War years. As a form of victorious expression, it is imposed in absolute terms as the *indisputable road* to a new world order and as the *sole doctrine* for the organization of production, imposing market liberalization in all areas and on a global scale. The advantages and promises of adhering to the principles and guidelines of the "Washington consensus" implied a new era of world progress, the fruits of which were to be shared by all. Those promises appeared to be solidly rooted in a macroeconomic rationale that, more-

over, did not provide room for denial or objection, since such acts would be considered deviations from good behavior and punished with exclusion from the established order. These promises have either not been kept or have been selectively kept—generally at the expense of the developing countries. After 15 years of adjustments and reforms, most of these countries in Latin America and, generally, others throughout the world, seem to find themselves in a relatively worse situation today. In some cases, countries are absolutely worse off than before. Globalization, however, has infiltrated all dimensions of life, creating new situations and conditions that appear to be permanent, or at least, to have long-lasting effects.

Below are some aspects particularly relevant to living conditions and health, which primarily affect the Latin American and Caribbean countries.

a) Science and Technology

Globalization is based on unprecedented progress in science and technology. Productivity and competitiveness are based largely on that progress, including improvements in management that have reduced the importance of the traditional comparative advantages associated with natural resources and cheap labor, since the principal strategic input is knowledge, technology, or information. This fact further encourages the selective concentration of research and technology development toward solving the problems of the core countries; toward market preferences, toward fields that provide greater profit potential, and it also favors the strengthening of intellectual property protections. This hinders access by poor countries to the resulting services and technology products, thus increasing their dependency on the core countries. Moreover, all of this is sanctioned in multilateral agreements. However, science and technology are also promises of social redemption if put to the service of human development and the values that sustains it. Consequently, these inputs are critical factors for progress in health and should be applied in ethically and socially correct ways. Information and technology constitute essential elements for the development of public health; since they expand its effectiveness and capacity for intervention, provided they are appropriate and used in a rational manner.

b) Information and Culture

One of the basic instruments of globalization, in both the modern and postmodern era, is the enormous expansion of the information and communications media, including transport media. In fact, today's economy and all the conveniences of modern living are possible due to the extraordinary capacity for managing information—compiling it, processing it, using it, and disseminating it for different purposes and circumstances. Today's virtual realities parallel factual realities and are increasingly replacing them. More financial capital due to the speed of its universal circulation, the expansion of markets through the marketing of expectations and representations of real, derivative, and future assets, and Internet transactions represent the very essence of current globalization. The strength of that process reaches all sectors of human society, exerting influence over culture, values, and the practices that form society. Values that can be exploited for market purposes are dis-

seminated universally, resulting in cultural breakdown and promoting a certain degree of cultural homogenization. This is a process of critical importance, although it has yet to be fully assessed.

The explosion of information and advertising has broadened consumption habits, which are the expectations and behaviors required by markets. This is accelerating the pace of a large-scale cultural breakdown, capable of destroying or substituting values and diminishing cultural diversity and identity. The result is a loss of moral and ethical parameters for the sake of a materialistic hedonism, whose models lie far beyond the reach of poor societies. Cultural breakdown and unmet expectations are important determinants in the origins or incentives of socially destabilizing behaviors, including self-aggression, aggression toward others, and mistrust. On a collective scale, the replacement of positive values such as solidarity and cooperation by other interests contributes to the corruption, domination, and marginalization of the weak. In other words, freedom without control of the powerful in society amounts to a denial of justice and fundamental human rights for many. The risk of social fractures increases with the development of the behavioral sciences, which offer more powerful analytical tools and interventions in that area.

As in other fields of science and technology, information can also be the most powerful instrument of liberation, as well as of individual and social progress; it can facilitate individual and collective training and the building of citizenship, as well as social participation and control in the public sphere, which are essential for deepening and

expanding democracy and strengthening the rule of law. Thus, information can be used to evaluate the cultural diversity and identity of nations, which is indispensable to their ability to build their own futures, working together for a unified and just humanity.

c) The Market, the State, and Society

In keeping with the principles of the new world order, the three entities listed in the title of this section appear in order of their importance. The market is affirmed, despite its occasional imperfections, and has sufficient virtues to provide all the necessary answers. The role of the State is to facilitate market activities by creating favorable conditions for its full operation, while abstaining from intervention, except when warranted by market interests or in very specific situations. And society is the substratum through which the market and State exist and are justified, and thus should be organized and act accordingly in the hope that in the final analysis, the market-State alliance will also prove to be socially beneficial. Nevertheless, the obvious limits and the failures of the extreme liberal—or neoliberal—model have led to the realization that there is a need to modify some of its characteristics.

A strong State with the capacity for balanced regulation reduces excessive instability, uncertainty, the undesirable destructive effects of competition, and untempered private interests. Furthermore, the State should also have the capacity to effectively meet its state obligations (i.e. defense, public safety, and justice), provide the necessary incentives for private enterprise, and create the conditions to address complex social needs that involve major uncertainties and externalities in circumstances where market mechanisms have serious imperfections, such as in education and health. This contributes to stability, legitimization of the political regime, improvements in the distribution and exercise of power, as well as the strengthening of the market itself, and by extension, the sustainability of the process. But this review should go farther and deeper. It is increasingly recognized that a system of positive values, expressed in organized social relationships and practices and backed by solid, effective institutions (social capital), is essential for market expansion, well-being, and the development process.

Moreover, the management of goods whose generation, use, benefits, and production are destined for regional or worldwide consumption—known as *global public goods* (i.e. knowledge, peace, some natural resources, international regulations and standards, and aspects of health)—requires international cooperation, which is virtually impossible without the input of capable governments. Hence, the major social entities mentioned in the title are placed, at the very least, on equal footing, opening up the possibility of their proper re-articulation: the primacy of the society served by its main instrument or institution (the State), and by the principal mechanism or form of production (the market).

Nevertheless, the terms of this debate are still in the theoretical phase of development. For the most part in practice, the liberal—or *neoliberal*—concept still prevails in a more pure form, with some incidental limitations.

For example, the modernization of the State has largely been reduced to the privatization of public enterprises and delivery of services, often done with the immediate end of obtaining additional fiscal resources to subsidize financial capital through debt servicing and contract guarantees. The reorientation of the State toward fulfilling its own "specific functions," including its social responsibilities as well as health, has either not been done or done with many limitations. In many cases, in fact, the capacity of the State has been undermined in these areas by the devaluation and *demoralization* of public service, the lack of incentives for public employees, heightened uncertainty, and the slashing of resources. It is interesting to note that the claims of a State with no role in production activities that private market initiative does a better job, do not apply to financial intervention: despite the resources obtained from privatization and an increased tax burden, the public debt has swelled in most countries; debt servicing has greatly reduced the power to allocate resources for social spending and has also compromised their economic futures, particularly as a result of external dependence.

Another dimension, perhaps more important than scaling back the public role of the State, is the decline in its influence as an agent of social cohesion and as a means of reinforcing a sense of national identity. In the case of peripheral countries, once the State submits to the rules of multilateral interdependence, thereby placing itself in a position of inferiority, it often gives up the sovereignty to defend the interests of its own people. State reform that seeks to safeguard the public interest, democracy, justice, as well as national identity—and therefore resist corruption and its own "privatization," and be able to guarantee free enterprise and stable markets—has still not been achieved in most countries.

d) Inequities and Injustice

The inequities between countries and within developing countries themselves are increasing visibly. The initial distributive effects of successful stabilization policies are offset many times over by the social injustice of regressive macroeconomic policies, and those that place special emphasis on capital. According to Wolfensohn,[1] without taking China into account, in the 10 years between 1991 and 2001, the number of poor in the world has increased by at least 100 million. Inadequate growth or recession increases unemployment and reduces wages; with the reduction in income, relative poverty (and in some cases, absolute poverty) increases. This situation brings about an increase in the need and demand for public services—including health services—precisely at a time when public response capacity has fallen. Poverty, inequality, and social exclusion threaten the stability of the new order and thus, gain priority in the discourse. This increases possibilities for change with a social orientation and a human face. Social inequalities between countries are, for the most part, unjust and avoidable and affect significant segments of the population. Such inequalities are not only ethically inexcusable as an assault on human rights, but also impose severe restrictions on the possibilities of expanding production and, indeed, on all development. The poor living conditions of those affected by these inequalities constitute the primary risks and health problems of public health.

---

[1]President of the World Bank; prologue of *The Quality of Growth*. PAHO; 2002. (Scientific and Technical Publication No. 584)

e) Management Models and Organizational Tools

Globalization also has an obvious impact on behavior in all areas—from the "style" of governance to the managing of the programs and productive units of social services. The undeniable contribution of business management tools to public administration is understood as a substitute or universal solution for all problems. In government, the situation of ill-defined public and private functions leads to the uncritical adoption of management methods and to a diverse mix of interests and actors, almost always with disastrous results: corruption, privatization of public concerns, institutional weakening, social insensitivity and ineffectiveness. The dogmatic application of market principles to the organization of health care systems has resulted in costly and socially painful experiences in the Region of the Americas and worldwide. The sectoral reforms promoted by many Latin American countries in recent decades have suffered the consequences of that approach, including distortions in health objectives, socially perverse subsidies, increased inequalities and real social costs and, as a result, reduced social effectiveness of their health systems. In the case of such reforms, public health has either been marginalized or overlooked entirely.

f) Missed Opportunities

There is no humanist who does not yearn for a united humanity in which opportunities to realize the human potential are available to all, where all humanity is free to exercise its fundamental human rights. Globalization, thus understood, would be an objective worthy of pursuit. Without a doubt, this includes the intensification of capital flows and trade on a worldwide scale in order to take advantage of productive opportunities everywhere and increase production, with a more equitable distribution of profits and protecting our common natural heritage now and in the future, respecting the essential diversity of cultures. This definitely embraces the idea of a single humanity with different cultures and complementary ways of being and living.

On the other hand, the current model of globalization, which is predominantly geared toward financial and trade concerns, is not contributing to this end, but instead seems to be widening gaps and divisions. Capital flows follow highly profitable immediate interests, sometimes with disastrous consequences for the weak economies at the periphery, as well as their customs, social practices and government. Trade is governed by a set of asymmetrical rules and double standards. Transactions are liberalized on goods for which the rich countries have comparative advantages, namely, those of the industrial and service sectors, while transactions in markets that poor countries are able to compete in with some measure of success are protected or restricted, such as agriculture and mining. Generally speaking, the result in either case is an increase in the exposure and weakness of poor countries externally, hence the increase of dependency and reduction of the possibilities of development.

Moreover, international cooperation is seriously distorted. At international forums there is no shortage of promises or commitments. However, they are subsequently met only partially, generally only when it is convenient for the core countries. Flows, transfers, or voluntary assistance from central governments are, in most cases, only a fraction of the amount promised (on average, 0.3 as opposed to 0.7 of GDP) and appear to be declining. And worse still, the selective protectionism practiced by wealthy countries harms poor countries by reducing their income on the order of US$100–150 million annually. This represents huge losses—two to three times the volume of the cooperation assistance received, which additionally, is subject to diverse conditions.[2]

The use of global public goods, particularly environmental goods, involves a regressive distribution of costs and risks to the world's population living in poverty.

These, as well as other symptoms of the asymmetrical world power structure represent the loss of many opportunities for reducing poverty, for supporting real development, for strengthening democracy, and for promoting respect for human rights. They stand in the way of a world where all humankind can live in peace, freedom and safety.

In short, globalization has ignored the importance of social and human capital in the poor countries, the strength of their cultures, the stability of their institutions, and the requisite human resources necessary for their comprehensive and sustainable development. Consequently, these conditions create instability, uncertainty, fear and mistrust, which is exactly the opposite of what is needed for investment decisions and a healthy market.

In addition, all of these aspects have a negative impact on the development of

---

[2] Alonso, J.A. "Sin respuestas de Monterrey". Madrid: El País; 3/22/2002.

health and public health. Nevertheless, many people still adhere to the dogmatic belief that the market is the primary model for health system organization in all situations, and that the State should only intervene when the market fails or is not interested. This belief, which tends to overlook market deficiencies in health and the need for public intervention, puts at risk the indisputable advantages of market mechanisms for the provision of many goods and health services and as a corrective complement of public action, although always under the direction, regulation and monitoring of the State.

2.2 The Political Processes

The phenomena mentioned in the previous section are also reflected in the political sphere. The great convergence and common ground between economic liberalism and liberal representative democracy is the greatest strength of both processes. Over the past two decades, almost all countries of Latin America and the Caribbean have upheld, returned to or acquired a representative democratic regime, thus opening channels for mobilization and participation that are indispensable for effective social progress and for the assertion of democracy in the Region. Growth of the *non-State public sphere* [3] accelerated, resulting in a more pronounced presence of new and existing social agents. The wide range of direct participation forums, mechanisms and initiatives of society and communities reinforces the possibility of expanding and intensifying democracy and of en-

---

[3] The term *non-State public sphere* is understood as the nonprofit civil society organizations that do not seek to defend special personal or private group interests.

hancing the legitimacy of representation and political institutions.

However, there are troubling signs that the political process is being affected by distortions in current models and practices:

- The totalitarianism inherent in market ideology, like most ideologies, is controlled neither by the liberal doctrine nor by representative democracy—the political regime that legitimizes capitalism. It subordinates the political process to the economic rationale and, frequently, to the special interests that represents it. This inversion or subversion of hierarchy between the two camps is facilitated through a process of cultural breakdown and the predominance of interests over values. This natural corruption affects not only policy, but management as well.

- Simultaneously, such distortions increase the legitimacy gap or deficit of the political process to the point where there is no correlation between decisionmakers and the people affected by their decisions. In such circumstances, the institutions, authorities and their decisions lose the public trust and, at the same time, hinder development. Consequently, political power becomes more concentrated, placing more distance between society and the fulfillment of its real needs.

- The political parties of some countries are merely ad hoc groupings of personal interests or alliances of convenience that are not guided by programs or principles and have a vendor-client relationship with the population. The social illegitimacy of their practices contaminates the en-

tire political process, corrupting the representativeness of the representatives, who, on numerous occasions, literally purchase their mandates to defend their own interests.

- There is a growing popular perception that public institutions and the State exist only to serve a few; that the system places too much value on the interests of capital and obeys the dictates of the market at the expense of society and country. That perception includes the meting out of justice, which threatens democracy and the rule of law. Moreover, examples abound in this regard.

- At the international level, interdependence often operates asymmetrically against the weak countries, especially at economic forums. The *mandatory* or necessary surrender of national autonomy is not sufficiently accompanied by just and effective international mechanisms that offset the disadvantages to the weakest. The imbalance of power reinforces the influence, often directed, of the multinationals and financial capital. This is a particularly important point in a "unipolar" world in which the unilateral decisions of a dominant country—which are difficult to foresee because they are frequently based on national interests and situations, or under the nonnegotiable label of "national security interests"—affect all; the nonexistence of equitable, universal standards increases the insecurity of the weak and, consequently, of all.

- Undoubtedly, all this is much more troubling because the normalcy and strength of democracy, and of the rule of law, are fundamental for socially responsible economic freedom and for health, especially public health.

2.3 The Environment and the Population

The role of the environment in health is crucial and, consequently, has been recognized since ancient times. At the same time, environmental conditions have been priority and irrefutable objectives of public health. The experiences of recent decades have offered proof of the importance of the environment to sustainable development and to solving many environmental problems at the global and regional levels. This topic has been debated at several international conventions (Oslo, 1968 and Rio de Janeiro, 1992), which have approved recommendations and even a detailed plan of action (Agenda 21, Rio de Janeiro) for universal protection of the environment.

At the national level, progress has been made in the delivery of basic and general services. On the other hand, with regard to air, water and soil pollution, the rational use and protection of biosphere resources, and urban problems, less progress has been made and, in many cases, setbacks have been observed. Numerous and substantial threats to health persist, which end up becoming priority public health concerns. At the international level, the lack of action is frustrating. Ten years after the Rio de Janeiro Summit, ratification of the primary instrument developed for implementation of Agenda 21—the Kyoto Protocol for limiting the emission of greenhouse gases—was undermined by the withdrawal of the United States, the main greenhouse gas polluter. However, the proposal to consider the global aspects of such assaults and their environmental solutions as global and regional public

"bads" or goods, has a great deal of conceptual strength and enormous potential to influence multilateral development policies and international cooperation. However, this will require extensive development of instruments and institutional reorganization, which the international community has not demonstrated any enthusiasm for taking on. In view of the foregoing, the environment will continue to be a primary source of health hazards and a key concern both for public health and the international community.

Because the population is the central concern of public health, demographic characteristics are strategic for its practice. The countries of the Region of the Americas are completing—although to different degrees and at different rates—the final phase of the demographic transition, one of low fertility and mortality. Accordingly, the natural increase rate is declining, although it remains high in some countries. The total population of the Region in 2001 was estimated at 841,254,000, some 317,195,000 of which are found in the English-speaking countries of the Americas, whereas 524,099,000 are distributed throughout Latin America and the Caribbean. In spite of lower and declining rates of natural growth, by 2020 there will be 174 million more inhabitants in the Region: 52,600,000 in the English-speaking Americas and 121,400,000 in Latin America and the Caribbean.[4] In the case of Latin America, that additional population represents more than 50% of its total population in 1950. The regional population is already mostly urban (>80%) and will be even more so in the future. With regard to the need and demand for health services, the rural pop-

---

[4] Encyclopedia Britannica, *Yearbook,* 2002.

ulation of the past will all but disappear. But perhaps the most significant demographic change is the rapidly aging population of Latin America, and by extension, of the entire Region. The combined effect of the decrease in birth rates and increase in life expectancy is inverting the proportion of young to old and economically active to inactive in the regional population. The population pyramid of the recent past is rapidly becoming pear-shaped: after one more generation, the proportion of the population over 60 will exceed 15% of the total population, rising to 25% by mid-century. In addition, declining fertility and the proportional reduction in the number of women of childbearing age will lead to birth rates below the necessary minimum for maintaining the population, as is already occurring in some countries of Europe and Asia. The impact of this new demographic revolution will be profound and affect all areas of human society. In fact, it is a significant characteristic of the new society that is already taking shape, and constitutes one of the principal challenges for public health and for social security systems in general.

2.4 Necessary Development

The backlash of societies against liberal dogmatism or market fundamentalism is growing and even welcomed by unexpected actors and authors. This is not a matter of a return to previous situations; what is needed is to establish the necessary balances that will not only allow the creative capacity of individuals and companies to flourish, but also ensure their just contribution to social progress through an achievable and essential complementary synergy. Thus, the development of social capital is a fundamental condition, and health is one of its instruments: an essential component and a desirable outcome. The five guiding principles for necessary development are: an objective centered on human well-being and security; equilibrium in the concentration of all assets—physical, financial, human, social and natural; equitable distribution of benefits that also takes the intergenerational perspective into account; participation; and an institutional framework for implementing these principles that includes guarantees of good governance.

The search for a new concept of the State, including its functions and responsibilities and their relationship to civil society and the market, are fundamental tasks designed to strengthen the rule of law, the distribution of justice and security, and also to expand and deepen democracy. This is especially true with respect to guaranteeing levels of social justice and equity that are ethically desirable and necessary for true human development. In this regard, the rhetoric of consensus should find its expression in public policy and through effective instruments of action that can be fully implemented in the countries of the Region and worldwide. This is development that links vital economic growth under stable conditions with adequate social development, implemented under conditions that ensure social and environmental sustainability.

All the foregoing should take place under the basic principle of the preeminence of society, which is served by the State and the market in a complementary fashion.

3. Health and Public Health in Today's World

The change occurring in the economic, cultural, and political framework coincides with changes in other external determinants of health, specifically in health care systems, and thus, in the health problems and status of the population. Despite the spectacular advances of recent decades in terms of the usual health indicators, the health situation is still considered unsatisfactory in most countries of the Region. Consequently, this poses old, new and evens some re-emerging challenges. In fact, the countries of the Region show an alarming gap between what has been done and what could be done with the available resources in terms of the levels of development attained. For example, unjustifiable and avoidable mortality still accounts for more than 1 million deaths annually. In addition, health services systems reveal several shortcomings and deficiencies, reinforced by a context that is many times more adverse than favorable.

Accordingly, the challenges for public health are numerous and far-reaching; they are found in the external factors that can affect the context, in health care systems, in risks and threats, and in the health status of the population.

3.1 Challenges in the Context

Each topic discussed in the previous section involves risks, problems or opportunities for public health. Generally speaking, the contextual determinants of health have collective dimensions and, consequently, are inescapable issues for public health. The general proposal to effectively incorporate health into all dimensions of the development process, and the resulting intersectoral intervention, is the primary strategy for responding to challenges from the context. This also entails expanding the field of public health, from concern over specific aspects of disease etiology and health threats, to the general mechanisms for producing health and the risks that threaten it. These issues will be addressed in more detail, in the following chapters, without being concerned with examining them categorically as yet.

3.2 Related Challenges to Health Systems

Insomuch as the organization, policies and strategies, management, financing, supply and management of health care systems are matters of public interest, they are also challenges for public health. The public demands socially effective health systems—capable of producing health—that generate social satisfaction, under the guidance of a structured set of basic principles, ethics and politics, and are established rationally. Included among these principles, on which there is consensus in Latin America and the Caribbean, and possibly throughout the Region, are equality for the universality of care, social participation, collective financing, efficiency and decentralization.

One particularly significant aspect involves the adequate definition of functions and relations between the State public, the non-State public, and the private spheres, and preparing the State to exercise its functions, especially those it assumes as the steering authority of the health sector. These functions include regulation of the entire health care system, the identification of financing mechanisms, providing insurance coverage for care, performance of EPHFs, and the organization and management functions associated with the generation of resources, knowledge, and information.

Also important is how public health is defined in health and health care systems and the mechanisms through which it operates, which is the main focus of the next chapter.

Another challenge facing health systems is how to make use of the potential offered by science and technology so as to take maximum advantage of their problem-solving capacity in each situation, while adhering to the ethical principles of respect for human dignity and fundamental human rights.

The ethical challenges involve much more than the ones found in the fields of science and technology and include everything from basic research up through the application of knowledge and technology. These are present in all health care processes and activities. These challenges are also considered beforehand, during decision-making processes geared to the development of public policy and other standards that affect health. Yet they go much further; they are present in the behaviors and relationships of persons and groups in society, to the extent that the corresponding social practices have an impact on health. In short, the ethical considerations reveal the human values attached to public health.

Furthermore, all of these challenges are linked to the greater challenge of incorporating health into truly sustainable human development for the benefit of all peoples and countries, where health must be at the same time both component and purpose, and thus becomes one of the principal indicators of development.

It is also time to modify many of the current sectoral reforms to make them more responsive to these challenges, which in itself poses a significant challenge to public health. Table 1 summa-

---

Table 1 Health Sector Reforms

Shortcomings of Reform Processes
- Incentives are centered on economic factors;
- Equality and public health continue to be treated as second-tier priorities;
- Quality of care and the redefinition of care models are marginal; and
- The role of the State is far too limited.

Primary Lines of Action for a New Generation of Reforms Focusing on the Health of the Population
1. Expand social protection in health and ensure universal access and equality;
2. Develop efficient forms of collective financing;
3. Emphasize quality and effective care;
4. Incorporate health promotion as the primary focus of the comprehensive care model;
5. Strengthen public health through the reorganization of health systems;
6. Strengthen the steering role of the health authority;
7. Develop human resources; and
8. Promote social participation and control.

---

rizes definitions of current processes and desirable lines of action for a new generation of reforms.

3.3 Health Status

Due to changes in health determinants at the individual country level, the health of the population in the Region of the Americas is in different stages of epidemiological transition. In many countries, infectious diseases and illnesses associated with poverty are still significant problems, whereas the incidence of chronic degenerative diseases, generally associated with the developed world, is also on the rise. Added to this are new health problems, including AIDS; the resurgence of old problems, such as tuberculosis; and the serious and growing risk of violence, drug abuse, and environmental degradation. The repeated individual harm takes on collective dimensions and ends up by reducing the differences between personal and population-based care—or, put differently, by revealing the collective potential of personal health care due to the cumulative effect.

In addition, advances in science and technology provide more and better instruments for intervention and new methods and possibilities for their use. Progress is being made, from the prevention and diagnosis of diseases, to their treatment and control, to health promotion and the prediction of risks and, subsequently, to the actual creation of healthy conditions. In fact, the primary focus of health is promotion, which is increasingly relevant to the organization and management of health care and corresponding systems, as well as public health.

3.4 Need for Definitions (or Redefinitions)

Conventional public health by itself is no longer able to meet these challenges. There can be no doubt that disease control, the recognition and production of public goods, or those with significant externalities, as well as the organization of activities recognized as responsibilities of the State, continue to be important elements in the work of public health. Strategically, they should even serve as the platform from which public health expansion is promoted, until it embraces other significant aspects, both within and outside the health sector, in order to improve the health of the population.

A review of public health concepts, its linkage with significant social practices for health, the identification of its essential functions, as well as the instruments for carrying them out, will be analyzed in Part II, Chapters 4 through 7. These aspects, including their operational characteristics, will be examined in greater depth and detail in Parts III and IV of the book.

3.5 Recent Initiatives

"Public Health in the Americas" is not the only initiative where effort has been directed in this area. Many other initiatives with similar intentions have been formulated in recent years, and several are currently being implemented. Thus, there is a general need for this review. However, we will cite only the initiatives that have more directly inspired or adopted the ideas that we wish to analyze:

a) Canada's experience with the formulation of its health policies and reorientation of health care and health promotion systems;

b) The work currently under way in the United States, especially a study on the future of public health by the National Institute of Medicine, and a project of the Centers for Disease Control and Prevention[5] to evaluate the performance of essen-

tial public health services, which have served as the basis for developing the methodological component of the SPA, with a view to evaluating performance of the FESP;

c) The Delphi study, coordinated by WHO, on essential public health functions; and

d) A series of debates promoted by PAHO/WHO in the early 1990s that were taken up again in 1998, giving rise to this project in which the Association of Schools of Public Health (ALAESP) has played an important role.

The Initiative is based on these earlier efforts and experiences and benefits from the abundant and growing debate, as well as the work on *necessary development*, health promotion, equity, and the struggle against poverty—especially from the agreements expressed in declarations or resolutions of the international community and its principal agencies.

Bibliography

Alonso, JA. Sin respuestas de Monterrey. Madrid. *El País*; 22/03/2002.

Amartya, S. Address to the International Labor Conference. 87th Session. Ginebra. In Decent Work, ILO.

Aristotle. Poética, Organon, Política e Constituição de Atenas en Os Pensadores. São Paulo. Editora Nova Cultural Ltda. 1999.

Bambas, A. et al. (ed.) Health and Human Development in the New Global Economy: The Contributions and Perspectives of Civil Society in the Americas. Washington, D.C. PAHO 2000.

Bezruchva, S. Is Globalization Dangerous to our Health? *West Journal of Medicine* 2000. 172: 332–334.

Burckhart, J. Historia de la cultura griega. Vol. III. Parte VIII. Sobre la filosofía, la ciencia, y la oratoria. España. Editorial Iberia S.A. 1965.

Camdessus, M. Speech to UNCTAD-10. Bangkok. 12/02/2000.

CEPAL y UNICEF. Panorama social de América Latina, 1998. Santiago, Chile. 1999.

Chauí, M. A pastoral de Florença e a guerra de Seattle as fantasias da Terceira Via. Caderno Mais. Folha de S. Paulo. 19/12/1999.

Douglas, N. Globalization and Health. Washington, D.C.: Global Health Council. 2000.

Douglas, WB. Sapirie S. y. Goon E. Essential Public Health Functions: Results of the International Delphi Study. WHO, *World Health Statistics* 51. 1998.

Drucker, P. The Next Society. *The Economist*. Nov. 1, 2001.

Encyclopedia Britannica, Macropaedia. Vol. 11 History of Medicine. Pp 823–841. 15th edition. 1980.

Encyclopedia Britannica, Macropaedia. Vol. 15 Public Health Services. Pp 202–209. 15th edition; 1980.

Evans, R., Barer, M. Marmor, T., De Grayter, A. eds. Why Are Some People Healthy and Others Not? New York. The Determinants of Health of Populations. 1994.

Fee, E. The Origins and Development of Public Health in the US. Chapter I of Oxford Textbook of Public Health. 2nd Edition. Oxford Medical Publication. 1991.

Fuentes, C. Democracia latinoamericana: anhelo, realidad y amenaza. Madrid. *El País*. 15/05/2001.

Fukuyama, F. The Great Rupture. The Free Press. 1999.

Garison, H. x fielding. Historia de la medicina. 4a edición. México. Editorial Interamericana. 1966.

Gianotti, JA. Nossa Barbárie. Caderno Mais. Folha de S. Paulo. 3/03/2002.

Giddens, A. 5 clases: Globalization, Risk, Tradition, Family and Democracy. Reith Lectures Home. BB.C. Homepage. 1999.

---

[5] NPHPSP: National Public Health Performance Standards Program. CDC, Atlanta, U.S.A.

Habermas, J. Nos limites do Estado. Caderno Mais. Folha de S. Paulo. 18/07/1999.

Health Canada. Strategies for Population Health Investing in the Health of Canadians. Ottawa, Canada. 1994.

Hippocrates. The Genuine Works of Hipocrates. Birmingham, Ala. The Classicals of Medicine Library. 1985.

Hutton W. Como será o futuro Estado. Brasilia. Linha Gráfica e Editora. 1998.

Jaramillo, AJ. La aventura humana. San José. Editorial de la Universidad de Costa Rica. 1992.

Kaul, I., Le Louven, K. Global Public Goods: Making the Concept Operational. Mimeografiado. New York. UNDP. 2002.

Kaul, I., Grungberg, I., Stern, MA. Bienes públicos mundiales — cooperación internacional en el siglo XXI. New York. UNDP. Oxford University Press. 1999.

Kliberg, B. ¿Cómo reformar el Estado para enfrentar los desafíos sociales del 2000? Instituto Interamericano para el Desarrollo Social. BID. 2000.

Krugman, P. Globalización e globobagens: verdades e mentiras do pensamento econômico. Editora Campos. 1998.

Kurz, R. Totalitarismo Econômico. Caderno Mais. Folha de S. Paulo. 22/08/1999.

Lawrence, G. Public Health Law in a New Century. Three parts. *JAMA*. Vol. 283. Núm. 21, 22 y 23. June 2000.

Legowiski, B., McKay, L. Health Beyond Health Care: Twenty-five years of Federal Health Policy Development. Health Network, Canadian Policy Research Networks, Inc. October 2000.

Macêdo, C. Notas para uma História Recente da Saúde Pública na América Latina. Brasil. OPS. 1997.

Macêdo, C. A Globalização e a Saúde nos países do Mercosul, apresentação no Seminário A Globalização e a Saúde e o Lançamento do Mercosul, mimeo. Brasilia. Ministério da Saúde. August 2000.

Nalón, JJ. Antecedentes y desarrollo de la salud pública en los Estados Unidos. Capítulo 2 del libro Principio de administración sanitaria, segunda edición en español. México. La Prensa Médica Mexicana. 1963.

OPS. Sobre a teoría y práctica de la salud pública: un debate, múltiples perspectivas. Washington, D.C. OPS. 1993.

OPS. La crisis de la salud pública: reflexiones para el debate. Washington, D.C. Publicación Científica Nº 540. 1992.

Padovani, H., Castagnola, L. História da Filosofia. 4ª edición. Edições Melhoramentos. 1961.

PAHO/IDB/World Bank, Investment in Health—Social and Economic returns. Washington, D.C. PAHO. 2001. Scientific Publication Nº 582.

PNUD. Informe sobre el desarrollo humano, 1998 (Cambiar las pautas de consumo). New York. 1998.

PNUD. Informe sobre el desarrollo humano, 1999 (Una globalización con rostro humano). New York. 1999.

PNUD/Chile. Desarrollo humano en Chile, 1998: Las paradojas de la modernización. Santiago. 1998.

Putman, RD. Comunidad y democracia — a experiencia da Italia moderna. Fundação Getúlio Vargas. Rio de Janeiro. Editora. 1996.

Sachs, J. Helping the World's Poorest. Web: The Harvard Center for International Development. 2000.

Sapirie, S. et al. PHC and Essential Public Health Functions: Critical Interactions. Geneva. CIOMS International Conference. 1997.

Savater, F. Elegir la política. España. Letras Libres. Feb. 2002. pp. 12–15.

Sigerist, H. Historia y sociología de la medicina. Bogotá, Colombia. Edited by Gustavo Medina. 1974.

Stiglitz, JE. O que eu aprendi com a crise Mundial. Folha de S. Paulo. 14/04/2000.

Stiglitz, JE. International Financial Institutions and Provision of International Public Goods. European Investment Bank. Papers, Vol. 3, nº 2; 1998.

Stiglitz, JE. La grande Désillusion. Les Echecs de la Mondialisation. París. Ed. Fayard. 2002.

Taylor, L. Stabilization, Adjustment and Human Development. UNDP. Paper N.º 12. 1999.

U.S. Institute of Medicine, Division of Health Care Services, The Future of Public Health. Washington. National Academy Press 1988.

Veronelli, JC., Testa, A. La OPS en Argentina: Crónica de una relación centenaria. Argentina. OPS. 2002.

Vinod, T. et al. La calidad del crecimiento. Washington, D.C. Banco Mundial y OPS. Publicación Científica y Técnica. Nº 584. 2002.

Wade, RH. The Rising Inequity of World Income Distribution. *Finance & Development*. Vol. 38. Nº 4. 2001.

Webster, C. Medicine as Social History: Changing Ideas on Doctors and Patients in the Age of Shakespeare, in Celebration of Medical History Editor Lloyd G. Stevenson. The John Hopkins University Press. 1982.

WHO. Bulletin of the World Health Organization. Vol. 79. Nº 9. Special Theme—Globalization 2001.

World Bank. World Development Report, 1998/99 Knowledge for Development. Oxford University Press. 1998.

World Bank. World Development Report 1997 The State in a Changing World. Oxford University Press. 1997.

World Bank. World Development Report 1999/2000 Entering the 21st Century. Oxford University Press. 1999.

World Bank. DC/2002-16 Poverty Reduction and Global Public Goods: Issues for the World Bank in Supporting Global Collection Action. Sept 2000.

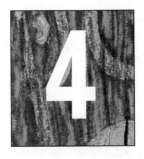

Foundations of the Conceptual Renewal

Public health is understood as the health of the population and, hence, encompasses all collective dimensions of health. This notion of public health stems from the concept of health itself: the absence of disease, injury and disability, as in a complete state of well-being.[1] However, identifying health with well-being poses operational difficulties in terms of delineating health sector responsibilities since at the same that it establishes the responsibilities of other sectors in health and the need for intersectoral action. Viewed from a more sectoral and operational standpoint, health is the fulfillment of the biopsychic potential of the individual and of populations in accordance with their particular living conditions, without the limitations of injury, disability or disease. However, when these limitations do exist, there must be the possibility for prompt recovery or for functional adaptation in cases of irre-

versible disability. Public health, understood as the health of the population, constitutes the fundamental reference point for all efforts to improve health, from which it derives its most complete expression.

While the traditional cornerstones of public health—the prevention and control of communicable diseases or environmental sanitation—continue to be important areas of activity, the current definition of public health includes much more. It is no longer sufficient to define public health in terms of what the government does. Although with the premise that the State must serve the interests of the population, there has been greater correlation between the actions of governments in the health field and public health activities. Government should in fact play a central and fundamental role in public health today. However, not everything that government does in terms of health can be regarded as public health, just as public

health cannot remain limited to government action. From an economic perspective it may be useful to view public health as the production of public health goods and services, or as the generating of important and socially beneficial externalities, however, this definition falls short of covering all the necessary aspects for achieving effective and efficient public health, which is understood as the health of the population.

In light of current public health challenges, there is a need to further expand and clarify what public health means today. This chapter will focus on the conceptual analysis of public health, whereas subsequent chapters will discuss its contents.

1. Objective and Focus

The main objective and primary focus of public health is the health of the population. This includes all elements of collective interest that contribute to

---

[1] WHO, Constitution of the World Health Organization.

improving people's health. Consequently, its specific focus should not be limited to so-called public goods and services, significant externalities, or actions considered responsibilities of the government or the State. As already mentioned, there is an existing consensus that this constitutes an important part of public health and it can and should be its overall strategic core. However, if public health is thus limited, it cannot fully serve the public interest. Consequently, its reach and concern must extend much further, toward the external determinants of health and the collective dimensions of the health care systems, while never losing sight of its main objective the health of the population, even in circumstances where the instruments of public health are in themselves insufficient to effectively change these factors. Two primary consequences reult from this concept: on the one hand, the need for joint action with other sectors; and on the other, concern for the health of the individual, to the extent that some of these aspects take on a collective interest and are essential to public health or that the operative tools, like health services and human resources, are shared.

The argument can be made, and justifiably so, that such a broad understanding of the focus of public health could jeopardize its effectiveness and the operational definition of its responsibilities. Even though the main criterion for this analysis, namely the health of populations, should be the central objective of public, these arguments must also be taken into consideration. Insofar as public health—understood as the health of the public—is determined by living conditions for example, and that the activities of public health itself are also determined by the conditions of its context, its activities cannot be effective and

may sometimes be impossible, unless it seeks to influence these conditions. Logically, the function of public health with respect to many such factors is not to decide or intervene directly but rather, to promote and coordinate, with the express aim of protecting the health of the population. Thus, for public health to be effective, it must expand its focus as a function of its main objective. As for defining specific responsibilities, the problem can be solved by identifying the direct and shared responsibilities of public health and the different performance indicators for the two categories. The first demands more precise indicators for measuring the structure, processes, production capacity and outcomes related to health, whereas the indicators in the second category focus on measuring performance and evaluating processes and outcomes—that is, the impact on direct responsibilities, the factors that determine public health, or the health of the population itself.

2. Sphere of Activity

The objective and focus determine the sphere or spheres of activity of public health.

First, it is important to note that public health implies a field of knowledge, and especially, a field of practice that can be defined and organized. However, it is neither a science nor a discipline. Consequently, the body of knowledge required for its exercise comes from a number of disciplines, articulated in terms of the objective and focus of public health. This articulation of the knowledge that the practice of public health comprises an interdisciplinary dimension, is the epistemological essence of public health, which often transcends the disciplines that contribute to it, even though it is not a specific discipline in

and of itself. Furthermore, there is a need for an instrument or method for coordinating information, since public health draws on knowledge from diverse disciplines, depending on the specific focus of the public health practice that is required for a particular situation. However, one discipline that appears to hold a great deal of potential for public health and which, likewise, frequently serves its purposes, is the field of epidemiology. This has to do with the kind of epidemiology that is broad enough to include all the determinants of health and aspects of health care, one that is not limited solely to the study of disease. In fact, this combination of epidemiology and demography constitutes the science of population; the focus and methods are consistent, in terms of structure and outcome, with the concept and focus of public health. Since epidemiology evolves together with public health, it is not surprising that the history of epidemiology is sometimes confused with that of public health. Ultimately, the epidemiological method is the more powerful and general instrument, but it is by no means the only one for coordinating the inputs of the many disciplines that contribute to public health.

Inasmuch as public health involves both knowledge and practice, it also generates knowledge that enriches the various disciplines that it draws from or that are specific to it. Thus, we are correct in speaking of public health knowledge, public health research, as well as the functional fields that are specific to it.

The spheres of activity are a functional reflection of the focus of public health, namely, its main concerns, health determinants, risks, etc. Accordingly, they cover all facets of the social process associated with the production of public health. Responsibility for the corresponding public health activities lies with a specific actor or actors or is shared among several actors, as explained further on in section 4 of this chapter. Nevertheless, it is possible to identify a core set of functions and responsibilities belonging to the health authority, the fulfillment of which is, without exception, necessary in order to ensure good public health. This set of basic public health functions make up what the initiative considers the "Essential Public Health Functions" (EPHFs), which are the primary operational focus of the project. The EPHFs will be examined in subsequent chapters, especially in Chapter 5 and Parts III and IV.

3. Public Health, the Health System, and Health Care

Public health's sphere of activities covers the field of health in general, encompassing all of its components from the standpoint of the health of the population. Public health functions are carried out within the broader context of health actions, so that no analysis of the concept of public health is complete unless it is done within the context of the health system, health care and medical care, with which it is so intrinsically linked.

Public health is an integral part of the health system which is understood to be the interventions carried out in society with health as the primary goal.[2] This concept of the health system includes care for people and the environment, with the purpose of promoting, protecting and restoring health, or reducing or compensating for irreversible disability,

[2] WHO, "The World Health Report 2000—Health Systems: Improving Performance"; 2000

Figure 1 Spheres of Health and Social Components

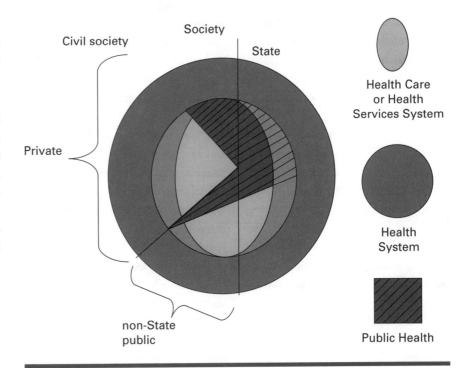

and it includes provision of the necessary means, resources and conditions to accomplish this. This definition also includes actions affecting the general determinants of health, undertaken to improve health or facilitate care, regardless of the nature of the agents—whether public, State, non-State, or private—who carry them out. The health system is much broader than the health care system or health care services, which include medical care. Figure 1 illustrates these health areas and their relationship to the primary social components—civil society, the component with a basically private operation that includes the market, the non-State public or "community" sector,[3] and the State.

The larger circle, which is society, represents the health system, which in turn

[3] *Non-state public sector:* non-profit public and social services-oriented civil society organizations, such as charities and community organizations.

contains the health care system (dotted oval), both containing their State, private, and non-State public components. The irregularly shaped shaded area represents the field of public health, which covers part of the health care system area, but also some additional areas outside of it. Thus, as will be seen in section 4.1 and subsequently in Chapter 5, the concept of public health encompasses some aspects outside the health system that are important to the health of the population. Nevertheless, it is appropriate to limit its extension to the health system.

The operational side of the concept adds another dimension to the scheme—that of the health sector. In every institutional setting or political/legal/administrative system, there are institutionally formalized organizations whose main purpose is to advance health. This group of institutions, including the relationships among themselves as well as between them and other institutions, is conventionally known as the health sector. The concept of the sector, to be conventional and utilitarian in administrative terms, adjusts to each set of circumstances. In the case of the health sector, it also generally includes the public State and public non-State subsectors, as well as private subsectors of public or private interest associated with the market or other groups. The sector is ordinarily delimited within the scope of the health system, but rarely corresponds with it; it corresponds more with the health care system, but is not consistent with the fields of public health at the present time. Moreover, albeit designed for administrative purposes, in reality, a well-established, functioning organizational structure does not necessarily exist. Often, certain health-related institutions and organizations are, from an administrative standpoint, part of other sectors, such as basic environmental sanitation, the production of health equipment and supplies, food security, and health insurance. Thus, the nature of a productive organization and not its purpose is the test for determining which sector it belongs to.

The proportions of the elements presented in Figure 1 do not reflect any concrete situation nor are they intended to serve as a model. They do, however, generally reflect the most common situation found in the Region of the Americas, which is the fact that most health and health care systems are private, although the State participates in these to a large extent, and that the field of public health is largely public, where the State is the dominant contributor to the health system and only a small part comes from the private sector.

Given the above considerations on the general organization of health actions, a brief analysis of the main objective, general contents and universal basic functions of the health system is in order, in an effort to link them with the objective and fields or functions of public health, with a view to establishing public health actions, responsibilities and relationships within the health system.

The basic purpose of the health system and the health care system that comprises it is to produce health in the best possible way in keeping with each specific situation. This constitutes the primary focus of the social process of health generation—to produce health for people, but especially for the population as a whole. The social effectiveness of the system is, therefore, its main performance indicator. However, it is not enough to be effective and produce health collectively; the system must do so by generating individual and, especially, social satisfaction. Satisfaction is not just an attribute or a result of the quality of care but also something that is necessary for its effectiveness. In democratic societies, governed by human rights and real humanitarian values, satisfaction is an essential value for enjoying a full quality of life and has significant political importance in terms of legitimizing the political system and exercising the rights of citizenship. Thus, the level of satisfaction constitutes the second global performance indicator of health and health care systems, especially when complemented with an evaluation of its primary factors—quality of care, as defined by problem-solving capacity and the types of services; and response to the population's expectation in health or some other sphere. The two final goals—effectiveness and social satisfaction—are always present in health and health care systems, whether explicitly or implicitly.

Health systems are based on values, some of which constitute the structural principles of these systems, influencing their organization and operation, as well as their final goals. As such, they constitute complementary and/or intermediate objectives of the final goals and, in some cases, are justifiable and sought after in their own right. Currently in the Americas, the following values are included in this category:

a) *Equity.* Equity is viewed as an essential value for correcting the unjustifiable inequalities and social injustice that exist in health, as well as for attaining effectiveness and social satisfaction. Equity is also a necessary and strategic condition for achieving universal access to care, based on existing needs and available resources.

b) *Social participation.* Social participation is considered the right and capacity of the population to participate effectively and responsibly in health care decisions and their implementation. Social participation in health is one facet of general civic participation, a condition for exercising freedom, for democracy, for social control over public action and, hence, for equity. It is also an essential condition for ensuring effectiveness and satisfaction, and, in terms of health actions, constitutes a desirable end in itself.

c) *Efficiency.* Efficiency is understood as the use of resources in terms of the objectives and principles established. Efficiency is especially important, given the scarcity of resources.

d) *Decentralization.* This maintains the most appropriate balance of complementary responsibilities among the different levels of government. It also helps to facilitate the aforementioned principles, as well as the final goals of health systems and health care.

e) *Comprehensive care.* This means health care that attends to needs in keeping with the seriousness of the illness or harm and problems that require progressive care, which constitutes a requirement for effectiveness, satisfaction and equity.

f) *Solidarity.* There is a need for solidarity to counter the uncertainty and complexity of health problems associated with risks and diseases and to mount responses to these challenges. Solidarity is fundamental for balancing financing—defined as the distribution of financing efforts based on fair criteria and collective coverage of costs for the delivery of equitable, universally accessible services. Solidarity is the recognition of common situations and interests and organization for joint efforts to protect health—that is, for the organization and delivery of necessary health services. Solidarity is therefore a characteristic that includes equity and participation, and it contributes to efficiency and productivity, which makes it a key factor in the effectiveness of and social satisfaction with health systems.

Health systems and health care must have resources and conditions in place to facilitate the realization of their final goals, as well as to apply the structural principles adopted. Because the characteristics of such resources and conditions are critical for system performance,

they constitute immediate objectives for management. This situation leads to the risk, which is quite commonplace, of disassociating these resources and conditions from the objectives, values or principles they should be serving and of being transformed into independent objectives themselves. This has certainly been the critical mistake of many recent sectoral reforms. Among these resources and conditions, we will cite five that are particularly important:

a) *Leadership.* Leadership is understood as the capacity to formulate and implement plans and projects. This includes the ability to set up agreements and support mechanisms; effectively bring opposing parties together; mobilize willpower and resources; and ultimately, to bring about the most favorable conditions and situations for realizing system objectives, principles and functions. Leadership, then, is the most essential attribute for properly exercising the management function.

b) *Information.* Information is considered vital input for appropriate decisions and actions, provided that the information is produced and used properly to generate the intelligence required.

c) Sufficient *human resources* and appropriate *physical capacity for production;*

d) Appropriate *knowledge* and *technology;*

e) *Financing.* Because financing is an instrument that makes all other resources and conditions feasible, and ordinarily depends on decisions made outside the health system, it

takes on special meaning. The following factors are important: the level of financing in relation to the wealth of a country. which reveals the extent of societal efforts and the degree of sufficiency or production that is possible; its origins or sources, which determine the level of solidarity—or absence thereof— and equity in the distribution of that effort; and its use (process of allocation and distribution and production generated), which represents the essence of the management model, its level of efficiency, and the final destination of resources—that is, which needs are met and who are the beneficiaries.

The objectives, basic principles, and the required conditions and resources guide the definition of system functions, as well as its organization and operation. In this document, we only consider the global functions as a frame of reference for public health functions. WHO identifies four global and universal functions of health systems:[4] stewardship; provision of services; generation of resources through investments and development of human resources; and financing, which includes collection, incorporation and purchasing. With respect to the dimensions of the steering role in health, PAHO[5] also identifies four global health system functions: stewardship, service delivery, financing and health care insurance. The EPHFs form part of the steering role, together with heath system management and regulation, harmonization in the delivery of services, the distribution of financing, as well as oversight and insurance.

---

[4] WHO, op. cit.
[5] PAHO, "Steering Role of the Ministers of Health in Health Sector Reform Processes," 1996.

Among the functions subsumed under the steering role, and considered in part an essential public health function, is public information. This is not a matter of information for management in the broader sense, which would be part of the requirements of other functions, nor does it have to do with the propagation of institutional information, as called for by the steering role or other auxiliary functions. Rather it is a matter of information directed at the public for empowerment pusproses and to ensure the public's co-participation in taking responsibility for health and taking control over public action. It is information for building citizenship, for affirming values and institutionalizing them through the development of social practices. All this is part of a wider process under the essential responsibility of the public sector but is specifically manifested as a basic function of health systems. The concept of transparency in public administration is included here as well, which facilitates ongoing and effective oversight by society.

The foregoing analysis makes it possible to position public health within the health system and to regard it as a part, or rather, as a manifestation of the health system, from the perspective of population health. It is more than just a health system function; it is about its fulfillment in the collective and social dimensions. The final goals of the health system and health care, particularly those pertaining to social effectiveness, are also public health objectives. Values and basic principles make up the parameters of public health, which are applied as a specific focus to achieve to the main objective—which is the health of the population. The essential conditions and resources of health systems are also a public health concern to the extent that they are necessary for the health of the

population as well. Global health system functions, as they relate to the health of the population, are references for public health functions. Public health, through its essential functions (EPHFs), supports and integrates the steering role, even directly assuming responsibility for some of its tasks and transforming them into public health functions. Public health is concerned with financing as a requirement for collective health; it shares responsibility for the creation of productive capacity in order to ensure that it addresses the health needs of the population; it is concerned with the collective aspects of service delivery, with a view to social effectiveness (i.e. organization, quality, coverage and access); and finally, it assumes responsibility for providing the public with information, which is a collective function *par excellence*. In this way, public health contributes to the organization and execution of health system functions; it is not simply a component, even though its limits and contents can be delineated.

This vision of public health makes it possible to understand the interdependent relationships between it and medical care and, at the same time, their differences and complementary nature. Medicine, then, becomes one of the sciences that contribute to public health, but it neither defines it nor is confused with it. The practice of medicine itself is not part of public health, although the sum of its activities and contributions to collective health are indeed. Thus, an individual vaccine may not be considered part of public health, whereas repeated vaccinations aimed at protecting the population and controlling disease certainly would be. This same kind of relationship can also be seen if the basic health system or health care functions are defined from the most narrow and traditional standpoint of the natural

history of disease, according to the phases of promotion, prevention, recovery and rehabilitation.

Consequently, it comes as no surprise that public health also acts through the resources allocated to the operational elements of personal health care and even through that same care system. In fact, the nature of the two fields and their complementarity warrant the use of common resources and taking advantage of the opportunities created by health services and personal care to carry out public health interventions. Physicians' contact with patients, for example, provides significant opportunities for health promotion and disease prevention, in addition to other public health activities geared to the individual and the family, as well as to their relationship to the environment and the communities in which they live. The same holds true for other types of health workers. This joint action enhances personal health care, while extending the social reach of public health that would not otherwise be possible. In the case of environmental health, such action is more than a matter of articulation or complementarity; it is public health itself at work.

4. Actors

Many actors are involved in the work of public health. Given its very broad and varied sphere of activity, public health demands the participation of practically all the actors.

4.1 Society

The population, organized into society, is the fundamental and permanent focus of public health. The public constitutes not only the main focus of public health but also its primary actor. Public health is the health of the population, for the population, and by the population. Society's activities to promote health are reflected in its institutions and social practices, and are represented in socially recognized values that shape the attitudes and social behavior in support of life and health. These are also reflected in the recognition of health needs and demands, and in collective efforts aimed at satisfying them. The activities of the population as a public health actor are reflected through the work of organized groups in society, informal or formal public support networks, community interest groups, and even specific or vague feelings of satisfaction or dissatisfaction. All these manifestations of the population in society and of the non-State public sphere constitute the social foundation of public health and its recipients, as well as its instruments of action, inspiration and strength.

4.2 The State, the Non-State Public Sphere, and the Private Sphere

Societies establish legally recognized institutions to perform functions of common interest or of interest for socially significant groups. The State constitutes the most important of these institutions, and one of its priority responsibilities is to monitor the performance of public functions, including those pertaining to public health. The State, acting on behalf of the population, plays a central role as a public health actor, given its direct responsibility for ensuring that its functions are carried out. In some cases, the State performs these directly and exclusively—for example, the functions associated with formal political power (i.e. mandatory observance of legal values through legislation and other general regulations); with the coercive power of justice, through the

legal use of force or the implementation of formal international commitments; or with the defense of national sovereignty and integrity. In other cases, its functions are carried out by means of delegation, promotion, complementarity, or subsidiarity. The primary responsibilities of the State in public health include mobilizing, coordinating, orienting, and supporting the actions of society—particularly those of its non-State public sector actors. This synergy between the State and civil society is the key to achieving effective public health.

The action of private social agents helps to further expand the reach of public health, as well as the capacity of the State, and is consistent with the concept of public health that is being studied. Notably, the role played by social organizations, the non-State public sector, offers undeniable opportunities for the health system in general, and for public health in particular. These public interest organizations are not limited by some of the shortcomings of State action, their behavior does not follow the rules of the market, and they tend to operate at the grassroots and community levels. This is not, however, an alternative to State action and does not excuse the State from its public health responsibilities.

Moreover, private agents also have functions, although limited, in public health. Generally, the shortcomings or imperfections in the health market are magnified when it comes to public health, where, by definition, public goods or goods with significant externalities prevail and where there is greater asymmetry of information, complexity, and uncertainty, and where moral hazard and adverse selection are even more inexcusable. The market is an additional mechanism available to public health that can

be used in special situations or to correct certain shortcomings in public administration. However, some market agents, such as companies and corporations, can assume responsibility for issues of public interest that are in keeping with their nature and can even achieve social legitimacy, and at the same time make important contributions to public health. There are some situations that offer opportunities even for typically private entities, like companies, to act as public health actors—for example, in the field of occupational health, environmental protection, or in a voluntary capacity in other fields.

As mentioned earlier, this societal vision of public health draws individual care and collective care closer together. In fact, many collective public health actions stem from individual care. For example, the entire population can be protected by protecting a number of individuals or by common individual behaviors. Personal care also requires conditions that are public in nature, such as financing, organization and regulation. Adopting a public health perspective in personal health care complements it and promotes greater quality and effectiveness while expanding the capacity of public health by offering opportunities for action at all levels of care.

4.3 Professions and Professionals

Public health, as a separate field of knowledge, depends on the services of specifically trained agents, namely, professions and professionals. The public health professions consist of disciplines that contribute to its realization, whose exercise is differentiated according to their specific purpose—the health of the population. Some of these professions are more widely identified with public health insofar as their respective disciplines are more committed to the objective and focus of public health. Such is the case with epidemiology, which is closely integrated into all facets of public health, running the gamut from etiological research to communicable disease control, and from policy formulation to health systems and services management and evaluation. It can even be argued that the quality of public health is directly proportional to the quality of the epidemiology practiced, and vice versa. In addition, it is possible to identify professionals working in the contributing disciplines who are committed to the task of coordinating knowledge to further the objective and focus of public health. These professionals devote themselves exclusively to the exercise of public health and can be characterized as "holistic" public health professionals. That fact exemplifies the scientific, technical and professional nature of public health, which is essential for its exercise, although the field is always immersed in the context that shapes it and is at the service of the values which sustain it. However, scientific and technical excellence is strategically important to the quality of public health and can only be achieved by taking all the other dimensions into account. The work of public health cannot be limited to the work of public health professionals, but must be expanded to incorporate the work of all workers in health and related sectors, especially at the primary level of care. In fact, one of the main challenges for public health workers is to make others understand the focus and actions of public health and to incorporate them into their own behavior.

In short, there are many actors in public health, and its core lines of action are found within society itself, in the form of different organizations and particularly the State—in its role as the dominant social institution in the public sphere. The key to success in the practice of public health lies in understanding how all the different actors contribute to the common goal and in facilitating these contributions in an articulated and synergistic manner so that they respond efficiently, responsibly and in a socially controllable way to the needs of the population. This is also fundamentally a task of the public authorities.

5. Construction Process

With such deep roots in the social sphere, health and public health are the result of a complex social process that has been constructed over the ages—a process that entails the generation and regeneration of values, as expressed through public health institutions and organizations or through those that contribute to its practice. This fact is essential for understanding public health in each situation and culture, and also for understanding general aspects related to its theory and practice.

6. Values and Principles

As a sociocultural and historical process, and as a humanistic activity *par excellence*, public health is the union of knowledge and technology in a practice that is at once subordinate to and based on certain values. At the extreme of these values is the concept of health and life as the supreme goods of human beings who are endowed with rights and responsibilities, including among others, the higher right to social protection of their supreme goods and the shared responsibility to take care of them. There is also acceptance of the concept that it is the function of an organized society to join the efforts of its members in solidarity in order to fulfill that responsibility in favor of health for all—i.e. public health. As society's main institution, it is also the duty of the State to lead the way towards that social aspiration. Arising from these fundamental values are others such as solidarity, the efficient use of available resources, social participation, social control and equitable access to health-generating goods and services.

This concept seems too obvious, since it would be difficult for anyone to dare to dispute it. However, it has conceptual and operational implications, and defines, albeit in general terms, the final goals for action, for the development of knowledge and technology, and of course, for public health. From the perception and identification of needs, to the definition and implementation of responses to address them, values should precede the rationale; in other words, the rationale must be constructed on the foundation of those values. Accordingly, public health as a scientific and technical exercise places value on identifiable and measurable evidence and endeavors to base its decisions and interventions on such evidence. However, there is awareness in public health of the limitations of scientific evidence when it comes to social realities, especially in conditions of underdevelopment, and the importance of values in shaping public health. Likewise, public health will always try to reconcile scientific evidence with values, while recognizing, in principle, the origin of those values.

Viewed from another perspective, the erosion of values undermines consideration of the final goals of human practices and, ultimately, of the nature of humankind and the value of life and its protection through health. Under these circumstances, science ceases to be an "episystem" and basically shifts its focus to building real world models, without examining the valueswhich would legitimize them and which should shape the practices promoted by the models, a shift that runs counter to the objective of public health.

The risk of abuse in the name of values is always less than the risk of abuse posed by formal rationality that has the appearance of science in order to justify opinions and even interests (i.e. imposing values on others). The assertion of unquestionable truths has frequently been observed in the social sphere, only to be proven false or altered by the real conditions later on. Deficiencies in the definition of objectives and methods of observation in the data compiled, in the observation itself or in the observer, are all too obvious in the social sphere. As a result, it is difficult to have complete confidence in such evidence, especially if it is divorced from the basic purpose and principles that should govern health systems and especially public health. This warning call is not meant to belittle the importance of evidence; on the contrary, it aims to increase its importance by allowing values to place conditions on it.

In an approach that emphasizes the importance of values, public health is associated and inspired with ethics, and spreads it out in all its spheres of action—throughout society, the State, for specific and shared tasks, and even in the consideration of individual needs. This is an ethical framework with social dimensions that reinforces the primacy of society and the population.

From this perspective, one value that has been especially lacking in the Americas—that of equity—actually acquires significant importance and serves to integrate the value-added dimension of public health. In the context of health care, the concept of equity calls attention to the value of human life and the absurdity of rules of conduct that allow privileges based on ethnic differences, economic status, gender, culture or place of residence. Thus, equity works towards and calls for universal access to health care and demands that the State fulfill its social obligation to see that this is extended, especially to disadvantaged groups. Equity also demands comprehensive, quality health care and, ultimately, the most efficient use of available resources. In public health, the equity principle is the core line of action for modeling health financing, the organization and management of the health care system, and the generation of real resources to ensure full exercise of health system and public health functions. Equity is more critical since reality reflects major inequalities and injustice in the health situations of and between countries. Moreover, it has been demonstrated that a lack of equality in the way people are treated is one of the main contributors to the unsatisfactory social performance of health systems.

7. Politics and Legislation

To a large extent, public health is subservient to and depends on politics, and in many ways the corresponding actors need to operate with reference to it.

7.1 Democracy, Participation, and Healthy Public Policies

The expansion and deepening of both democracy as a frame of reference and the actualization of civic participation constitutes the main political determinant of public health and the social conventions that shape it. The socially legitimate political process and institutions are in turn the prerequisite and the result of effective democracy and salutary public policies that adequately respond to the health needs of the population. In essence, these elements are related to the characteristics of the process and the political system, and to the democratization of power through the empowerment and participation of citizens, thus legitimizing the process and conferring on it the capacity for socially correct public action.

From this perspective, public health improves with democracy and civic participation. It is this context that makes it possible to have genuine social integration of public health values with real empowerment (even political empowerment) of the people, enabling them to assume co-responsibility in matters pertaining to the health of everyone in society, and to the actual socially charged role of the State in the health of the population. This essential condition compels health systems to incorporate the strengthening of the process of democratization and social participation as part of their global functions, as set down especially in the steering role, and which must be assumed operationally by public health.

All of this lays the foundation for the formulation, adoption and implementation of healthier public policies. Public health is responsible specifically for promoting and advocating these healthy public policies in all the sectors, and for evaluating projects related to these policies in order to determine the impact of adopted or implemented policies on the population. Likewise, it is incumbent upon public health to promote and prepare the necessary legal instruments for organizing its functions and to promote behaviors aimed at their adoption and implementation.

7.2 Legislation and Democracy

Public health is the recognition and implementation of socially accepted values for protecting life and health, and the promotion of health-related values in society. This effort requires legal norms and their compliance by a lawful society in which the monopoly of institutional political power exercised by the State produces the necessary laws and ensure their equal enforcement for all. Only under such conditions can the neutrality of the law and its impartial application for the health of all be guaranteed. The work of preparing, proposing and advocating the necessary legislation for health protection, of ensuring that it complements the health authority's sphere of competence and is appropriately applied—even going as far as using supervisory powers conferred by legislation—constitutes the essential regulatory component of the steering function of the health system, and public health serves as its main beneficiary as well as executor.

7.3 Viability of Public Health Practice

The viability of public health practice is determined by the degree of acceptance and support for the proposed measures that culminate in effective fulfillment. Creating that viability is essentially a political process that entails the creation of consensus-building, the forging of partnerships and the neutralization of opposition in civil society, in the various state institutions and the health system itself. The effort required is part of the steering role function of the health system and is especially important for public health.

The viability of public health practice is assured with the viability of the conditions and resources that are necessary for carrying out its functions. Thus, achieving political and cultural viability is of practical significance.

7.4 Public Health and Politics

The importance of politics in public health can be deduced from the above. Obviously, it is not a matter of politicizing public health in the sense of subordinating it to political ideologies or partisan interests, although the importance of some ideologies and interests should not be discounted. What is needed is deliberate and consistent action, with a view to achieving the desired political results. At the very least, this requires:

a) Understanding the political process and its relevant aspects and actors with respect to the decisions desired and the capacity to prepare effective strategies in this regard;

b) Analyzing policies from the standpoint of the health of the population in terms of their merits, defects and contribution toward developing healthy policies;

c) Promoting public health interests by using the power of science and technology and the capacity for mobilizing society and the most effective alliances according to the situation and the moment;

d) Contributing to citizenship-building and the capacity for social participation, especially through information, health education, and the organization of community participation; and

e) Building alliances and mobilizing politically significant support.

If we understand politics as the exercise of power, both real power exercised by society with its capacity to influence, and formal or institutional power that is substantively on a par with the powers of the State, then the essence of the political process consists of channeling the demands of society to the State for consideration and fulfillment. This is not to ignore the importance of the private decisions of some actors in civil society, but these decisions are voluntary, and their effects are hardly evident for those who believe that these decisions belong to the restricted domain where they operate and are respected, without forgetting that some of these decisions indirectly affect other actors found outside this domain. The State is the only institution that society entrusts with the power to decide for all. Nevertheless, the problem lies in the enormous concentration of real power in society, which distorts the political process, causing governments to make socially detrimental and non-salutary decisions at times. Hence, one important task of public health is to actively contribute to citizenship-building and the democratization of power in society. This is based on the principle that a well-informed citizenry, conscious of its rights and responsibilities and organized for democratic participation, is the most effective guarantee of a democratic and socially beneficial exercise of real power as well as political or formal power, including in the sphere of health. Accordingly, the main political instrument of public health consists of having at one's disposal a reform process that can strategically mobilize society and be supported by it, and which can, as occasions arise, help to develop alliances and political support that would make it viable. In addition, it is crucial to be able to demonstrate the capacity for effectively implementing reforms and realizing the benefits that can be obtained as a result.

8. Social Practices and Public Health

All of this underscores the close link between public health and health-promoting social practices. As already mentioned, this relationship can be used as a matrix for identifying essential public health functions, which is the topic of Chapter 5.

9. Intersectoral Approach and Public Health

It makes sense that the multisectoral nature of the factors that determine health also affects public health, while the importance of intersectoral action is reinforced by the diverse facets of the concept of public health that we have analyzed. Indeed, areas such as nutrition, environmental health, citizen participation, and ultimately the creation of better living conditions and healthy public policies, depend on cooperation with other sectors. However, even specific aspects of health care services such as inputs, transportation services, communication, etc., are contingent on support from other sectors for accomplishment or quality improvement.

Public health is not only a multidisciplinary and interdisciplinary field of knowledge, but also a social practice that is necessarily intersectoral. All public health functions require cooperation with other sectors to one extent or another. Hence, ensuring this type of cooperation is one of the challenges facing public health.

10. International Dimension of Public Health

The risks and determinants associated with health are not confined to national borders. The fact that disease has no respect for borders was established long ago. In a world immersed in globalization, the threats and possibilities for solutions in the matter of health related to this phenomenon are more likely to become important issues than those related to the transmission of disease. Many of the key decisions regarding health determinants are often made or developed abroad, especially in the case of developing countries. Some of these global influences were mentioned in Chapter 1, where we examined globalization, its manifestations, and modern public health networks. Examples include the global effects of environmental pollution, the AIDS pandemic, the resurgence of tuberculosis, the commercial interests of transnational corporations in the health industry, as well as a socially perverse concentration of the means of production in the areas of knowledge and technology. There are also natural and man-made catastrophes, as well as criminal organizations linked to drug abuse and other forms of violence. On the other hand are the promises of science and technology, the intense and progressive interdependence

and solidarity between countries and peoples, regional and universal agreements, international organizations—whether intergovernmental or private, all working to analyze the problems of humanity and to find solutions.

The aspects mentioned in the preceding paragraph constitute public goods or "bads" that affect the global or regional population with a supranational scope. This necessitates that their production and many of their regulatory considerations be managed at the international level, which requires an institutional framework that ensures the requisite decision-making capacity for their implementation. Moreover, the profound differences between countries in terms of development and the capacity to exercise essential public functions—including those in public health—require a growing level of international cooperation in health, based on the development of public health.

The world has become integrated, and the health of populations is increasingly influenced by events and processes occurring outside countries, or that are common to some or all countries. International health is thus a universal component of a public health that is also becoming increasingly universal, or "the health of humankind".

11. Toward a Definition

It is impossible to synthesize in a brief definition all the conceptual aspects that have been analyzed. This means that a consensus on the notion of public health is virtually inconceivable. Nevertheless, the reality is that a definition that aims to integrate these conceptual components will facilitate the dissemination of the concepts and help strengthen public health practice.

Several definitions can be found in the literature, all of which have positive and negative aspects. Perhaps the most accepted and complete of all is the definition offered by Winslow in 1920: "Public health is the science and art of preventing disease, prolonging life, and promoting health and efficiency through the organized effort of the community for: 1) the improvement of environmental sanitation; 2) the control of community infections; 3) the education of the individual in the principles of personal hygiene; 4) the organization of medical and nursing services for the early diagnosis and treatment of disease; and 5) the development of social mechanisms that will guarantee everyone a standard of living adequate for the maintenance of health, organizing these benefits such that each individual will be in a position to enjoy his innate right to health and longevity".[6]

This is a very broad definition and covers most contemporary elements of public health, even though it was proposed more than 80 years ago. Its emphasis, however, is still on disease and based on the dominant hygienic/sanitary paradigm of the day, although it incorporates the social dimension of health and the collective nature of public health action.

A more recent definition (Piédrola Gil *et al*, 1991), which further simplifies Winslow's, holds that public health is the science and art of organizing and directing collective efforts designed to protect, promote, and restore the health of a

community's inhabitants. This definition at once simplifies and expands the sphere of public health activity, specifically incorporating the area of restoring health. Nevertheless, the emphasis on the collective is connected more to the method of operation through collective efforts than to the targeted goals of that action.

The idea of basing the concept of public health on the health of the population has been gaining strength and consensus and is contributing a lot to the new conceptual framework in this regard. This concept includes all the essential elements of the previous definitions, is compatible with the current understanding of the course of health and disease, and has the potential for addressing the complexity of public health in today's world as well as demonstrating how it can be put into practice in response to the challenges that all this entails.

The concept of public health has been evolving throughout the history of humanity in accordance with our understanding of reality and the instruments available for intervention. The necessary complexity of public health in today's world has turned it into a multifaceted concept that is in constant flux. All the different facets of this concept deserve to be examined carefully from all possible angles, as they manifest themselves through the many different ways in which they are defined and acted on. Indeed this also includes the use of alternative or complementary expressions in reference to tn the use of terms like social medicine and community health.

Therefore, as already pointed out, building a definition that might be considered appropriate and unanimous is not possible. As such, the definition that we propose below combines com-

mon elements from the many previous definitions and tries to adjust for the concepts analyzed in this chapter:

"Public health is an organized effort by society, primarily through its public institutions, to improve, promote, protect and restore the health of the population through collective action."

Bibliography

Berkman L and Lochner K. Social Determinants of Health; Meeting at the Crossroads, Health Affairs, Book Review Essay; March/April, 2002.

Claeson M et al. Public Health and World Bank Operations. Washington: HNP/ World Bank; 2002.

Cordeiro H. "Sistema Único de Saúde," Ayuri Editorial Ltda., Rio de Janeiro; 1991.

Escuela de Salud Pública del Ecuador y OPS. "Salud pública — Ciencia, política y acción," Quito; 1993.

Frenk J. "The New Public Health," in: Annual Review of Public Health, Vol. 14, pp. 469–490; 1993

Frenk J. "La salud de la población — Hacia una nueva salud pública," Fondo de Cultura Económica, México; 1994.

Glonberman S. "Towards a New Perspective on Health Policy," CPRN Study no. H/03, Renouf Publishing Co, Lrd, Ottwawa; 2001.

Granda E. "Salud pública e identidad," presentación en el Foro "Modelos de Desarrollo, Espacio Urbano y Salud," Santafé de Bogotá; April 1999.

Guimarães R e Tavares R. "Saúde e Sociedade no Brasil — Anos 80," Relume Dumará, Rio de Janeiro; 1994.

Hanlon JJ. "Principios de administración sanitaria," Parte I — Introducción, 2ª edición, La Prensa Médica Mexicana, México; 1963.

Hartge P. "Epidemiologic Tools for Today and Tomorrow," Anal of the New York Academy of Sciences, 954: 295–310; 2001.

---

[6] Winslow, C.E.A. "The Untilled Field of Public Health," Modern Medicine, 2: 183, March; 1920.

Henderson H. "Paradigms in Progress," 1994. Healthier Communities Summit, Anaheim, CA; 1994.

Hertzman C. "The Social Dimensions of Public Health" in World Science Report 1999, pp. 341–351, London; 1999.

Kawl I and Faust M. "Global Public Goods and Health: Taking the Agenda Forward," Bulletin of the World Health Organization, 2001, 79: 869–874.

Koplan JP. "From Anthrax to Zyban: 20th Century Triumphs and Implications for the New Millenium: 1999 Fred T. Foard Memorial Lecture, University of North Carolina School of Public Health; April 1994.

Last JM. "Public Health and Human Ecology," Appleton & Lange; 1987.

Legowski B and Mckay L. "Health Beyond Health Care: Twenty-five Years of Federal Health Policy Development," Canadian Policy Research Networks, IN; 2000.

Londoño JL and Frenk J. "Structural Pluralism: Towards and Innovative Model for Health System Reform in Latin America," in Health Policy, 41:1–36; 1997.

López-Acuña D et al. "Reorienting Health Systems and Services with Health Promotion Criteria: A Critical Component of Health Sector Reforms," Technical Paper for the Fifth International Conference on Health Promotion, Mexico; June 2000.

Maxcy-Rosenau. "Preventive Medicine and Public Health," Ninth ed., Edited by Phillip Sartwell, Appleton–Century–Crofts, New York; 1965.

Milio N. "Promoting Health Through Public Policy," Canadian Public Health Association, Ottawa; 1989.

Mullan F. "Public Health Then and Now—Don Quixote, Machiavelli and Robin Hood: Public Health Practice, Past and Present," in American Journal of Public Health, Vol. 90 no. 5, May 2000, pp. 702–706.

Musgrove P. "Protecting Health in Latin America: What Should the State Do?," (mimeo), World Bank, Washington, D.C.; 2001.

Musgrove P. "Public Spending on Health Care: Are Different Criteria Related?,"

The World Bank Institute, World Bank; 1999 (mimeo).

OPS. "El desafío de la epidemiología," Públicación Científica nº 505; 1988.

OPS. "La crisis de la salud pública: reflexiones para el debate," Públicación Científica, n.º 540, Washington;1992.

OPS. "La rectoría de los ministerios de salud en los procesos de reforma del sector de la salud', Documento presentado al cuadragésimo Consejo Directivo; 1996.

OPS. "Las condiciones de salud en las Américas," Edición 1994, Vol. I, Públicación Científica, n.º 549; 1994.

OPS. "Las condiciones de salud en las Américas," Edición 1998, Vol. I, Públicación Científica, n.º 569.

OPS. "Promoción de la salud: una antología," Públicación Científica n.º 557, Washington, DC; 1996.

OPS. "Sobre la teoría y práctica de la salud pública: un debate, múltiples perspectivas," Washington; 1993.

PAHO. Division of Health and Human Development "Principles and Basic Concepts of Equity and Health," October; 1999.

Paim JS e Almeida Filho, N. "A Crise de Saúde Pública e a Utopia da Saúde Coletiva," Casa da Qualidade Editora, Salvador, BA; 2000.

Piedrota G et al. "Medicina preventiva y salud pública," 9a edición, Ediciones Científicas y Técnicas AS, Barcelona; 1991.

Preker A, Harding A, and Girishauker. "The Economics of Private Participation in Health Care: New Insights from Institutional Economics," World Bank, Washington; 1999.

Rebecca S. "The Policy Process: An Overview," Overseas Development Institute, London; 1999.

Restrepo H. "Increasing Community Capacity and Empowering Communities for Promoting Health," Technical Report 4, presented at the Fifth Global Conference on Health Promotion, Mexico City; June 2000.

San Martin H. "Administración en salud pública, Parte I: objetivos de los sistemas

de servicios de salud," La Prensa Médica Mexicana, México; 1988.

Schaeffer M. "Salud, medio ambiente y desarrollo," OMS/EHE/93.1, OMS/OPS; 1994.

Solimano G e Isaacs S. (EE): "De la reforma para unos a la reforma para todos," Editorial Sudamericana, Santiago; 2000.

Strategies for Population Health—Investing in the Health of Canadians," Ottawa; 1994.

The Belmont Vision for Health Care in America," Institute for Health Futures, Alexandria, VA; 1992.

The Core Functions Project Steering Group. "Health Care Reform and Public Health: a paper on Population-based core functions," Journal of Public Health Policy, Vol. 19 no. 4, pp. 394–418.

UN/Committee on Economic, Social and Cultural Rights, Twenty-second Session: "The Right to the Highest Attainable Standard of Health," Geneva; 2000 (unedited version).

US Institute of Medicine. "The Future of Public Health," National Academy Press; 1988.

Whitehead M. "The Concepts and Principles of Equity and Health," International Journal of Health Services, Vol. 22, No. 3, pp. 429–445; 1992.

WHO. "The World Report 1999—Making a Difference," Geneva; 1999.

WHO. "Health a Precious Asset, Accelerating Follow-up to the World Summit for Social Development. Geneva; 2000.

WHO. "The World Health Report 2000—Health Systems: Improving Performance," Geneva; 2000.

Why are Some People Healthy and Others Not? The Determinants of Health of Populations," Editors Robert Evans, Morris Barer and Theodore Marmor, Aldine de Gruyter, New York; 1994.

Wilkinson R, and Marmot, M. (EE) "Social Determinants of Health: The Solid Facts," WHO/EURO, Copenhagen, 2000.

Winslow CEA. "The Untilled Field of Public Health," Modern Medicine, 2: 183; March

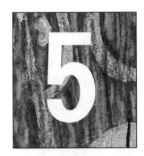

Social Practices and Public Health

1. Culture, Social Capital, and Social Practices

The concept of public health encompasses not only a population's health, but also the health generated by a population. Society, understood as an organized population, is the principal actor in public health and, in the final analysis, is responsible for the collective means to protect the health of its members, including the actions of the State, its main institutional structure. However, the population's role in public health is not exercised solely through the formal organizations in its society. It is also exercised through society's actions and interactions, formally organized or not, which may have a positive or negative, direct or indirect impact on health. To be effective, these actions and interactions do not have to be guided by or have goals specifically related to health, but their positive impact increases when they are carried out conscientiously for this purpose. Health is part of a population's daily life, both as individuals and

as a group, and results from its actions and interactions in society.

The actions and interactions of a society are usually a reflection of its values, customs, beliefs and standards, which govern the attitudes and behaviors of its members. These values and standards guide and condition individual behavior through explicit and implicit rewards and punishments. Moreover, they also define the organizational structure of the society and the relationships between it and other groups, as well as the relationships within the society. In other words, institutionalized values shape the social organizations and relational networks through which a society functions and meets the needs of its members. This is also the principal means of societal renewal and creation, which determine the form, capacity for self-generation, and sustainability of societies. When the dominant values place special importance on life and lead to the establishment of conditions, situations, and behaviors that favor health, public

health is then strengthened and improved. The most communal societies are geared more toward sociability and association, have higher levels of trust among its members and organizations, and thus exhibit a greater degree of cooperation. Hence, these communal societies are more inclined to expand public forums in social activities and to favor the development of civic spirit and the value of common goods. By extension, they develop human resources and protect the environment through the rational use of natural resources and better utilization of artificial capital, both financial and technological. In these societies, sustainable human development is more likely to engender greater equity, well being, and health for all.

This set of positive values converted into social institutions and manifested in active social organizations and relational networks is what current thinking on development has called social capital. Its importance is being increasingly recognized as fundamental to development itself. Social capital is built on culture and consists of values or institutions and other cultural components such as beliefs, the arts, and language that define the identity of peoples and nations and sustain the desired cohesion, stability, and change in a society. These conditions are essential to dynamic and sustainable integral development.

In theory, social capital and culture define the social processes of decision making and, by extension, the orientation and characteristics of development. A well-structured society with a high level of social capital and a strong cultural identity will be cohesive enough to define its needs and the means to meet them to reach a consensus on its own development projects. This consensus, based on effective social contracts, will extend to controlling the distribution and exercise of political power, including of course the State, its principal instrument. The public policies formulated under these circumstances will necessarily be healthy and generate health and be geared toward making the best use of development potential in a sustainable manner that benefits all. Assertion of the basic values of social solidarity and responsibility will help create stability and reduce uncertainty, stimulate creativity, and reduce transaction costs, among other things. These conditions are essential to increasing production in regulated markets and employing a certain degree of social responsibility. The balance and complementary relationship among society, the State, and the market will be the foundation and, thus, the reference point and purpose of the entire process.

Democracy, expanding into everyday life, borne out in the permanent participation of citizens, and based on a complete state of law, is the political system needed in this situation. Political representations and governments, whose legitimacy is a true reflection of the will of the people, adhere to the mandates and expectations of the people by means of ongoing and effective social control carried out using multiple and convergent instruments and mechanisms. The trust provided by the awareness of its identification as a society, solidarity among its members, and procurement of future projects give a society the willingness and ability to make the changes needed for renewal and sustainability.

This summary is provided merely to emphasize how beneficial social capital can be when it is based on its own positive culture. In reality, it is nearly impossible to achieve this utopia in marginalized countries where there is a stronger trend toward heterogeneity than toward cultural autonomy. Social capital is weak and can even have negative manifestations. The basic values of trust, solidarity and civic spirit are drowned out. Society disintegrates, and uncertainty and insecurity increase, weakening basic institutions, such as the family and religion. Social and political organizations lose credibility and legitimacy. The modern world is compromising the chance to achieve the development needed precisely because it does not take into account the importance of social capital and culture.

In public health, culture and social capital are even more important, because, in addition to the impact of their general importance and consequent development, they directly affect health. Favoring the development of conditions and behaviors that reduce public health risks, culture and social capital increase the health potential of people and populations and the capacity and effectiveness of the social response to health needs. Promoting the development of these favorable conditions and of healthy and the subsequent health-generating behaviors is at the core of public health. There is sufficient evidence, experiences, and analyses showing that communities or populations with similar material resources can differ with regard to health conditions as a result of their culture and especially of their specific values, beliefs, institutions, organizations, and social processes. We will not analyze this evidence and examples here; suffice it to state that public health is very dependent on culture-based social capital. Technical interventions, doubtlessly very valuable, provide opportunities and specific solutions whose full benefit and effectiveness depend on how a society uses them. The integrity and sustainability of public health can only be achieved when a population permanently incorporates health protection measures into its everyday routines, including the appropriate use of health care through interventions based on science and technology.

Culture is an amalgam of the values, traditions, customs, beliefs, and social standards formed throughout history, and it makes it possible for use to perceive reality, interpret it, and act on it. It is the perspective through which we see life and take part in it. Culture is also the result of its application throughout history incorporated into the lives we lead and into the future we build. In turn, social capital is the established capacity to take action, built on the foundation of culture. It is a structure composed of the key values, institutions, organizations, and relationships that shape societies' nature and capacity for action. This type of social action provides populations with the sense and purpose of culture and social capital. It is this type of social action, reflected in the practices that characterize social processes, that truly shows the dynamism or inertia of accumulated culture and social capital. Ultimately, it is what really defines a society's possibilities in public health.

In other words, the social values attributed to culture set the guidelines for understanding and building reality, and guide or determine the behavior of individuals or social groups. In essence, they define the means by which societies and their components endeavor to meet the needs of all and of each of its members, including the formation of institutions, organizations, and social relationships, and the use of social capital in their general operations. This set of facts and actions that are socially recognized and carried out by societies, whether individually or collectively but always for the public, is what have come to be known as social practices. In other words, there is an obvious manifestation of culture and social capital in action; Social practices encompass all aspects of life in a society, and serve their different reasons for existing, including the improvement of the health of populations.

As can be seen, public health achieves its full potential when its purposes and practices are accepted by society and incorporated into social practices. As was pointed out in chapter 3, the combination of positive values that are geared toward health and institutionalized by a society, and the availability of socially effective knowledge and technology has been the driving force for public health progress. Moreover, the effect of this combination is increased by powerful, convergent interests, favorable political circumstances and adequate leadership.

Like human and physical capital, social capital can be produced and accumulated, as well as produced in an economic sense. The production of social capital, however, is essentially indirect and normally is expressed in externalities and public property, such as a general reduction of production costs, shared knowledge, trust, association, and cooperation. Social capital thus becomes a public good and the production of it tends to be spontaneous within a society and to be the result of social interaction, imitation, and cultural continuity by means of socialization. It is slow in forming, but its existence and effects tend to be lasting.

From another perspective, social capital is very important for governance and the social performance of governments, as demonstrated by R. Putman[2] in his extensive study on the process of regionalization in Italy. In many ways, social capital mingles with the concept of citizenship, an indispensable condition for creating a full democracy and state of law. It is in opposition to political corruption, and to the subordination of the State to private interests. Instead, it promotes the renewal and social legitimization of the significance and accountability of public organizations and governmental authorities. Social capital, however, can also be used to negative ends, as is the case with human capital when it is used for oppression and torture or with physical capital when it

[2] Putman, R. Comunidade e Democracia — a experiência da Itália moderna. Rio de Janeiro: Editora Fundação Getúlio Vargas; 1996.

is used to produce illegal weapons or drugs. In addition, negative values and standards can promote unnecessary conflict, violence, and destruction.

These initial theoretical reflections are geared toward facilitating comprehension of the two following sections, which address social practices with regard to health and public health.

2. Social Practices and Health

Given the nature of health, the social practices that affect it are multiple and encompass the broad spectrum of its determining and deciding factors, as well as health care itself. Thus, specific health practices are not the only factors that should be identified. The scope of this document, however, does not allow for an exhaustive study of all the social practices relevant to health. We have limited ourselves to a set of social practices pertinent to health in broad spheres of action, defined in terms of the large general goals on which societies base their efforts to improve the health of populations.

Four groups of social practices are set forth according to their main goals.

- Development and strengthening of a culture of life and health.

- Attention to health needs and demands.

- Development of healthy environments and control of risks and threats to public health.

- Development of citizenship and the capacity for social participation and control.

The four groups and the end goals that define them also correspond to a possible system for classifying the challenges affecting health today and in the immediate future.

Various practices within each group and among groups continually complement and reinforce each other, blurring the boundaries among them. Moreover, a social practice can serve more than one end goal, but will be included in the most relevant group.

2.1 Development and Strengthening of a Culture of Life and Health

The purpose of the practices in this group is to make life and health fundamental human values, rights, and responsibilities in a society. A culture of life guarantees the sustainability and development of the society where it flourishes. The culture of life includes values essential for coexistence, mutual respect, and cooperation among social actors. It is also the source of certain related values, such as peace, solidarity, and democratic participation. A culture of life does not negate the concept of self, but rather demands an awareness of others, in the same way that the projection of the self in the existence of the other is needed to protect the development of life in the community. This clears the way for recognizing the unity of life and the codependence of all life forms, where death is only a contingency of biological necessity or the imposition of the survival of the species. Within this perspective, the structure is built for peaceful coexistence based on cooperation among all members of society.

The culture of life is associated with quality of life and the constant attempt to improve it, as well as with the well-being of individuals, groups, and the entire population. A culture of life demands true human development, which ultimately have the same objectives. In many ways, quality of life and well-being determine health and, at the same time, are shaped by health. In essence, health, in the broader meaning given by WHO, mingles with well-being and is indispensable to quality of life and social development.

A culture of life is necessarily also a culture of health, and thus becomes the main condition for the protection and quality of life. It is not merely a matter of survival, but of living a full and healthy life. The culture of health adds other values to the culture of life that are linked to the promotion and protection of health, recovery of health if it is lost or affected, and the elimination or mitigation of all disabilities. A culture of health is a permanent and basic foundation for fully developing public health.

In addition to its importance in the structure and functioning of societies and in the health of populations, a culture of life and health is one of the highest universally recognized ethical mandates. The rights to protection of life and to health are part of basic and universal human rights, and are recognized as the first of all rights. Unfortunately, reality is far from reflecting this recognition, and human life from economic and political perspectives has different values depending on national or social situations. Moreover, the lives of many people, sometimes even the majority of people, have very little value. Today's basic rejection of the culture of life and health should not, however, be an obstacle to defending and promoting it, but rather an incentive.

In addition to positive values and beliefs, a culture of life and health requires appropriate institutions, organizations, and social relationships, i.e. adequate social capital that will be reflected through the healthy and health-generating behaviors of individuals and societies. Some institutions that can promote a culture of health and life include, among others, the family in particular, religion, general education, and other socialization mechanisms. These organizations play a key role. In particular, they transmit the values that reinforce life and health as basic human rights and, moreover, they instill life with a transcendental aspect that goes beyond the simple results of biological processes and, therefore, has a higher value than material things. The transmission of this concept, be it a matter of faith and ethical principles or the simple belief in the special destiny of humanity, is essential to strengthening a culture of life and health.

The culture of life is the most basic expression of humanism, and is the convergence of faith, beliefs, and hope in the future of humankind. In this context, the agents of public health are not merely instruments that contribute technical solutions. Above all, they should be the transmitters of values and hope, co-builders and even Quixotes of projects designed to protect and improve life.

The social practices of and for a culture of life and health precede and are the root and basis for other groups of practices; they inspire these other practices that complement and strengthen them.

2.2 Attention to Health Needs and Demands

This group comprises the specific social practices needed for health care. It includes the way in which society and its members recognize health problems and the need for care, which are the basis for the demand for health services, including informal and alternative services. It also encompasses efforts to create, organize, and implement health care services. Basically this group deals with the social demand and supply of services that respond to the problems, needs, and the demands of health care. At the convergence of these two actions are the practices of self-care, the demand for and use of organized health services, and, in general, the ways in which a society shapes and uses health systems and heath care.

The practices of this group are largely derived from the practices of other groups. The culture of life and health is the main determinant of the way health is understood, how disease and the need for care are recognized and the demand for health care, including self-care. Sickness and disease are the result of living conditions, environment, and the risks in and with which a population lives. Thus, the needs, perception, and demands basically stem from ways of life and living conditions. Even when the extent of health services, specifically the offer of health services, is largely based on science and technology and the rational use of available resources, the use of these services is very dependent on culture. Moreover, the same rationality based on science and technology, particularly in regards to the allocation of resources and of public resources in particular, are also political in nature. Thus, they are dependent on the distribution and use of power in a society and on the values that regulate the use of power. Essentially it is a question of the social capacity to participate in and control political power and, by

extension, to make use of the decisions that have been made and of resources that have been allocated. In many respects, it is also a matter of regulating the operation of health markets and of the spontaneous generation of demands.

These observations are not intended to downplay the importance of specific social practices in the health care field that are truly vital to public health. However, the importance of specific social practices is related to their dependency on other groups of practices. If the latter were not taken into account, understanding of the former and of their role in public health would be seriously prejudiced.

2.3 Development of Healthy Environments and Control of Risks and Threats to Public Health

The origin of society is the need for collective protection of life in order to ensure the survival of society's members. This same motivation still holds sway in today's societies and is even more pronounced when the culture of life is stronger and more structured. Adherence to this principle and the consequences of doing so are what lead to the protection of public health, which necessitates non-aggressive environments and favorable living conditions.

In analyzing health and public health, all social practices should be taken into account if they help improve living conditions and protect the environment, as should any actions of and within the society if they modify external health conditions and determinants. Of particular importance are social practices related to environmental health and

those geared toward meeting basic needs. They include the production of goods and services, their distribution and use, and, consequently, income generation and distribution, and social protection mechanisms, i.e. the model for and dynamism of the development process.

This group of social practices is the juncture of the other three. The culture of life encompasses a culture that favors the natural and social environment, and its values require that basic levels of social equity and solidarity be met in a society, thus preventing extreme need among the population. Essentially, public well-being is the principal raison d'être of societies and their institutions, especially the State. This becomes a basic political matter, which is dependent on the distribution, relationships, and the exercise of political power. This matter is resolved through effective citizenship and the existence of true democracy and a state of law. Finally, a clear demand for health needs, which garners the most attention and the best possible response, is an essential part of living conditions and a healthy environment. Social practices related to health care share the same goal of controlling risks and harm. Reduced risks and harm as a result of healthy environments go hand in hand with specific actions to protect individual, group, or environmental health.

Although the social practices in this group almost always relate to health, they are of interest in other sectors, reinforcing in a society the multi and intersectoral nature of the process of health production, especially in the communal aspect of public health.

Within this group of social practices, acculturation and socialization mechanisms play a key role, particularly education and social communication, organizations related to production and labor, networks stemming from social and solidarity movements, and, logically, the institutions of the State through public policies in particular. Actually, the role and responsibility of the State as the basic driving force behind and guarantor of these practices are even more important and decisive than in other groups.

The practices in this group are almost always carried out with regard to public goods (or evils), making them particularly relevant to public health. Many phenomena, such as the disappearing ozone layer, the greenhouse effect, pollution in oceans, the conservation of species, hazardous waste, peace and world security, drug consumption, international terrorism, and equity in world trade, are international public goods and evils. Addressing them necessitates a great deal of cooperation among countries and true international regulation, i.e. the need for universal healthy, social practices.

2.4 Development of Citizenship and of the Capacity for Social Participation and Control

This group of practices is fundamental for endogenous social strategies or those imposed on societies, is the principal driving force of a society in movement, and lends dynamism to the creation and development of the organizations and institutions through which the society operates. Most important, these social practices are able to preside over and control these organizations and institutions, and can even prevent specific groups from owning them and thereby reducing their social character.

Effective, aware, and participatory citizenship is the basis of real democracy and of the creative or regenerative power of a society. Actually, citizen participation expands a society's power of cultural assertion, and makes use of strong and effective institutions and organizations through which its values are implemented. It modulates the distribution and exercise of power, keeping the State faithful to its social commitments. It can be said that citizenship, as reflected in participation, is the determining factor of integrated development that necessarily encompasses public health or health in general at both the individual and collective levels. Thus, citizenship is the expression of and a factor in culture and social capital. It is the driving force behind health and health-generating social practices. If culture is the foundation and social capital is the productive structure, then citizenship is the motor for healthy social practices.

Development of citizenship results from knowledge- and experience-based training, contributing to learning-by-doing. It is also a product of the cultural heritage that shapes social learning. The existence of effective mechanisms of participation within social organizations and the State translates into measurable citizenship, while at the same time favors its development.

Mechanisms of information and education, and community organizations are very important in this process. Exchanges with formal political powers are indispensable in two ways: toward civil society as a conduit for demands that strengthen participation by establishing channels to make them more effective; and toward political representation and

the government as a means of legitimizing processes, authority, and decisions. However, citizenship and citizen participation go much further; they are the permanent source for creating and expanding the social capital needed to increase the productivity, stability, and predictability needed for the sound operation of markets. At the same time, they automatically regulate market operations and correct many related shortcomings. In turn, the market can be a permanent means of learning about citizenship, with regard to the economic rationality needed to make decisions about consumption and investment.

Citizenship and participation also have an extensive and profound impact on public management, from the approval of policies and plans to the management of services, through demands, contributions, and requirements for transparency and regulation that limit unwanted and socially detrimental deviations. In the final analysis, citizenship and the capacity for participation must be developed to completely achieve democracy and the dominance of a state of law, in turn guaranteeing social cohesion and stability and creating real possibilities for true human development.

In health and particularly in public health, citizenship and social participation are the foundation for best meeting the goals of health and ensuring that it is sustainable.

3. Development of Healthy Social Practices

Social practices are the result of the social process and, at the same time, one of its manifestations, which implies that they simultaneously act as an instrument for consolidating culture and for changing and renewing it. The slow, repetitive, and evolutionary process of history, as seen in concrete social practices, also creates the stimuli, needs, and changes in values, standards, beliefs, and institutions that set the guidelines for these same practices. Essentially, this process is endogenous to a society. Still changes can be introduced and accelerated by what begin as external factors and eventually lead to cultural ruptures and even cultural revolutions. Social practices are not actually constructed, rather they are elements of the culture and social capital that produce them. Social practices are the same actions made possible by social capital within a cultural context. However, changes in culture and social capital are manifested through social action, that is, through social practices. So completes the practical and conceptual unity of this trinity.

In other words, the culture and social capital that serve as a foundation and structure of social practices can be deliberately constructed or destroyed, giving rise to new practices that in turn will change the culture and social capital. Today, a market-based, globalized culture is imposing itself on national cultures and changing them in fundamental ways. The strength of modern communication technology, especially marketing and the effects of demonstration and imitation, has universalized consumption and social organization patterns, changing expectations and behavior and favoring material hedonism, exaggerated individualism, destructive competition, and the objectification of human life. The negative results of this phenomenon are the marginalization or exclusion of the weak, neglect of the values of solidarity and cooperation, the de-

creased importance of basic institutions like the family and religion, and the erosion of the meaning of "public" or "social." In the structurally most mature societies, the cradle of globalized culture, the extensive, complex, and stable network of institutions and social organizations has softened the impact of cultural rupture, guaranteeing the stability needed for their social renewal and for the formation of the required new values and standards. In marginalized societies, cultural rupture without substitutes and without strong established social capital often implies a loss of their ethical referents, manifested by increased uncertainty, insecurity, and all forms of corruption and violence. In these cases, the societies are less communal, in terms of having common shared goals and values, in spite of the recent surge in social organizations. The rate of decomposition is greater than efforts to develop or maintain goals and values. The social practices resulting from this process are often not healthy and the construction of social capital does not meet the needs of the development needed and in certain instances or situations yields a negative balance. In this way, public health is developed to a much lesser degree than would otherwise be possible.

However, the mechanisms used in this cultural downgrading can also be used to assert the values of a culture of life and of health in order to develop conditions and situations, which, taking into account the cultural identity of populations, instill the trust needed to create social capital through solidarity and cooperation. In turn, they sustain true human development to the benefit of all. The goal is not cultural isolation or intractability, rather it is a matter of using the external stimulus of interac-

tion among cultures to initiate endogenous and indigenous, and therefore socially legitimate, processes of change. The appropriate balance between autonomy and heteronomy will result in societies that are more sustainable and have a greater capacity for self-renewal, within a culture and social capital that produce healthy and health-generating social practices.

In the four groups mentioned, specific practices can be exercised by organized groups or by individuals that reproduce socially established models. But what is important for public health is the presence of a collective meaning, even in repeated and aggregate individual actions. The link between the social practices of a population and those of the individual lends a social dimension to the aggregation and organization of individual practices and justifies the actions of individuals or groups in promoting healthy social practices and their contribution to public health.

The construction and development of social practices can be analyzed in the following phases, which are always present in society and continuously occur and complement each other: a) the construction, accumulation or assertion of values and knowledge, and of the operational contents that sustain them and through which they are manifested; b) the formation of the institutions, organizations, and actors that apply the values and knowledge, and the relationships they establish among themselves, ranging from the most simple to the most complex; c) the mobilization of efforts within and by means of social practices as such; and d) the strengthening, expansion, renewal, and modification of the entire process.

This overview of the construction of social practices shows the importance of the combination of values, knowledge, and institutions that influence the development of social practices and their importance in public health. Education, in all its forms, as a means of citizenship training is one of the main driving forces in the process. Essentially, it is an instrument for transferring training information, which should be complemented by the creation of mechanisms to use it effectively. The fourth group of practices, the development of citizenship and of the capacity for social participation, thus becomes the principal strategy for promoting the desired social practices.

The construction of citizenship is, in essence, the process of procuring power and the conditions for effectively exercising it. Accordingly, it is basically a political process where preparation is needed to consciously select individual yet shared projects that thus have a certain potential to create change. According to the definition of Savater, it is the capacity to do, more than simply to be.[3] In other words, it is the capacity to assert cultural, group, and community identity and ownership (the being) as the basis for participation (the doing), which becomes the main goal of the entire process. Citizenship can only be complete through participation by sharing values, rights, and responsibilities, and action projects to build the future, i.e. to change the present.

The foregoing does not imply only ideas and thoughts. On the contrary, it means strengthening multiplicity through the homogenization of rights, duties, and

possibilities, so that each actor can participate in the formulation and execution of shared projects, while maintaining the specific, individual goals of the individual or group. Developing citizenship in a less than ideal social context generally implies working to change and transform. By extension, the resulting social practices are geared toward the same goal. Developing citizenship and the capacity for participation also means building and accumulating positive social capital. At the same time, it means creating socially endogenous mechanisms to correct distortions or problems within social and collective acts: negative opportunism seen in the personal gain of individuals or of closed groups, corporatism, and antiquated political practices, such as political patronage or nepotism, passivity, and corruption.

Logically, social practices are not consistently uniform among themselves; nor are they always associated with common and good purposes. In the vast complexity and diversity of social processes, there are divergent and conflicting processes. What matters is the possibility of establishing viable courses of action to meet the goals accepted by the majority of a society and shaped by good, socially hegemonic practices. Public health can and should take advantage of the high degree of consensus about the value of health and life in order to take part in the necessarily intersectoral effort of promoting the development of conditions that produce healthy social practices. In this regard, the human actors especially, i.e. public health professionals, should also act as messengers and promoters of cultural change and of the formation of social capital that leads to healthy and health-generating practices—the development of citizenship and the capacity for participation. This

is, without a doubt, their most important mission in public health.

The process is simultaneously dynamic, thanks to the continuous evolution of society, and sufficiently stable, thanks to the values of sustainability, making it possible to develop strategies within reasonable time frames. In all of this, and particularly in public health, the role of the State is fundamental as the principal social institution. Despite the basically endogenous character of the process, the State can stimulate and promote it by recognizing its importance for governance, all levels of education, information for public training, and the creation of adequate institutional mechanisms. The last item not only makes participation effective, it also makes it possible to view participation in terms of quantifiable results and benefits. Perhaps the most important of the State's specific roles, in this field and in today's world, is expanding public actions by mobilizing and bringing together social actors from the non-State public arena so that they can play a synergistic role in achieving common purposes. Nonetheless, it should be borne in mind that the State has certain direct responsibilities that cannot and should not be delegated, or that would be very difficult to delegate in practice. When the State fulfills this role, power over the state reverts to society, and state interventions are subject to social control through citizenship. In terms of public health, this means expanding its reach and making it more effective by sharing responsibility with its principal actor—the population.

Bibliography

Borsoti CA. In: Planificación social en América Latina y el Caribe. Chile: ILPES-UNICEF; 1981. pp. 47–117.

---

[3] Savater, F. "Elegir la Política", Letras Libres, Spain, 2002.

Borsoti CA. La teoría sociológica y la planificación social. Diferentes paradigmas y sus consecuencias. pp. 97–117.

Carin E. The Social and Cultural Matrix of Health and Disease. In: Why are some people healthy and others not? New York: Aldine de Gruyter; 1994. pp. 93–132.

Casas JA, Dela Casco, R., and Torres-Pasodi, C. Toward Health and Human Development. In: Health & Human Development in the New Global Economy. Washington D.C.: PAHO/WHO, University of Texas Medical Branch; 2000. pp. 251–255.

CEPAL. Equidad, desarrollo y ciudadanía. 28º Período de Sesiones. Mexico, D.F.; 2000. See in particular chapter 14: "Ciudadanía, igualdad y cohesión social: la ecuación pendiente".

Coleman J. Foundations of Social Theory. Harvard University Press; 1990.

Collier P. Social Capital and Poverty. World Bank, Social Capital Initiative; Nov. 1998.

Evans T et al. Desafío a la falta de equidad en la salud — de la ética a la acción. OPS; 2002. (Publicación Científica y Técnica 585).

Cardoso FH and Lanni O. Homem e sociedade — Leituras básicas de sociologia geral. Companhia Editora Nacional, 7ª Edição; 1972.

Fukuyama F. Social Capital and Civil Society, IMF. Washington D.C.: Conference Agenda; 1999.

Health Canada. Salud de la población, conceptos y estrategias para políticas públicas saludables. Washington D.C.: OPS; 2000.

Kliksberg B. Capital social y cultura; claves olvidadas del desarrollo. www.worldbank.org/poverty; 1999.

Etzioni A and E. Los cambios sociales — fuentes, tipos y consecuencias. Mexico: Fondo de Cultura Económica; 1968.

Pancer M and Nelson G. Enfoques de la promoción de la salud basados en la comunidad: guía para la movilización comunitaria. In: Promoción de salud: una antología. OPS; 1996. (Publicación científica 557).

Mcalister A. Cambio de conducta de la población: un enfoque con base teórica. In: Promoción de salud: una antología. OPS; 1996. (Publicación científica 557).

Milbrath LW. Envisioning a sustainable society—Learning our way out. State University of New York Press; 1989.

Milton T. Conceptos de la promoción de la salud: dualidades de la teoría de la salud. In: Promoción de salud: una antología. OPS; 1996. (Publicación científica 557).

PNUD. Desarrollo humano en Chile — 1998: las paradojas de la modernización, Santiago, Chile; 1998.

Prats J. Gobernabilidad, globalización: los desafíos del desarrollo para después del 2000. In: Gobernabilidad y salud — políticas públicas y participación social. OPS; 1999.

Prats J. Liderazgos, democracia y desarrollo: la larga marcha a través de las instituciones (ponencia a debate). prats@campus.uoc.es, Barcelona; 1999.

Putman RD. Comunidade e democracia — a experiência da Itália Moderna. Rio de Janeiro: Editora Fundação Getúlio Vargas; 1996.

Restrepo HE. Increasing Community Capacity and Empowering Communities for Promoting Health. Technical Report 4 to the Fifth Global Conference on Health Promotion. Mexico D.F.; June 2000.

Rex J. Problemas fundamentales de la teoría sociológica. 2ª ed. Buenos Aires: Amorrotu; 1971.

Rodrigues-Noboa P. Programación del cambio social. En: Planificación Social en América Latina y el Caribe. Santiago, Chile: ILPES/UNICEF; 1981. pp. 141–175.

Savater F. Elegir la política. España: Letras Libres; 2002. pp. 12–15.

Wright Mills. La imaginación sociológica. 3ª ed. México: Fondo de Cultura Económica; 1971.

Essential Public Health Functions

In this chapter we begin the transition from the concept of public health to its implementation. This idea will be explored further in the next chapter for the same purpose: to define how the conceptual elements and aspects analyzed in chapters 3, 4, and 5 can be reflected in operational instruments and in their application in the practice of public health.

As per our analysis, the breadth of the concept of public health, and the resulting complexity of this field, as well as the many and varied aspects taken into account, make it difficult to implement. An operational proposal needs to be adopted based on a well-defined functional core that is well-designed and manageable, but of sufficient breadth and trategic significance to address all public health comprehensively. Fortunately, it is easy to identify this strategic functional core of public health in the Americas: the functions under the direct responsibility of the State. Three reasons

justify and even necessitate arriving at this conclusion. First, the State is the main institutional actor in public health, and is an individualized entity from an operational point of view, with legal status and its own powerful means for carrying out actions. Identifying operations, particularly the delegation of responsibilities and the idea of accountability, is easier if it is centered on institutions of the State that are directly responsible for the health sector (the health ministry or secretariat); these will be denoted as the national health authority (NHA), the regional/provincial health authority (RHA), and the local health authority (LHA). Second, the objects of public health are largely public in nature, e.g. public or socially meritorious goods, and therefore are also the responsibility of the State. Lastly, as we have already seen, one of the State's most important functions in public health is the mobilization of civil society and the training of the population for social participation. Thus, using the

state functions carried out by the health authority as the starting point not only makes it possible to reach all other actors and the entire public health field, it is also the most appropriate and, strategically, the most powerful way to do so. Using the State's instruments for taking actions is the mandatory and best foundation for the most effective practice of public health.

Parts III and IV will analyze certain operational aspects of this approach in detail. This chapter will focus on more general considerations of public health functions from the point of view of the responsibilities of the health authority. The goal is to specify the concept and make it more operational with regard to the following four points:

- The concept of essential public health functions (EPHF).

- Essential public health functions and social practices in health.

- Institutional responsibilities in public health.

- The essential public health functions in the Americas.

1. The Concept of Essential Public Health Functions

By virtue of its objects, actors, and fields of knowledge and practice, public health is an identifiable functional and operational part of the health system with a specific operational and functional identity. Thus, not only is it possible, it also necessary to identify public health functions to view them as an operational part of the health system and to optimize their performance.

Public health functions are understood as the set of actions that should be carried out specifically to achieve the central objective of public health: improving the health of populations. In other words, within the set of public health actions and responsibilities, it is possible and advisable to define more homogeneous specific subsets—public health functions—based on the objectives or tasks needed to achieve the end goal of public health.

The operation of a function depends primarily on a sufficient definition of its contents, objectives, and activities and on assigning responsibility for implementing it. If responsibilities are not precisely identified, it is impossible to verify, monitor, and assess operations, and to plan or program strategies and activities. Hence, an operational definition is needed, which identifies public health contents and responsibilities in concrete situations.

Based on the conceptual framework described in chapter 4 and on the reasons mentioned at the beginning of this chapter, we have adopted as the operational definition the responsibilities that the State should undertake in public health, or, more precisely, the responsibilities of official health authorities within governments, i.e. the group we generically refer to as the health authority. This includes not only the responsibilities for directly carrying out specific public health activities and actions, but also the strategic priority areas of mobilizing, promoting, orienting, and articulating other social agents and the support needed from them in public health actions. In other words, it is a matter of making other agents carry out these actions, rather than doing so directly. In this regard, promoting healthy social practices is particularly important. The work of promoting these practices as the principal means for promoting and protecting health is a basic structural component of good public health.

In this way, the State acts through the health authority to mobilize the general public and various social agents in all pertinent sectors to ensure that public health functions are carried out. Public health is thus perceived as a social obligation, which, nonetheless, is particularly manifest in the realm of the specific responsibilities and operational definition of the health authority. The latter is the institutional instrument capable of mobilizing all the relevant actors and carrying out its own executive functions.

The broad and social nature of public health thus is channeled into specific operations that make possible public health planning, follow-up, and evaluation. The concept of responsibility as being "responsible for" is articulated with the idea of assuming responsibility in the sense of being "responsible to" or being "accountable through responsibility." Diffuse general social responsibility and impractical "accountability" are substituted with the specific and extensive operational responsibility of the health authority, which is manifested as a public health indicator. Basic public health functions viewed as being the responsibility of the health authority are thus functional indicators for the entire public health field. Thus, these functions need to be identified and defined.

However, even with the operational limitation discussed, public health actions can help identify numerous functions, depending on the criteria used. The greater the number of functions, the more complex it is to articulate putting them into operation to achieve the ultimate objective of public health. Exaggerated aggregation decreases the specificity of the function in terms of its own determined and quantifiable objectives, meaning that certain important, practical referents are ignored. The concept of the essential public health function offers a very useful alternative. Thus, the focus is on grouping public health interventions into limited and defined functional groups from the operational point of view, with the identification of their the end goals, objectives, activities, resources, and organizational forms that are essential to the overriding goal of public health, i.e. the health of populations, and are sufficient for addressing public health as a whole.

Essential is understood as being fundamental and even indispensable to meeting public health goals and to defining public health. This term is also makes reference to the definition of the responsibilities of the State, through health authorities, considered essential to the development and practice of public health. Consequently, the EPHF are at the core of the functional definition of the entire public health field and, in turn, are indispensable to improving the health of populations. Other functions may or may not be added, but the essential functions should always be present. The latter also shape the matrix for building an operational infrastructure, within the circumstances and possibilities of each environment: national, regional and local.

The complexity and variety of social situations and health systems help identify many public health functions. Different perspectives and situations will give rise to different lists of public health functions. However, the previously agreed-upon criteria can be used to identify a limited number of essential public health functions, which are manageable from an operational perspective, fulfill the characteristics previously noted, and are based on a large enough consensus to be applied internationally, like in the case of the Americas, particularly in the countries in Latin America and the Caribbean. A list of this type makes it possible to develop common instruments to analyze the situation of public health in the Region and even to carry out a comparative analysis of compliance with these functions, as well as to design the necessary corresponding interventions, always bearing in mind a country's specific situation.

Section 4 of this chapter provides a list of the EPHF, adopted as part of the "Public Health in the Americas Initia-

tive", and the main criteria that were used to identify them. Part III of the book details the characteristics of each EPHF as a base from which to evaluate their completion or performance.

The main goal of the initiative is to develop the institutional capacities of health authorities to carry out sound public health practices. The leading criterion for identifying EPHF is the functions that make these capacities possible. Public health actions are carried out through the substantive aspects of its field of action, including environmental health, occupational health, child and maternal health, and chronic diseases. Applying the generic functions to the diverse field of specific or programmatic actions makes it possible to intervene in these actions. These generic functions are thus the core of the capacity for action in public health. Examples of these functions include monitoring health status, public health surveillance, and regulation and control. When these essential functions are properly defined and encompass the capacities needed for the sound practice of public health, appropriate operations are assured in all and each of the work areas. Table 1 provides a schematic.

The distinction between structural functions and programming or areas of action is very useful in selecting the essential functions to develop institutional capacities in public health. However, this does not imply absolute mutually exclusive concepts. Rather structural functions also have their own programming areas of action, and specific fields of action have an obvious functional significance. Some of them are so important to public health in concrete situations that they are deemed to be essential.

Actually, there will always be a balance between these two types of action, even though structural functions dominate. This balance generally depends on the scope and importance of the specific problems addressed by public health and on the level of societal development and institutional public health structure. In well-structured societies, that have a consolidated and effective health infrastructure, the generic or structural functions that make up the necessary public health infrastructure are, generally, sufficient for responding to the needs of specific interventions to solve public health problems. In societies facing major and priority public health risks and harm and that have a weak and ineffective institutional base, the generic or structural functions are the core of the public health infrastructure and are generally sufficient for meeting the need for specific interventions to resolve public health problems. In these societies, there may be a need for more of the specific or programming functions that shape the direct response capacity of public health to meet the priority needs of the population. Some of these aspects will be addressed in greater detail in chapter 7.

In terms of the end goals of the health and public health systems, functions can be considered final or instrumental. *Final* functions directly assist in meeting these goals, including the promotion of health, the control of risks and threats, the protection of the environment, and the quality of care. *Instrumental* functions are the means to meet these goals, creating or contributing to the creation of the conditions or other elements for meeting the final goals, such as monitoring and analyzing the health status, developing human resources and public in-

Table 1 Essential functions and spheres of activity of the public health

EPHF \ Areas EPHF are applied	Environmental health	Occupational health	Maternal and child health	Chronic diseases	Etc.
1. Monitoring of health status	Monitoring of environmental risks	Monitoring of risks in the workplace	Monitoring of health risks to mothers and children	Monitoring of health risks for chronic diseases	
2. Regulation and control	Establishment of regulations and monitoring compliance with them	Monitoring of legislation on workers' health	Monitoring of compliance with laws to protect mothers and children	Monitoring of compliance with regulations promoting healthy behaviors	
3. Etc.					

formation, and regulating public health matters.

Another dimension of the concept of essential public health functions relates to the collective aspect of personal health care. It is difficult to establish a clear separation between the health authority's public health responsibilities in disease prevention and health promotion among population groups and in its responsibilities in the organization of individual care services. This last item is obviously important in a different way, but the essential responsibility of public health is to focus on the first of the functions previously mentioned. In terms of the second function, essential public health functions point more toward concern for equitable access to services, the guarantee of their quality, and the incorporation of a public health perspective into individual health services. Thus, one of the EPHF is geared toward reinforcing the capacity of the health authority to ensure the population's equitable access to health services,

but delivery of such services is not part of the essential functions.

2. Essential Public Health Functions and Social Practices in Health

Essential public health functions are not synonymous with the social practices that affect health. Social practices shape much broader areas than do essential public health functions and are the actions of an entire society, even though they are specifically carried out by certain sectors or actors. The essential functions are the actions of a specific and functional segment of the health system. Social practices in health and essential public health functions are closely linked, however. Both are part of the society, and social practices are the principal matrix for shaping the functions that in turn should act as an instrument for developing the former. In effect, essential public health functions need to be viewed and identified as functions born of social practices and

also as being geared toward promoting and reinforcing healthy social practices. They integrate and promote social practices at the same time. One of the main strategic goals of public health is specific comprehension of social practices and how their benefits aid in developing health. The practice of public health through its essential functions thus has become part of the social practices in health, which ultimately determine and, at the same time, are affected by it.

Earlier in this chapter, analysis of the operative concept of the essential functions showed that the EPHF are instruments and indicators of social practices, understood as social responsibilities toward public health. Thus, essential public health functions need to be considered in relation with groups of social practices, regardless of whether correspondence between the two is exact or unique. It depends on the criteria and conventional limits employed; they do not eliminate overlapping or obscure the extensive, common and complementary areas that exist. Below are some examples of these relationships for each of the groups of social practices.

2.1 Development of a Culture of Life and Health

It should be borne in mind that this group of social practices, in keeping with its end goal, has the task of incorporating knowledge and forming socially shared cultural values reflected in the institutions, organizations, and social relationships that comprise social capital and form the basis for generating social behaviors with regard to life and health.

The EPHF most typically related to this group are the fostering and promotion of health and social participation.

2.2 Development of a Healthy Environment and Control of Risks and Threats to Public Health

The EPHF related to this group of social practices could be health promotion, public health surveillance and control of risks and threats to public health, reducing the impact of emergencies and disasters on health, and regulation and enforcement in public health.

2.3 Development of Citizenship and the Capacity for Social Participation

Examples of the corresponding EPHF would be social participation and training in health, health promotion, and development of policies, planning, and management in public health.

2.4 Attention to Health Needs and Demands

The EPHF related to this group of practices could include quality assurance in health care, promotion of access to health services, and regulation and enforcement.

Some EPHFs are directly related to a set of social practices. This particularly true in the case of generic or structural essential functions. Examples might include monitoring and analysis of health status, human resources development, and fostering research and developing technology in public health.

Public health in the context of healthy social practices seems have an extraordinary potential for developing public health, especially under the conditions seen in Latin America and the Caribbean. However, comprehending and managing it are still in the beginning stages. Increasing systematic efforts to implement the functions and better manage them is one of the objectives of the Public Health in the Americas Initiative.

3. Institutional Responsibilities in Public Health

The State has the primary institutional responsibility in public health. It is the basic social institution that should interpret the needs of a society, respond to them, and work to meet them in the most effective way possible. The State's responsibility should not eliminate or inhibit the responsibilities and actions of other social institutions or organizations. The State should not look to monopolize public health, even though its main re-

sponsibility is to serve society. On the contrary, meeting this responsibility in the best possible way necessitates the mobilization, orientation, articulation, and support of various social agents and of society itself. Adherence to this idea is justified by its importance to public health.

This responsibility is distributed among the various powers that constitute the State and among the sectors of the government covering public health-related areas, but is concentrated in the health sector and more precisely in the institution or organization with the responsibility for the steering role in the sector— the ministry or secretariat of health, what we have called the national health authority (NHA). The State confers on the NHA, as part of the government, the legal responsibility to monitor public health. But, it is much more than a formal responsibility; it is also the moral and ethical commitment to attend to the interests of society and of the population in the area of health and the obligation to make them its own. This commitment implies seeking the best results from the direct actions for which the NHA is responsible and maximizing the effectiveness of various social actors to improve public health. Thus, it is a commitment to technology and science, as well as to management. However, it is primarily a political and social commitment originating from the agreement that infuses life into and supports a society and the State representing it. In carrying out its responsibility, the NHA answers to the government under which it operates and in whose name it acts, including other non-executive powers, and above all to the society it serves.

However, the main public health responsibility of the NHA is not a monopoly within the State. Each branch of the State has its own specific province of responsibility where it exercises non-transferable functions. The legislative branch is responsible for legislation, regulating policies, and general management of the government in name of the people it politically represents. The judicial branch is responsible for compliance with laws. The public ministry or its equivalent (e.g. prosecutor's offices) is responsible for other mechanisms to defend rights; more and more often, this is the fourth branch in modern democracies and its responsibility is to monitor respect for legally recognized rights. Within the executive branch, i.e. government in the strict sense of the word and of which the NHA is a part, other sectors have a very significant presence in public health, even though their specific or overriding goal is not to protect the health of the population. Within the so-called health sector, there are normally institutions and organizations that do not formally answer to the NHA, but that carry out public health interventions. All these actors and institutions should be coordinated to promote public health through synergistic actions; this is an important part of the NHA's mission and responsibility.

The actions of the State, coordinated by the NHA, are geared toward civil society and articulated with and complemented by the intervention of non-governmental social agents, such as institutions and organizations, in the effort to mobilize all of society to promote public health, as subsequently reflected in healthy and health-generating social practices. This brief description of the process once again highlights its integrated, social nature and the broad scope of the health authority's responsibilities set out in the EPHF.

The health authority's functions are variables related to corresponding national and subregional situations. However, certain generic conditions seem to be common to the majority of these situations and can be considered as referents for specifying the conditions of each case. We will now briefly review the most important characteristics and will address this matter in greater detail in chapter 7.

1) Complementary relationships among relevant state sectors in accordance with the legal framework needed, including the definition of interventions, NHA regulations, and intersectoral actions in comprehensive health care for the population.

2) Effective inclusion of public health in an integrated development project, thereby favoring effective and very politically significant actions for public health and the NHA.

3) Distribution of responsibilities among the levels and components within the health authority, among the political/administrative levels in the State, and the organizational components of the NHA, and their effective articulation in a common project. The result of this is integration of public health as an essential component of health systems.

4) Development of effective capacities for the real participation of the population, which implies, among other things, development of adequate social capital, transparency, communication, participatory management, and acceptance of control exercised by the people.

5) Optimizing use of the scientific and technical instruments designed for better recognition of the realities and the selection and implementation of the best possible solutions. As already pointed out, this is the basic strategy for taking maximum advantage of the NHA's ability to facilitate creating other conditions, because it lends the NHA recognition, prestige, and authority in its actions. This also implies developing the institutional capacity to strengthen public health practices.

A simple review of these conditions highlights the complexity of the NHA's mission in meeting its responsibilities in public health and its essential functions. Aside from availability of resources and legal instruments, there are four basic requirements for satisfactorily carrying out this mission.

a) Optimization of the inherent or specific functions that form the basis for recognizing the NHA's capacities and promoting the completion of related functions (also see requirement (5)).

b) Capacity to understand the reality and base its proposals on irrefutable tests.

c) Ownership of a *consistent project that is never finished and always changing,* even though there are sufficiently stable and executable basic referents such as the purpose, strategies, and operational structure.

d) A capacity for dialogue, persuasion, and negotiation, making it possible to mobilize support and neutralize opposition, i.e. a true capacity for political action.

The four requirements demand effective and productive leadership. It is not merely a matter of personal or charismatic leadership in the Weberian sense, but rather of a capacity extending beyond this. It is leadership multiplied through the actions of various leaders and sustained by common values and goals. Charisma, authority, and tradition do not disappear, but neither is there an exclusive or overriding dependence on them. Based on shared ideas, values, and the participation of many actors, it is even possible to renew leaders in positions of power without interfering with the process. It is the leadership of a true democracy, which is also reflected in permanent participation.

Institutional responsibilities in public health are part of the aggregate responsibility toward the well-being of a population. This holds true not only because health is the product of living conditions and quality of life, but also because public health is a component and strategy for improving them. In this way, the responsibility for public health implies being part of the greater responsibility for comprehensive human development, which becomes a basic aspect for developing public health policies and strategies that are very dependent on development policies and strategies.

The NHA's institutional responsibility in public health and its essential functions are part of its overall steering role in public health. This does not mean that the NHA directly carries out each function. The EPHF are the instruments the NHA uses to oversee health,

and they help carry out specific functions of this task, including management, the organization of the delivery of health services, regulation of financing, guarantee of the social protection of health, and regulation of public health. They also act as criteria for orienting the other global functions of the health system, which were mentioned in Chapter 4. Actually, the health of a population and health promotion and protection should be a basic guiding criterion for the entire health system and especially for the health care model comprising it, which is definitely the principal referent of its organization and operation.

In civil society, the public health responsibilities of private or nongovernmental social institutions can be specific, i.e. their main facet, or secondary and can be either formal or informal. The main responsibility of specific private, social health organizations is the health of people or of a population. Other social organizations with broader goals or that are related to health assist in the field of public health as part of these responsibilities. Both are formally bound by the society's legal strictures not to threaten health, but the activities they carry out are basically the result of voluntary decisions. These institutions and organizations can make a profound contribution to public health. From the family to the community or nongovernmental organizations working in health or related to it, from religion or churches to the press, and from schools to unions and political parties, all these organizations comprise an expanding universe of actors that bond together forming relationships and action networks that make a decisive contribution to improving public health. This variety of social agents is the

organized manifestation of civil society that completes and even shapes the actions of the State and the NHA. Mobilizing and articulating this group effectively are fundamental to the essential public health functions so that, under the responsibility of the NHA, they reach society, are effectively linked with social practices, and comprise indicators suitable for the entire social sphere of public health.

4. Essential Public Health Functions in the Americas

The Public Health in the Americas Initiative has prepared a list of 11 essential public health functions. The number of functions was not determined a priori, but rather is the result of the analysis, definition of basic criteria, discussion, and field tests carried out to establish them.

Below is a summary of the basic criteria adopted to identify the EPHF, which would best respond to circumstances in the Americas, and to validate these functions. The entire process will be described in greater detail in chapters 8, 9, and 10 of part III.

1) Since the principal goal of the initiative is to promote the permanent infrastructure of public health, priority has been placed on selecting generic or structural functions from a purely functional view of specific functions in determined fields of action. The generic or structural functions are the basis of a functional public health infrastructure and are applied in various spheres of activity.

2) Comparing the three previous studies that specifically addressed identifying essential public health shows

Figure 1 EPHF defined in the NPHPSP,[2] the WHO Delphi Study,[3] and the PAHO position paper[4]

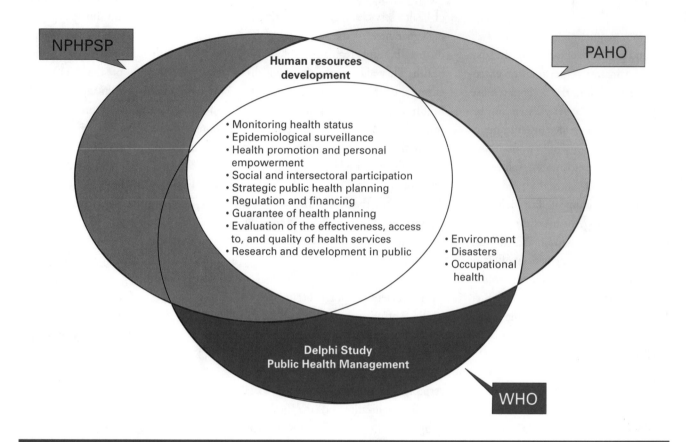

that there is a high degree of confluence among the functions identified. The following schematic reflects this idea. (Figure 1)

Nine of the functions appear in all three studies. One of them, human resources, appears in both NPHSP and PAHO documents. Three appear in both PAHO and WHO documents. Only one function appears solely in the WHO study. This overlapping helped indentify functions and was used to prepare the rough draft on an instrument for measuring the performance of the EPHF. This draft also includes the definition of all the 12 essential functions selected and the indicators and standards for evaluating their performance. Different groups of experts and public health professionals evaluated the draft, and this

process culminated a meeting of the network of institutions and experts, convened by PAHO.[1]

3) It was also important to define the functions as groups of actions that could be carried out adequately. This necessitated a certain degree of homogeneity to identify specific goals, components, and production

[1] Expert consultation on the performance measurement of essential public health functions, Washington, D.C., September 9 and 10, 1999.
[2] National Public Health Performance Standards Program, Centros para el Control y Prevención de Enfermedades (CDC), EE.UU.
[3] WHO. "Essentials Public Health Functions: results of The International Delphi Study", World Health Statistics 51, 1998.
[4] OPS. "Las Funciones Esenciales de la Salud Pública: documento de posición", 1998.

processes that could be verified and evaluated, and responsible operating mechanisms for accountability.

4) The initial list of 12 functions set forth in an instrument to measure the performance of essential public health functions was pilot-tested in Colombia, Jamaica, and Bolivia. These tests were analyzed, resulting in a list of 11 essential functions. (Table 2.) Obviously, this list it is subject to improvements. It was not designed to cover all the public health perspectives in the world; nonetheless, efforts have been made to minimize biases and include the relevant aspects determined by the experts and actors that help make health policy decisions. Their opinions were taken into account in all instances.

Table 2   Essential Public Health Functions

EPHF 1	Monitoring, Evaluation, and Analysis of Health Status
EPHF 2	Public Health Surveillance, Research, and Control of Risks and Threats to Public Health
EPHF 3	Health Promotion
EPHF 4	Social Participation in Health
EPHF 5	Development of Policies and Institutional Capacity for Planning and Management in Public Health
EPHF 6	Strengthening of Institutional Capacity for Regulation and Enforcement in Public Health
EPHF 7	Evaluation and Promotion of Equitable Access to Necessary Health Services
EPHF 8	Human Resources Development and Training in Public Health
EPHF 9	Quality Assurance in Personal and Population-based Health Services
EPHF 10	Research in Public Health
EPHF 11	Reduction of the Impact of Emergencies and Disasters on Health

Defining the EPHF is the first step in measuring public health performance in the Region of the Americas, and this activity will doubtlessly be perfected in the future.

EPHF 1: Monitoring, Evaluation, and Analysis of Health Status

Definition:

This function includes:

- Up-to-date evaluation of the country's health situation and trends including their determinants with special emphasis on identifying inequities in risks, threats, and access to services.

- Identification of the population's health needs including an assessment of health risks and the demand for health services.

- Management of vital statistics and the status of special groups or groups at greater risk.

- Generation of useful information for the assessment of the performance of health services.

- Identification of those nonsectoral resources that support health promotion and improvements in the quality of life.

- Development of technology, expertise and methodologies for management, analysis and communication of information to those responsible for public health (including key players from other sectors, health care providers and civil society).

- Identifying and establishing agencies that evaluate and accurately analyze the quality of collected data.

EPHF 2: Public Health Surveillance, Research, and Control of Risks and Threats to Public Health

Definition:

- The capacity to conduct research and surveillance of epidemic outbreaks, patterns of communicable and non-communicable disease, behavioral factors, accidents, and exposure to toxic substances or environmental agents harmful to health.

- A public health services infrastructure designed to conduct population screenings, case-finding and general epidemiological research.

- Public health laboratories capable of conducting rapid screening and processing of a high volume of tests necessary for identifying and controlling emerging threats to health.

- The development of active programs for epidemiological surveillance and control of infectious diseases.

- The capacity to develop links with international networks that permit better management of relevant health problems.

- Preparedness of the NHA and strengthening of local health surveillance to initiate a rapid response for the control of health problems or specific risks.

EPHF 3: Health Promotion[5]

Definition:

- The promotion of changes in lifestyle and environmental conditions to facilitate the development of a "culture of health."

- The strengthening of intersectoral partnerships for more effective health promotion activities.

---

[5] This function encompasses the definition of the capacities specifically required to implement, from the perspective of the NHA, the components of health promotion defined in the Ottawa Charter and reaffirmed in the recent Global Conference on Health Promotion in Mexico. Since it has been considered necessary to define another essential function to cover social participation, this latter has concentrated on defining capacities that largely facilitate health promotion.

- Assessment of the impact of public policies on health.

- Educational and social communication activities aimed at promoting healthy conditions, lifestyles, behaviors and environments.

- Reorientation of the health services to develop models of care that encourage health promotion.

EPHF 4: Social Participation in Health

Definition:

- Strengthening the power of civil society to change their lifestyles and play an active role in the development of healthy behaviors and environments in order to influence the decisions that affect their health and their access to adequate health services.

- Facilitating the participation of the community in decisions and actions with regard to programs for disease prevention, diagnosis, treatment and restoration of health in order to improve the health status of the population and promote environments that foster healthy lifestyles.

EPHF 5: Development of Policies and Institutional Capacity for Regulation and Enforcement in Public Health

Definition:

- The definition of national and subnational public health objectives which should be measurable and consistent with a values-based framework that favors equity.

- The development, monitoring and evaluation of policy decisions in pub-

lic health through a participatory process that is consistent with the political and economic context in which the decisions are made.

- The institutional capacity for the management of public health systems, including strategic planning with emphasis on building, implementing and evaluating initiatives designed to focus on health problems of the population.

- The development of competencies for evidence-based decision-making, planning and evaluation, leadership capacity and effective communication, organizational development and resource management.

- Capacity-building for securing international cooperation in public health.

EPHF 6: Strengthening of Institutional Capacity for Planning and Management in Public Health

Definition:

- The institutional capacity to develop the regulatory and enforcement frameworks that protect public health and monitor compliance within these frameworks.

- The capacity to generate new laws and regulations aimed at improving public health, as well as promoting healthy environments.

- Consumer protection as it relates to health services.

- Carrying out all of these activities to ensure full, proper, consistent and timely compliance with the regulatory and enforcement frameworks.

EPHF 7: Valuation and Promotion of Equitable Access to Necessary Health Services

Definition:

- The promotion of equity of access by civil society to necessary health services.

- The development of actions designed to overcome barriers when accessing public health interventions and help link vulnerable groups to necessary health services (does not include the financing of health care).

- The monitoring and evaluation of access to necessary health services offered by public and/or private providers and using a multisectoral, multiethnic and multicultural approach to facilitate working with diverse agencies and institutions to reduce injustices and inequities in use of necessary health services.

- Close collaboration with governmental and nongovernmental institutions to promote equity able access to necessary health services.

EPHF 8: Human Resources Development and Training in Public Health

Definition:

- The development of a public health workforce profile in public health that is adequate for carrying out public health services.

- Educating, training, developing and evaluating the public health workforce to identify the needs of public health services and health care, efficiently address priority public health problems and adequately evaluate public health activities.

- The definition of licensure requirements for health professionals in general and the adoption of ongoing programs that improve the quality of public health services.

- Formation of active partnerships with programs for professional development to ensure that all students have relevant public health experience and receive continuing education in the management of human resources and leadership development in public health.

- The development of skills necessary for interdisciplinary, multicultural work in public health.

- Bioethics training for public health personnel, emphasizing the principles and values of solidarity, equity, and respect for human dignity.

EPHF 9: Quality Assurance in Personal and Population-based Health Services

Definition:

- The promotion of systems that evaluate and improve quality.

- Facilitating the development of standards required for a quality assurance and improvement system and oversight of compliance of service providers with this obligation.

- The definition, explanation, and assurance of user rights.

- A system for health technology assessment that supports the decision-making process at all levels and contributes to quality improvement.

- Using the scientific method to evaluate health interventions of varying degrees of complexity.

- Systems to evaluate user satisfaction and application of its results to improve the quality of health services.

EPHF 10: Research in Public Health

Definition:

- Rigorous research aimed at increasing knowledge to support decision-making at the various levels.

- The implementation and development of innovative solutions in public health whose impact can be measured and assessed.

- The establishment of partnerships with research centers and academic institutions from within and outside the health sector to conduct timely studies that support decision-making of the NHA at all its levels and in all its fields of action.

EPHF 11: Reduction of the impact of the emergencies and disasters on the health[6]

Definition:

- Policy development, planning and execution of activities in the prevention, mitigation, preparedness, early response and rehabilitation programs to reduce the impact of disasters on public health.

---

[6] Emergency and disaster reduction in health includes prevention, mitigation, preparedness, early response and rehabilitation.

- An integrated approach with respect to the damage and etiology of any and all emergencies and disasters that can affect the country.

- Involvement of the entire health system and the broadest possible intersectoral and inter-institutional collaboration to reduce the impact of emergencies and disasters.

- The procurement of intersectoral and international collaboration to respond to health problems resulting from emergencies and disasters.

Bibliography

CDC/CLAISS/OPS. La salud pública en las Américas. Instrumento para la medición de las funciones esenciales de la salud pública — Prueba piloto (working document); April 2000.

Bettcher DW, Saprie S, Goon EH. Essential public health functions: results of the international Delphi Study. Geneva: WHO, World Health Statistics, n.º 51; 1998.

OPS. Funciones esenciales de salud pública: documento de posición. División de Desarrollo de Sistemas y Servicios de Salud, (draft); May 1998.

OPS. Funciones esenciales de salud pública (doc.). CE126/17 (Esp.), April 2000.

Secretary of State for Social Services. Public Health in England. The Report of the Committee of Inquiring into the Future Development of the Public Health Function. Londres: Her Majesty's Stationary Office; 1988.

The Core Functions Project. Health Care Perform and Public Health: a paper on Population-based Core Functions. Journal of Public Health Policy, Vol. 19, n.º 4, 294–418.

U.S, Institute of Medicine. The Future of Public Health. National Academy Press; 1988.

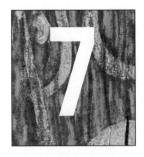

7 Framework for Action to Improve Public Health Practice

This chapter outlines the principal features of the interventions aimed at improving public health practice in accordance with the concepts and operational strategy of the essential public health functions. Although it seeks to cover the most important aspects of public health practice, the exposition hereby presented is more conceptual than operational. It identifies and provides a characterization of the factors that are important for good public health practice, without dwelling on how they are to be applied. Parts III and IV of the book delve further into operational issues and specifications for the application of some of these factors.

Given the number and variety of factors that must be taken into account it is recommended to group them within the sections that identify them. It is recognized, however, that the components overlap, both between and within groups. This calls for a holistic and comprehensive approach to the design

of effective strategies for action. Therefore, the groups of factors will be analyzed sequentially, the aim being to reproduce the reality as closely as possible, although this approach will entail some redundancy, which is unavoidable and at times may even be desirable. The last section will summarize the entire chapter, presenting a comprehensive overview of the process needed to develop public health practice.

1. Concepts and Practice

Unfortunately, evidence of a false contradiction between theory and practice continues to abound in the social sphere. Many who consider themselves pragmatic reject theory and theorists, whom they consider to be out of touch with reality and whom they label as academics or dreamers. On the contrary, some of the so-called theorists view the pragmatists with arrogance and even contempt. In general, the latter recognize their views as misleading because

they know that theory and practice, concepts and action, are interdependent. Indeed, theory that does not lead to practice is sterile, and all practice is, in turn, the manifestation of a conceptual representation of reality. The concepts that justify practice may not be explicitly stated, or they may not be perceived by the actors, who simply act on the basis of unanalyzed experience or they merely apply procedures and routines established by others. However, while an exercise carried out under such conditions may be effective in a specific instance—provided the conditions of the previous experience are replicated and the established rules followed—if it does not include some element of self-evaluation or cannot be adapted to different or changing circumstances, it will ultimately become less effective, if indeed it ever was. Practice, especially in the social realm, and in public health, in particular, both tests and validates theory. Most importantly, practice serves as the most effective mechanism for enhancing and broadening theory.

A similar situation may occur, but with a different argumentation: Concepts may be negated for ideological reasons. This occurs frequently in the area of health, especially in regards to its social determinants. There are no longer those who dare to deny that health and public health are influenced by social factors, but when the negative impact of the dominant economic models or political processes that lead to unhealthy public policies are analyzed, it is often argued that public health should confine itself to its own area of scientific inquiry—i.e., the biological and related sciences (classical epidemiology, statistics, etc.)—and not get mixed up in politics and economics. This risk involved in this type of argument is that it is used as justification for inaction in the social sphere under the guise of biomedical sciences which, in the final analysis, is an ideologically motivated political position that masquerades one of scientific neutrality. In advanced societies, in which basic social needs have been satisfied such position has negative effects mitigated by the fact that there is relatively little need for social change. This is so, particularly, with regard to political processes and practices. On the other hand, in those societies in which such changes are imperative for public health development the consequences are appalling.

In summary, a solid and well-defined conceptual framework—to guide action and which is validated and improved by it—is crucial starting point for public health development.

The transition from theory to practice in the production of goods is accomplished through the use of technology and the organization of production. In other words, real or potential unmet demand becomes the incentive to transform basic knowledge into the means to apply technology for the production of goods. It also encourages entrepreneurs to organize the production and sale of goods in the market to potential consumers. Public policies may help or hinder this process through fiscal incentives, credit, technical assistance, training, etc. However, in the field of public health, a very different process occurs. A significant portion of theoretical knowledge is the result of an analysis of reality and experience, and is therefore, to some extent already being manifested in practice. What needs to be done, then, is mainly to compile this knowledge, to organize it and make it more consistent, and to expand its application. In the case of public health, the goods in question are usually public goods or goods with great social value, which have high externalities and cannot be individually owned, leading to insufficient demand and scarce market supply. Thus public health is a State responsibility.

Hence, essential public health functions are a fundamental responsibility of the NHA, from the generation of knowledge to the development of technology and its appropriate implementation through the organization of its production. Similarly, the transition from concepts to action is basically an institutional process in which the NHA manages the participation of other actors. Accordingly, the essential requirement for carrying out this process is the institutional capacity to undertake such endeavor, the development and exercise of which will be discussed in the sections that follow. Institutional capacity means, in essence, the ability to ascertain the reality and to intervene to change it. It means, having the necessary information and intelligence and the ability to implement—i.e., actual resources, especially human resources, and adequate organizational and managerial capacity.

Public health practice is strongly influenced by the culture in which it takes place. The value placed on public health is an important factor in the application of technical instruments and limits or encourages their application, depending on the circumstances. The characteristics of social processes, including economic and political processes, determine the possibilities and opportunities for intervention. On the other hand, the availability and quality of resources will also influence the possibilities for action. It is therefore essential to consider specific factors that may affect interventions in the short term, structural factors in the broader context, and factors related to public health itself, as it relates to national and even intranational situations. Thus, implementation modalities are always specific and take place in a concrete situation. However, this does not negate the validity of general knowledge and the possibility of generalizing the use of some well-designed operational instruments in comparable situations, as long as care is taken to identify differences and variations in order to make the necessary adaptations. The possibility of generalizing may prove to be a very significant advantage for progress, given its potential usefulness for comparisons, mutual support, learning and shared development, etc. Hence, the process of developing public health practice will be based on national ownership and the willingness to cooperate and share achievements at the international level.

Chapter 6 described the basic functional strategy for public health development—i.e., performance of the essential public health functions for which the national health authority is responsible. This strategy is justified, not only because it represents a manageable functional interest in the field of public health, but also because of its potential to achieve overall health development of the population. Public health practice through the EPHF is the best way to address all aspects of public health, including health-promoting social practices. In this manner, the practical application of the concepts of public health will occur as a natural outgrowth of the adequate performance of the essential public health functions. The operational approach for assuring that this happens will be performance evaluation and development of the national health authority's capacity as an institution which enables carrying out the essential public health functions as effectively as possible, including the mobilization and involvement of other actors from the State and civil society.

2. Managerial Capacity as a Prerequisite

As was explained in Chapter 4, public health is part of the overall health system, and essential public health functions are part of the global steering function exercised by the NHA. This steering role includes, in addition to EPHF, management of financing, health care, and general organization of the delivery of services, as well as regulation and management of the entire system. The essential public health functions are

related to all these steering functions, sometimes overlapping or complementing them with regard to the objectives of public health—i.e., everything that has to do with the health of the population. The EPHF and public health are thus more than simply a component of the steering role and the health system; they are general reference frameworks and intervention instruments present in all actions that help enhance the health of populations. They are also, because of their objectives, necessary outcomes. Indeed, the steering role of the health system should be guided, first and foremost, by the fundamental objective of public health: the health of the population, which is also the principal and ultimate objective of the health system, and the EPHF, may be the best instrument to achieve such objective.

Stewardship is the central function of the steering role and defines it as such. Stewardship means guiding the health system from a given situation, which is considered partially or wholly unsatisfactory, to a better situation in the future, which is established as the objective to be achieved. In accordance with this view, stewardship entails an evaluation of the existing situation and the definition of the situation established as a goal—the vision of what is desired and possible—including the health objectives and determinants, which implies the design, implementation, and execution of strategies for achieving the proposed change. In the exercise of the steering role, stewardship performs or oversees other functions, including the EPHF, which are carried out so that the process of management can be accomplished effectively. Stewardship is thus central to the decision-making process that is part of the steering role. It is in

stewardship that the political and intersectoral dimensions of health, the health system, and public health are manifested most fully and obviously, and it is in stewardship that these dimensions are addressed in ways that will have repercussions and be replicated, to differing degrees, in other sectoral areas.

It is also in the stewardship that alliances are forged and support is enlisted for the implementation of the vision and proposed objectives, that the tasks of mobilization and cooperation are defined and organized, and that the greatest capacity for leadership and promotion should reside. It is here that general strategies for action are developed and articulated, that sectoral policies are formulated and negotiated, and that the characteristics of the planning, organization, and management processes are defined. Finally, it is in exercising the steward role that decisions are made about the general conditions that will lead to the effective execution of programs and activities within the health system—decisions about institutional organization, financing, assignment of responsibilities and allocation of resources, and monitoring and evaluation throughout the process. Without effective stewardship, it will be impossible to achieve good public health and the entire steering role and overall performance of the health system will be compromised.

The steering role should recognize and adopt public health as the basis for stewardship, with performance of the essential public health functions as its principal instrument, to be applied in the design of models of care, in insurance and quality assurance in the delivery of care, in the organization of systems of services, and in health systems performance assessment. Stewardship is, therefore, a prerequisite for—and, at the same time, benefits from—good public health practice.

3. Systemic and Specific Aspects of the Essential Public Health Functions

The previous chapter, in analyzing the concept of essential public health function, a differentiation was made between systemic or structural functions and specific or programming functions and the relationships between the two categories were established in a graph. This distinction is very useful for improving public health practice, and the selection of EPHF As noted earlier, if essential public health functions include all significant interventions of a systemic nature that define the essential capacity for public health action, and if those interventions are carried out satisfactorily, practice in the various specific or programmatic spheres of action will also be satisfactory.

Hence, a requirement for achieving good public health practice is proper selection of the essential functions and, especially, a clear definition of each function that identifies the principal activities involved and includes a comprehensive range of activities within the overall set of functions. A clear definition of the functions will make it possible to select the best indicators to measure their performance.[1] The first step is to assess the situation, as measured by performance of the EPHF, which is done by comparing it against optimal standards, established by consensus for the entire Region. This makes it possible to

[1] See Part III for more detail on the measuring instrument and process developed in the framework of the Initiative.

identify differences between the existing situation and the possible and desirable situation and determine the causal factors that explain the discrepancies.

The situation assessment will serve to identify weaknesses or deficiencies that need to be corrected, including their causes, as well as strengths that should be reinforced. The resulting strategies and programs for action will initially be centered on the essential public health functions as the structural matrix of the capacity for action in public health and as the basis for improving interventions in the specific spheres of action through public health programs. Later, or if possible simultaneously, the particular situations of those programs will be assessed and the necessary corrective or strengthening measures will be defined. Then, an effort will be made to deepen knowledge in regard to certain specific or complementary issues and expand the capacity for action with respect to social practices in public health.

Interventions aimed at improving the EPHF performance will involve specific actions for each function, but should place special emphasis on aspects common to several or all of them. These common aspects will frequently appear as features in the situation assessment and will usually reveal deficiencies in the overall public health infrastructure that are affecting some or all of the essential functions. The sections that follow will focus on this topic.

4. Complementarity and Comprehensive Development of the EPHF

Because its fundamental objective is the health of the population, public health requires a comprehensive vision. At the same time, owing to its complexity and the variety of objectives or spheres of action, it requires an analytical vision. The results of the overall action of public health are manifested in the specific outputs of its parts and in their joint contribution to the health of the population, which may be much greater than the mere sum of the partial results if the actions of the various components are guided by a common objective.

Essential public health functions, as the core of public health action, share individual and complementary traits as parts of the whole that is public health. Every EPHF has its own functional identity and specific processes and each generates specific outputs and results. At the same time, however, they share common resources and complement one another. There is also a question of efficiency involved: sharing resources and taking full advantage of the opportunities for synergy will increase benefits in relation to cost for each cost unit added. Optimizing the balance between the specificity of each function and achieving the most effective integration of their common aspects is thus the golden rule for the management of essential public health functions. The selection of functions (Chapter 6) was made to facilitate the achievement of that balance.

The EPHF 1 (monitoring, evaluation, and analysis of the health situation), EPHF 5 (development of policies and institutional capacity for planning and management in public health), EPHF 8 (human resources development and training in public health), and EPHF 10 (research in public health) are examples of systemic functions that support or complement the others and constitute areas that share capabilities common to all public health actions. EPHF 3 (health promotion) and EPHF 4 (social participation in health) require the contribution of some of the other functions but, especially through their results, they are also capable of changing the operational conditions of the entire health system and public health, amplifying the impact of their specific activities. EPHF 6 (strengthening of the institutional capacity for regulation and enforcement in public health) is instrumental and essential for ensuring adequate operation of the whole health system in its collective or public health dimensions. At the same time, the contribution of the other essential public health functions is needed to fulfill this function. Similarly, performance of EPHF 2 (public health surveillance, research, and control of risks and threats to public health), EPHF 7 (evaluation and promotion of the equitable access to necessary health services), and EPHF 9 (quality assurance in personal and population-based health services), which are directly linked to the ultimate objectives of public health, is aided by the other functions. Finally, EPHF 11 (reducing the impact of emergencies and disasters on health) is an example of a more specific function with a defined sphere of action, which receives support from the more systemic functions.

The foregoing examples point out the interrelationship between the individual essential public health functions, on the one hand, and between the EPHF and other areas of intervention in health systems. The specific approach, though necessary given the specificity of each function, entails significant risk of a loss of the synergism among them, unjustifiable duplication of effort, and, consequently, lack or reduction of effectiveness in public health.

The strategy that will achieve the best balance between specificity and integration of the essential public health functions is the development of a common

public health infrastructure and its articulation with the other functions associated with the steering role and with the related resources and activities of the health system. Thus, the principal strategy for developing public health and improving its practice will also be part of the strategies for making public health a fundamental instrument for strengthening the steering role with regard to health and enhancing the overall health system. In other words, another aim of the improvement of public health practice, or the integral development of public health, is to develop the steering role as an essential function for bettering the health system and increasing its effectiveness and raising the population's satisfaction with its services. If this aim is achieved, public health will be strengthened and its effectiveness in attaining its fundamental objective—the health of the population—will be enhanced.

5. Public Health Infrastructure and Development of Capacity for Action

The infrastructure for public health is the set of stable and interconnected means by which its activities are organized. In the broad sense, it is the permanent base of resources organized for action and defines NHA's capacity for performance of the essential public health functions. Accordingly, it is by establishing a sound infrastructure that institutional capacity for action in public health can be increased and the practice of public health can thus be improved.

The fundamental elements that make up the infrastructure are:

- Information, which implies the existence of adequate information systems and the capacity to turn it into intelli-

gence for action. Section 6 below analyzes this element in greater detail.

- Skilled human resources and satisfactory working conditions. Section 8 discusses this matter further and Chapter 15 (Part IV) explores the subject in depth.

- Organization, as the element that ties the resources together, endowing them with functional unity and enabling public health action. Organization, like infrastructure, defines the institutional characteristics of public health, specifically, those relating to the performance of essential public health functions. It comprises the legal basis for public health—i.e., the national authority responsible for public health, its functions and duties, the assignment of those functions and duties to the various elements and levels of the organization, and the mechanisms and processes for ensuring accountability and evaluation, among other things. Organization defines, in short, how the infrastructure is configured and how it can be managed to carry out public health actions. Organization also includes the fundamental technical processes through which scientific and technical activities are carried out in order to perform the essential public health essential functions and execute basic administrative and managerial processes. They are not technical manuals, but they do provide the basic parameters for the preparation of such manuals. The distinction between administrative processes and scientific and technical processes is important for the improvement of public health practice because it singles out scientific and technical tasks, differentiating them from management and administration, which makes it possible to tailor the infrastructure for these tasks to their specific characteristics.

These three functional elements operate on the basis of indispensable physical resources and essential support or auxiliary services. These support or auxiliary services are public health laboratories and, special research and training units. Public health laboratories, however, are essential structural elements for public health and for the performance of essential public health functions. In some situations, special research and training units may be so essential to the overall development of public health and serve as key structural elements for intervention in public health and for the effective performance of essential public health functions.

Functional infrastructure requires physical space, instruments and equipment in order to operate. This becomes even more necessary the more public health functions are not being performed. The most obvious examples are computer and communications systems for information management, laboratory facilities and equipment, and workspaces in which managerial personnel and public health workers can carry out their functions. In many countries these requirements are not being met, or the condition of the physical resources is extremely precarious. Public health development and practice require that these physical instruments and resources exist at least at a basic minimal level, which must be defined in each case.

In accordance with the conceptual basis adopted, the positive social capital that is produced by healthy and health-promoting social practices and manifested in citizen participation in health is, without a doubt, another kind of infra-

structure. In this case, the infrastructure is of a social nature, which corresponds to and is complemented by the institutional infrastructure that is the focus of this section. Section 12 will deal with the social infrastructure.

Articulation of the concepts and practice of public health is accomplished mainly by means of the institutional capacity for intervention, which is determined by the infrastructure, or by the social capacity for positive action, which in turn is determined by the social capital that is formed in the culture and manifested in healthy social practices and social participation. Creation or improvement of the institutional and social infrastructures for public health is therefore the principal condition and fundamental factor for achieving effective practice.

The institutional infrastructure is specific to public health, but public health action would be severely limited if it were restricted to the capacity of its own infrastructure. Therefore, the NHA should utilize the capacity of other areas of the health system and other sectors—especially those that have a hand in the steering function and in the delivery of care—to expand the capacity for action in public health. In fact, at one extreme of the health care system, public health activities are part of general health care for the population and often they are carried out by the same agents, especially at the primary care level. Similarly, the essential public health functions overlap with and complement all the functions of the steering role and depend decisively on the management function. Moreover, some important public health activities, including some of a systemic nature, such as regulation, risk and threat control, and human resources development, depend on the intervention

of other sectors or are carried out by them. For this reason, intersectoral action is also a means of expanding the capacity for action in public health beyond the possibilities of its own infrastructure.

The situation assessment and, especially, the evaluation of the performance of essential public health functions should be used to identify the weaknesses in the institutional infrastructure of public health. It will then be possible to design specific interventions to correct them within the conceptual framework presented here, which is the principal frame of reference for guiding the efforts needed in each case to strengthen the public health infrastructure. Use of the findings of the EPHF performance evaluation, coupled with a conceptual understanding of the characteristics and requirements of public health, will enable the development and implementation of strategies and plans to strengthen the infrastructure as needed and enhance institutional capacity for intervention in public health, in accordance with the possibilities and needs in each situation. Moreover, it will be possible to articulate institutional capacity with the contribution of the society. Chapter 13 in Part IV will address this subject in more detail.

In essence, the process of strengthening infrastructure and the consequent development of institutional capacity for action is the result of decisions made by the national health authority in the exercise of the steering role, through its stewardship function. Such decisions are political in nature and represent the exercise of institutional power. In the national arena, these decisions will have greater force and sustainability if the government assumes responsibility for them and if they become the responsibility of the State. Not only will the decisions themselves be reinforced, but all of public health, as much as it will be endowed with greater importance. The NHA, too, will be strengthened as its authority to exercise the global steering role in the health system will be augmented. Once a policy decision has been made, the process of implementing it becomes mainly a management responsibility with fewer political implications. In any case, it will be a slow and complex process, which will always depend on the existence of good sectoral management and the use that is made of it.

6. Information and Intelligence in Public Health

Information is the most generic input into the infrastructure of public health. It is also an indispensable input, since good public health practice cannot occur without information or if the information available is ineffective or insufficient. Indisputably, the improvement of public health practice depends on the availability of information, and it will only be as good as the quality of that information.

The information required for good public health practice is extremely varied and is related to a wide variety of topics, including objectives and areas of concern for public health, context, and external determining factors. Consequently, the processes by which the information is collected, analyzed, and used will also vary. To obtain an overview of all the complex processes involved in information management, it might be useful to construct a matrix indicating the relationship between the various categories of information, the principal subject areas, and the EPHF.

The suggested categories have great strategic importance because they de-fine not only the use or purpose of the information, but the users as well. The matrix also shows the variety of subject areas with which public health is concerned, including both areas related to specific public health objectives and essential functions, health risks and threats, and human resources for public health, as well as broader objectives, with information for exclusive public health use and for shared use in the performance of other functions related to the steering role and the health system. In general, the use to be made of the information will serve as a guide for the selection of the subject areas. Based on this simple and imaginary exercise, it is obvious that public health practice and the essential public health functions require information on both the specific areas of concern for public health and more general information, nonspecific to public health but essential to its capacity for action.

Nevertheless, it is not enough simply to have information; the information available must be of satisfactory quality, it must be timely, and it must be processed correctly in order to generate intelligence. Mechanisms and processes for evaluating and assuring information quality are just as, or even more, important than primary information collection, transmission, and processing systems. Intelligence is the parameter for measuring the use and valid of information. Knowledge of subject areas and situations is the first stage of intelligence gathering in public health, which facilitates or complements the wisdom and capacity to choose, carry out, or promote the most effective actions in relation to given objectives.

The concept of information used in this instance is quite broad, encompassing both objective, quantifiable, evidence-based information and qualitative information with a less rigorous formal basis. It is derived, preferably, from objectively observed and recorded facts, but it is also based on the perceptions and opinions of reliable actors. Fortunately, there are techniques for analyzing and minimizing inaccuracies, variations, and errors in such information, which makes it possible to reach reliable or acceptable conclusions on the actions to be taken. For example, to measure and evaluate the performance of essential public health functions in the countries, an instrument based on the opinions of groups with expert knowledge of the situation has been designed and utilized successfully. The limitations of evidence and the observations that produce it in the field of public health should be noted here, as should the importance of qualitative evidence, due in part to the limitations that may result from failure to include important variables that should be considered. Nevertheless, it should be reaffirmed that it is preferable to base public health intelligence on indisputable scientific evidence. Accordingly, there should be an ongoing effort to expand the evidence base.

Notwithstanding these considerations, the question of ownership of information systems in public health remains to be answered: Are they exclusive or shared? There seems to be no doubt that the answer is "both." To attain information that has to do specifically with the areas of concern of public health, there will be specific information systems that can delve into the particular area and components of each EPHF. For more general information, public health will coordinate with other systems to gain access to the necessary information. The guiding criterion for decision-making in this regard is to seek the most appropriate balance between specificity and integration in the steering role and in the health system. The ideal would be to design a health information system that is comprehensive in nature, but has components that will produce specialized information for particular uses, as well as a common information base for shared use. In such a system, public health and essential public health functions will have a specialized component, tailored specially to their needs, which will feed the information generated into the shared system in previously agreed formats. Such a system would permit access to the common information base and to other specialized components for the acquisition of necessary data and information, all of which would be available in usable formats.

In any case, public health should always have the capacity to analyze data for specific purposes and generate its own intelligence, although access to this intelligence should not be restricted or exclusive. One precaution that is frequently overlooked but that should be exercised in regard to information is not to go overboard in terms of the volume or variety of data and information produced, so that it does not exceed the capacity for use, which would not only waste resources, but could entail a risk of seriously biasing the entire process and, possibly, jeopardizing the generation of intelligence.

Information about public health proves its usefulness and becomes real intelligence when it serves for the formulation of plans and policies, planning, and effective and efficient management, including evaluations of sufficient breadth and depth. These matters will not be an-alyzed in detail here,[2] although they are essential for the improvement of public health practice.

In conclusion, the initial situation assessment of the essential public health functions through the measurement and evaluation of their performance also serves as a starting point for the management of public health information. Performance indicators are excellent guides for identifying the information needed, and application of the measurement instrument reveals gaps in the existing information, deficiencies in the available information, and even, in some cases, the fact that the available information is unusable or useless. It also reveals the strengths and weaknesses of the health services infrastructure in regard to information production. On the basis of this knowledge, interventions can be designed to remedy the weaknesses or reinforce the strengths and devise and promote strategies for the structuring, expansion, and enhancement of the corresponding systems.

7. Public Health Practice and Personal Health Care Services

As has been noted above, there is a close and complementary relationship between public health and personal health care activities, and this relationship is manifested in a variety of ways.

Both public health and personal health care are integral parts of the health system and share responsibility for contributing to the achievement of its objectives. Moreover, public health en-compasses some personal health care activities and is carried out through them, which blurs the distinction between the two fields. In the case of environmental health, the distinction disappears altogether because interventions aimed at the environment always have a public health connotation, whether or not they are carried out within the health sector or under the responsibility of the NHA. Environmental health, in all its practical manifestations, falls within the sphere of action of public health, owing to the public nature of the services rendered and the scope of their coverage in the population.

Definition and coordination of institutional responsibilities are basically the only issues that have to be addressed in relation to public health practice and the essential public functions. The relationship between public health and personal health care at all levels of the care delivery system, but especially the primary care level, has already been discussed, as have the simultaneous execution of public health activities in the course of caring for individuals, the shared support systems, and the complementarity of information. All these connections are crucial for public health practice and performance of the EPHF. Here, the focus will be on the influence of public health in the organization and operation of the personal health care system and the total health system, which may be a critical factor in the orientation of health sector reforms and also, be of great importance for the general orientation of public health.

The ultimate objective of a health system is to improve the health of the population and ensure that care provided provides social satisfaction. Both objectives—social effectiveness and satisfac-

---

[2] See Chapter 13 in Part IV for more information on this subject.

tion—have collective significance; they are related to the health of populations, and they are, therefore, public health objectives. The vision of public health should be the underlying criterion or basis for the formation, steering, and management of health systems and the delivery of personal health care. It is within the perspective of public health, understood as population health, which global health objectives and the desired health situation can be properly defined and the system and its resources and processes can be organized to produce the services that will make it possible to achieve those objectives.

The instruments of public health action, which are made manifested basically through the essential public health functions, also serve to achieve overall health objectives and fulfill the guiding principles of personal health care. For example, equity and universality of care are objectives of EPHF 7; quality of care and, therefore, its effectiveness and generation of satisfaction, are objectives of EPHF 9; and models of care that emphasize health promotion and disease prevention are objectives of EPHF 2 and EPHF 3. Public health and the essential public health functions, as has already been pointed out, are essential instruments for the NHA's exercise of its steering role in the health system, especially its management. Beyond the specific area of health care as such, public health, as it is understood here, is fundamental for the promotion of social participation in health (EPHF 4), not only for the protection of health and the appropriate use of health care services by the population, but also for the exercise of social control over public actions and for the promotion of social demands for healthy public policies that

will be consequential from a political standpoint.

Disregard for or failure to recognize the importance of public health in the organization and the operation of health care systems and health services has been, perhaps, the leading cause of the low social effectiveness of health systems, low levels of satisfaction among the population with the care received, and the failure of some of the sectoral reforms carried out in the last two decades. Now, however, a new generation of reforms designed to correct this deficiency is anticipated. It is not a question of reducing the importance of personal health care, since such care responds to perceived needs and urgent demands of the population and will always be a central priority in the health sector and, indeed, a specific response to the recognition of a fundamental human right: the recovery of lost health. Rather, what ought to be done is to organize the provision of this care in accordance with social effectiveness criteria in order to take maximum advantage of its contribution to the improvement of population health. Public health practice, from this perspective, takes on broader and more socially significant dimensions as it is situated at the center of decision-making and action by the sectoral leadership and is considered an integral part of the health care and health systems.

In short, public health and the essential public health functions, in particular, should never be considered in isolation from or in opposition to personal health care, including medical care. On the contrary, public health and EPHF coexist and their concepts and practices are intertwined with personal health care in health systems. They contribute decisively to the relevance, quality, and so-

cial effectiveness of personal health care; they also benefit from the opportunities that personal health care creates and from its resources to expand the scope and also the effectiveness of public health activities, without this implying any loss or weakening of the necessary specificity of these two spheres of action.

8. Human Resources[3]

Human resources are a fundamental and essential element for public health practice and constitute one of the pillars of its infrastructure; in reality, the practice of public health is no more than the sum of the practices of the personnel who work in public health. Nevertheless, the public health workforce is one of the most neglected and least valued resources within the health sector in the Americas, which is a reflection of the lack of regard for the importance of public health itself. Indeed, in most of the countries, the distinct nature of public health work is not recognized to the extent that would give rise to a differential approach to the development and management of public health workers.

The specific characteristics of the field and objectives of public health and the nature of its activities and relationships give the public health workforce differential characteristics within the health system. Because they deal with the collective dimensions of health, public health professionals utilize knowledge from multiple fields and employ intervention instruments that reach the entire population and address specific health risks and impairments, their direct causes and general determinants, social and instrumental responses for meeting

---

[3] See Chapter 15 in Part IV for a more thorough discussion of this subject.

collective health needs, health systems and social practices, political and management processes, and, ultimately, all the myriad, interrelated, and changing factors that have an effect on the health of the population. They are constantly combining various forms of knowledge and information and applying and revising the instruments available to them to solve public health problems. Owing to the variety of skills needed to cope with the complexity, diversity, and variability of the issues to be addressed, public health work—which relies on the management of knowledge—is basically an interdisciplinary field that calls for teamwork and requires the unique contributions of many professions and disciplines. Hence, public health work not only has objectives of a collective nature, it is collective in and of itself, and public health workers not only work with knowledge, they create knowledge and develop ways of applying it as part of their collective action.

The foregoing paragraphs underscore the need for a public health workforce composed of professionals from various fields. Although it continues to be assumed that training in the basic health professions, especially medicine, is advantageous for public health workers. Medical education, because of its biomedical orientation, can no longer necessarily be considered an indispensable requirement for public health work. In some spheres of activity and for some essential public health functions, training in other professions may be more helpful.

However, it is clear that specific training in public health, as a specialization, must take precedence over training in other professions in order to succeed in forming a distinct public health workforce,

thus creating a group of professionals devoted specifically to the practice of public health in its various manifestations. While this variety of manifestations requires professional specialization in the various spheres of activity within public health, it also requires an ongoing effort to link and integrate the various disciplines—which, in turn, requires special skills—in order to avoid the fragmentation and lack of focus that may result from an exaggerated division of public health into operational compartments and specialties.

Public health is not, however, restricted to the work of public health professionals or specialized workers. Because public health practice has repercussions on the work of other health professionals, especially those who care for people and the environment, and even the work of other sectors, one can speak of a joint work force, which should receive the necessary training and support to enable it to carry out its public health responsibilities in a satisfactory manner. Indeed, one of the skills or competencies that public health workers should have is the ability to raise awareness that public health is the responsibility of all, including both general health professionals and those who work in related activities and, ultimately, of all citizens. Public health workers are thus more than technical agents responsible for applying their knowledge; they are messengers who convey the social message of public health and promoters of healthy social practices and participation by all in the shared work of improving the health and well-being of the population.

Training in public health should therefore be tailored to these characteristics of its workers, its human resources,

which mean that one of the principal tasks of such training is to teach public health workers to continue to learn on their own. If this objective is achieved, the necessary continuing education will be assured, thanks to access to educational information and the creation of opportunities and environments for collective reflection, which will multiply individual ability to learn and collective capacity to create and produce. It should also be considerd, for all the foregoing reasons, emotional intelligence, a sense of social ethics, and the ability to work as a member of a team are often more important qualities in a public health worker than isolated technical skills.

Public health workers deal mainly with goods of a public nature or goods with high social value, and their work therefore earns very little recognition in the labor market. The organization and management of the public health workforce are an eminently public issue and a responsibility of the State. In general, public health work, especially in the case of public health professionals per se, requires total, full-time dedication, owing to the nature of the functions, the limited opportunities that exist on the market, and the numerous conflicts of interests that may arise. These circumstances require special management of the personnel who work in public health, including the creation of new occupational categories and careers specific to public health. In addition, incentives that will balance individual benefits with collective worth and incentives, so that individual performance and teamwork will be promoted simultaneously and there will be well-structured evaluation processes and general working conditions suited to the characteristics of public health interventions.

In sum, good public health practice depends on adequate consideration of the human resources who carry it out.

The instrument used to measure and evaluate performance of the essential public health functions in the Region of the Americas includes indicators relating to the availability of key human resources for each of the essential functions, in addition to the specific indicators used to assess the performance of EPHF 8 (human resources development and training in public health). The results of this initial exercise can be used to move ahead in this area and to significantly strengthen the work that PAHO is currently carrying out in support of the countries.

9. Public Health, EPHF, and Programs

Public health practice and performance of the essential public health functions, and the organization thereof, require a precise delimitation of each EPHF in order to identify the desired outcomes, the activities needed to achieve them and the necessary resources and organization to carry out the work. This, in turn, will make it possible to estimate expenditures and costs, establish the amount of financing and budget needed, and manage the financial aspects of public health work.[4]

In almost all the countries of the Region of the Americas, the essential public health functions are not identified as such. Their components, or some of them, are mixed in with other activities and are carried out by various agencies or institutions with little or no linkage among them. However, some typical

public health programs are more precisely defined, but they are also scattered throughout the institutional structure of the health sector or, sometimes, outside the sector. Reorganizing the essential public health functions as needed to give them functional identity and unity is a complex and difficult undertaking. In some cases, functional identity may be achieved without operational unity—that is, without a specific structural organization for all the EPHF. In other cases, a virtual structure may serve as a temporary solution. In either case, it will be imperative to carry out the process of functional identification and delimitation in order to improve performance. In this regard, it should be recognized that although the measurement and evaluation instrument and its application have led to progress, a great deal remains to be done.

Public health practice within the steering institution of the health system (the ministry or health secretariat) can be examined from the standpoint of four different components with structural significance:

- Specific practice of the essential public health functions—individually and together—which form the structural core of public health.

- Practice carried out in specific spheres of activity, usually structured in the form of public health programs, such as those pertaining to environmental health, health surveillance, control of diseases (AIDS, tuberculosis, malaria, etc.), and others.). It must be recognized that public health outcomes are achieved through the execution of programs, which are defined as a set of resources organized to carry out certain activities in order to achieve

defined objectives. Some of these programs, or parts of them, constitute an essential public health function, as is the case with programs on disaster preparedness (EPHF 11), health or epidemiological surveillance (EPHF 2), health promotion (EPHF 3), and health information (EPHF 1), etc.

- Practice incorporated into others areas of health care, particularly personal health care services at the primary level.

- Public health practice carried out by other institutions but subject to regulation and oversight by the NHA.

The fact of belonging to a structure or organization is part of the definition of the last two. Public health practice that is incorporated into personal health care is thus part and parcel of the delivery of those services, and only the support activities performed, and their respective costs, are counted as part of the corresponding EPHF. Similarly, public health activities carried out by other institutions are incorporated into the functions of those institutions, and only the regulation and oversight exercised by the NHA are part of the corresponding EPHF(s). The process of functional organization of public health thus remains limited to the essential public health functions themselves and to specific public health programs, which constitute the sphere of action for public health.

In the case of programs, the task of evaluating performance is relatively easy. The objectives and outcomes are defined, as are the activities, processes, and resource needed to achieve them. It is thus easy to assign responsibilities, establish monitoring and evaluation mechanisms, determine costs and expendi-

---

[4] See Chapter 14 in Part IV for more details.

Table 1 Organization of public health in the health system

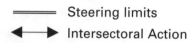

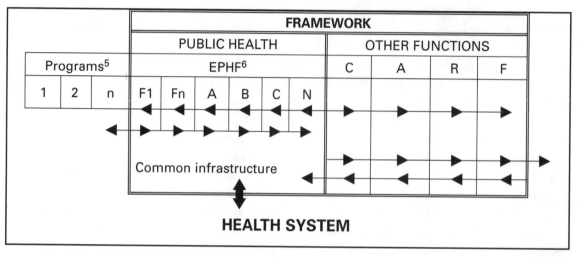

---

tures, and prepare specific budgets, such that the requirements for good practice or good performance are known or at least discernable. However, the situation is a good deal more complicated in the case of essential public health functions that do not correspond to programs or are not organized as well-defined functional units. First, it is necessary to establish that functional unity so that the EPHF can be carried out and, as mentioned earlier, this is not an easy, especially when it is necessary or desirable to have a common infrastructure for two or more functions. One of the crucial aspects that should be developed in public health practice is organization and management, for which the ideas presented in this book are only the beginning of a long process that will be refined through experience. However, it seems clear that

the organization and management of public health and of the EPHF should be included in the organization and management of the steering role, under the control of the NHA, with the necessary linkages and interaction with other areas of the health system, other sectors, and social participation mechanisms. Table 1 attempts to illustrate this situation with regard to the health system and the steering role.

10. Financing, Intersectoral Action, and Political Viability

These three major areas of action are decisive for public health development and practice. There can be no practice without real resources to carry it out and there can be no real resources without financing. Solving public health problems almost always involves some degree of intervention by other sectors, without which the effectiveness of public health will be jeopardized and it will

be impossible to carry out public health activities, a situation that is politically untenable.

Financing for public health is basically a matter of allocating resources, because it normally comes from the public budget, especially in the case of essential public health functions. There are exceptions, such as financing for the delivery of public services for which users pay in the form of charges, fees, or fines, as is the case with basic and urban sanitation services and those for enforcement of regulations on market goods. However, the majority of public health activities carried out in connection with the EPHF is the responsibility of the State, and attempts at cost recovery are ineffective because it is difficult and expensive to exclude some from the benefits. Moreover, such exclusion affects the effectiveness of interventions. There is also the possibility of external financing through loans or grants, which can substitute for or complement the resources of the State in some specific cases, but

---

[5] Specific programs that do not correspond to an EPHF are instrument for delivering care and as such are not part of the global steering function.

[6] F1 and Fn can be organized as programs.

this is an alternative that should be considered only in exceptional national situations or circumstances. In any case, the participation of the State is always crucial—even in cases in which the delivery of public services such as basic sanitation has been privatized—since it is the State that determines and approves the structure of rates and regulates and controls quality and other matters related to the provision of services.

Financing for public health and the EPHF is, in the final analysis, a government decision. In the Region of the Americas, the general impression is that EPHF and public health are insufficiently financed. The available studies, though they are few or incomplete, indicate that spending on activities associated with the EPHF is less than 1% of total public expenditure on health. When spending on specific public health programs or programs for care of the population is added to that figure, the percentage increases, but it is still very low. In reality, the true situation is not accurately known, because itemized accounts are not kept for basic activities (EPHF) and their exact costs therefore cannot be determined. As was noted in the previous section, this is a task that remains to be carried out,[7] and estimating financing needs is still an exercise in approximation. It may be possible initially to utilize standardized costs adjusted to the local price structure to obtain a more exact estimate of financing needs. Within the NHA's sphere of action, it is recommended that there be a reallocation of the available resources to whatever new organization is adopted, at least as regards current expenditure for EPHF activities. There is also the

possibility of raising the priority of public health and the EPHF, allocating to them resources from other areas, bearing in mind the constraints imposed by the availability of a finite amount of resources. The NHA, in exercising the sectoral steering role, should spearhead efforts to win an increase in the resources allocated to the sector, especially those intended specifically for public health functions. This is an eminently political process, which can be facilitated by technical arguments to support the proposal.

Intersectoral action can be encouraged and carried out at all levels of the health system, but it is facilitated when those responsible for the steering function and sectoral leadership embrace it as a preferential strategy. There are also more general ways of fostering an intersectoral approach, such as coordination of sectoral strategies and policies, sharing institutional conditions, etc., which must be dealt with at the national level. Promotion of the necessary intersectoral approach in public health is thus also a responsibility associated with the steering role, especially with respect to the exercise of the management function. Public health plays a key role in this regard, especially in identifying the areas in which an intersectoral approach is required and indicating how to apply such an approach. Public health can also support the process of negotiating and developing proposals for shared or complementary action and promote and support initiatives at the local or sub-national levels.

Public health, like health in general, enjoys a high level of consensus with regard to the values that underpin it and the objectives it pursues. On these points, there is virtual unanimity, at least

rhetorically. Among the many issues and interests that affect the living conditions of populations, public health is also deemed very important by public opinion. However, the importance attached to public health in the rhetoric and in public opinion is not necessarily expressed in concrete action, even within the health sector and among health authorities. Obviously, this constitutes a serious obstacle when it comes to making public health activities politically viable.

Assuring the viability of strategies and plans for strengthening public health and improving its practice implies the development of a political strategy that includes direct activities, as well as the creation of favorable conditions articulated among them. To this end, it is necessary, first, to convince the NHA to lead and oversee the process and, then, to build and project an image of effectiveness and efficiency and develop the capacity to gain support from political institutions and leaders, as well as civil society and the authorities of the State. Strategic instruments for achieving this must be chosen on the basis of specific situations, but the following seem to have universal application:

- Information on decision-making processes and on significant stakeholders and development of the capacity to utilize the information intelligently.

- Superior technical quality in the development of proposals and projects, carried out with the broadest possible constructive participation, but without detriment to the quality and timeliness of the outputs, such that maximum benefit is derived from the identification of the stakeholders of political significance to the process and the outputs.

---

[7] Part IV, suggests some methodologies for this purpose.

- Capacity to negotiate and build important alliances.

- Demonstration of ability to perform effectively and efficiently, so that results and benefits are perceived and recognized.

- Forging of relationships of trust and solidarity that will enable cooperation and support, which implies transparency, dedication, and productivity.

- And, perhaps most important, capacity for social mobilization and creation of conditions that foster effective social participation. The population will thus feel ownership of the proposal and demand formal political support from its representatives.

Clearly, building viability is a political process that is aided and strengthened by general technical and social aspects. It is also an ongoing process, since its principal purpose is not the approval of a single proposal or document, but the overall development of public health and public health practice. An important part of this process is the creation of sustainable and ever renewable structural conditions to enable full performance of public health functions, in particular conditions of an institutional and legal nature. The process is also ongoing because the conditions in which it occurs and the actors involved are constantly evolving and changing. It requires, moreover, formal and logical capacity, but also a special sensitivity to the variety and mutability of motivations and human behavior. This is, therefore, the most interesting of the dimensions of health and public health and the most remarkable of the institutional capabilities that ensure good public health practice.

11. International Cooperation

International cooperation can play a vital role in the development of public health practice and the performance of essential public health functions the in the Region of the Americas. From the formalization and promotion of ideas, to the development of concepts and operational instruments and the provision of support for countries and cooperation among countries, there is ample room for effective cooperation. The contribution of public health to the improvement of overall health and development is now widely recognized in international circles. The progressive restoration of the essential functions of the State, relative freedom in regard to the pressure of demand for medical care, and the failure of previous initiatives all necessitate the consideration of sectoral cooperation strategies that include public health as an important component. The "Public Health in the Americas" initiative thus is timely.

Cooperation strategies must take account of all possible factors and contingencies and must be adapted to national situations. Several strategies, however, are worth serious consideration:

- Enhancement and progressive expansion of the operational strategy of the essential public health functions, which include the improvement of instruments for deepening knowledge of the situation and for remedying any deficiencies detected, emphasizing their functional delimitation and characterization and strengthening of the infrastructure of public health services and the capacity for institutional action.

- Coordination of this strategy with the development of the steering capacity and with the rectification of the sectoral reform processes still under way.

- Construction of alliances among international cooperation organizations, especially the banks, as well as bilateral agencies, through joint or compatible projects in keeping with the internal positions adopted within each organization.

- Promotion of the Initiative in each country, as a fundamental and indispensable requirement for its success, so that the countries will take ownership of the Initiative, make it viable, and extend it to other sectors, as well as social practices and participation.

The combination of good ideas and suitable instruments for implementing them, with quality technical cooperation and appropriate and well-oriented supplementary financing, has great potential for success. This potential can be increased by means of promotion and support through cooperation among countries, taking advantage of their respective strengths and ability to complement one another, and intensifying the exchange of information and mutual support, especially among subregional groups. Advantage should also be taken of the public health-related concerns that currently occupy a priority place on the international agenda. The debate on global public goods and international cooperation, for example, can be a useful vehicle for promoting public health, which is an area that unquestionably deals in public goods. Analysis of the issue at the international level underscores the importance of public health as a field of cooperation and also strengthens the importance attached in the countries to public goods as a responsibility of the State and, by extension, public health. The increase in cooperation resources for control of preventable diseases—especially AIDS, tuberculosis, and malaria—reflects a shift in priorities that affords opportunities for highlighting the crucial importance of public health in controlling such diseases and, therefore, its importance for health in general.

In short, international cooperation can have a decisive influence on the development of public health practice in the Region of the Americas.

12. Towards Social Practices Centered on Public Health

Public health achieves its pinnacle when there is ownership by the people and communities, and when it is incorporated into social practices—i.e., when it is manifested in healthy and health-promoting practices. Accordingly, this is one of the aims of the operational strategy of the essential public health functions, which also offers the best means of achieving it. Each EPHF, in practice, contributes something towards that aim, and it is the fundamental purpose of EPHF 3 (health promotion) and EPHF 4 (social participation in health). Through these functions, institutional action is directed towards training and empowering people to participate in health and public health and in the exercise of their rights and responsibilities as the principal stakeholders, while also exercising control over the actions of the State. This does not eliminate or diminish the responsibilities and actions of the State, but it

shapes and guides them, giving them a true social dimension by transforming them into real instruments at the service of the population. The practice of public health and the EPHF, in particular, is strengthened in terms of its sphere of action, its purposes, and its social importance. Without doubt, approaching the essential public health functions from the perspective of social practices will increase their effectiveness as a preferential strategy for public health.

The considerations presented in Chapter 5 and expanded on in Chapter 6 provide a general idea of the concept of social practices and their application in public health, but we are only just beginning to understand the process and explore its potential for public health practice. Nevertheless, some modes of intervention are currently available to facilitate institutional action in public health in order to implement the process:

- Training and empowering the population for participation can be accelerated through information and organization, in which health institutions can play a key role. Health and public health, thanks to widespread consensus about their value, enjoy an undeniable social acceptance that can be an advantageous platform for mass communication and transfer of information and knowledge. It can also serve as the starting point for encouraging and supporting social organization processes, especially in communities, which can be utilized to join forces and actions, expand social relations, manifest collective demands, and consolidate the values of confidence, solidarity, and cooperation, thus increasing the social capital that can nurture public health practices

and facilitate projects for development and progress. But without organization, there can be no effective social will and participation.

- It is not enough, however, to train and organize. It is also necessary to create institutional mechanisms for participation that link health and public health institutions to the organized and involved society. Specific mechanisms for participation in health should be articulated with other forms of participation, both in other sectors and in general, and these mechanisms should allow for real participation in decision-making. This implies a substantive change in management models to open them up to participatory processes and at the same time benefit from their productive potential. Participation mechanisms should be representative of the diversity of society and should be organized and operate democratically, with the capacity to recognize and process the diverse interests and opinions represented, minimize corporate distortions, and resist manipulations of all types, so that they are subject to the interests of groups, parties, authorities, or ideologies. The process of promoting participation is complex, slow, and often frustrating, but it has potential that goes beyond health to the construction of a future characterized by greater well-being, freedom, and true democracy.

- Social participation has costs, of which the least and easiest to defray is the institutional cost of promotion and support. The cost to the population—in time, thwarted expectations, disillusion, etc.—is the social price paid in advance, which must be compensated for in the form of responses and results that reward the effort made. Indeed, the process of participation will not be sustainable if the stakeholders and the population do not acknowledge its usefulness.

- Promotion of participation and training of citizens as a strategy for fostering healthy social practices in public health is part of a broader process, as it is in regard to health in general. Indeed, citizenship is a broad attribute that has specific manifestations in the various fields of human endeavor, which means that it cannot be limited to one of those fields. Although public health should take responsibility, through its essential functions, for promoting the process in the field of health, this task, in order to be truly effective, should be accompanied by a solid attitude of support, political will, and intervention by the State, involving all sectors, or at least those with the greatest potential in this regard (education, labor, social development, public prosecutor, etc.). In addition, as a process of empowering the population—that is, the transfer or creation of power—the development of citizenship and social participation is a political process in that it changes the distribution and exercise of power in society. For that reason, social participation mechanisms should be incorporated into the formal political process, through these they can find appropriate channels for conveying social demands to the State and have a better chance of obtaining a reply.

- Information and communication comprise the principal input and most powerful instrument of action

in this area. Two types of information, in particular, are essential:

- Educational information that encourages citizen participation and prepares individuals, families, and communities to care for their own health and the environment in which they live, so as to enable them to make the best use of available health care services, monitor the performance of public authorities, and take part in the development and execution of joint projects to improve living and health conditions.

- Information on institutional activities that ensures the transparency of public action, enables social control, and provides greater safeguards against deviation or distortion of public functions.

- Communication that transmits information and thus makes it real, utilizing all kinds of media, from specific personal communication at the time care is delivered to mass communication, with emphasis on those media that will have the greatest reach and impact in each situation, and adjusting the format of messages to the target audience.

The summary provided in the preceding paragraphs gives an idea of the importance and the nature of the action needed to incorporate health into social practices and encourage public health social practices. It also gives an idea of the complexity of the process and the means available for carrying it out, emphasizing the development of social capital by building citizenship and social capacity for participation, for which

purpose educational information, effective communication, promotion of social organization, and creation of effective participation mechanisms are the principal intervention instruments. Consideration of social practices shapes and strengthens the practice of public health and the essential public health functions, while at the same time introducing extraordinary possibilities for progress that, beyond their contribution to health, will help foster sustainable human development.

13. Summary

The ideas presented in this chapter are elements that should be taken into account when developing a strategy for the improvement of public health practice. They constitute, as the title of the chapter indicates, a framework for action to that end.

The process begins with recognition of the importance of public health and the need to improve its practice. This should be manifested in a firm commitment by the NHA to adopt the strategy of essential public health functions for the development of public health and make those functions a fundamental tool for carrying out its steering role in the health system. Such a commitment implies the use of its stewardship function, especially to create the necessary conditions for the development of public health and for better fulfillment and performance of the EPHF and their use in the management of the entire health system.

The next step is to understand the current situation, which can be accomplished, at least initially, by measuring and evaluating performance of the

EPHF. Such an assessment will point out the weaknesses and strengths in the existing infrastructure and the way it works. The information obtained will guide the development of interventions targeting the strategy's fundamental component, which is to build institutional capacity for action by developing and strengthening the infrastructure of public health services and the components of that infrastructure: information and strategy, human resources, organization, and basic support processes and essential support services. To do this, it is necessary to deepen the analysis, expanding it to include other aspects, such as the study of relevant stakeholders, costs and expenditures, etc. The resulting proposal will be comprehensive in nature, encompassing the whole set of essential public health functions and the shared infrastructure of public health and their applications in specific spheres of action through programs, relationships within the steering role and the health system, requirements for intersectoral action, etc., but it will have as a unifying and supporting principle the development of institutional infrastructure and institutional capacity-building. The cycle is completed with the establishment of the functional organization for management and execution, including the assignment of responsibilities and allocation of resources such as financing and budget, as well as mechanisms and processes for monitoring and evaluation. The process also includes simultaneous and ongoing political action to enable intersectoral action. International cooperation helps catalyze and extend the process.

From the strategic standpoint, it is also important to incorporate the perspective of social practices from the outset, expanding the sphere of action of EPHF 3 and EPHF 4 to the utmost and marking the course of future development.

Doing all these things will set in motion a process of public health development, based on performance of the essential public health functions, that will lead to progressive and sustainable improvement of public health practice and enhance its contribution to the improvement of population health and the overall performance of the health system.

Bibliography

Atchison C. et al. The quest for an accurate accounting of public health expenditures. *Journal of Public Health Management Practice* 2000; 6(5): 93–102.

Claeson M. et al. *Public Health and World Bank Operations.* Washington, D.C.: World Bank; 2002.

Leppo K. Strengthening Capacities for Policy Development and Strategic Management in National Health Systems. Geneva: WHO; 2001.

Macedo C. Desarrollo de la capacidad de conducción sectorial en salud. Washington, D.C.: OPS; 1998. (Serie Organización y gestión de sistemas y servicios de salud 6).

Macedo C. Modelo de gestión y eficacia de las reformas de salud en América Latina. In: Solimano, G. Isaacs, S. *De la reforma para unos a la reforma para todos.* Santiago, Chile: Editorial Sudamericana; 2002.

Milen A. *What Do We Know about Capacity Building? An Overview of Existing Knowledge and Good Practice.* Geneva: WHO; 2001.

Organización Panamericana de la Salud. *Desafíos para la educación en salud pública. La reforma sectorial y las funciones esenciales de la salud pública.* Washington, D.C.: OPS; 2000.

Organización Panamericana de la Salud. *Educación en salud pública: nuevas perspectivas para las Américas.* Washington, D.C.: OPS; 2000.

U.S. Department of Health and Human Services. Public Health Infrastructure. In: *Healthy People—2010 Objectives.* Washington, D.C.;1998. (Preliminary report).

PART III

Performance Measurement of the Essential Public Health Functions

Rationale for the Performance Measurement of EPHF

8

The processes of State modernization and health sector reform have highlighted the importance of evaluating the performance of social systems and, in particular, of health systems, to make them more transparent and useful while providing a public accounting of their actions with respect to the allocation, utilization, and development of resources that society provides for the fulfillment of social objectives and public policies, including health policies.

In this context, a variety of actions and debates have unfolded regarding the direction, purpose, process, and utilization of health systems performance assessment in recent years, including, in the Region of the Americas, a series of consultations on the subject among participating countries. Performance measurement of the EPHF by national authorities fits within the framework of those interventions and debates.

1. Assessment and improvement of health systems performance

The regional consultations in the Region of the Americas on health systems performance assessment included a concerted effort to orient the debate toward the future and to contribute to the development of a clear definition of performance assessment and to improvements in the reliability and usefulness of the data collected for the participating countries. These consultations resulted in several conclusions that are summarized below.[1]

Health systems performance assessment should be linked to political, social, and

---

[1] Pan American Health Organization. *Health Systems Performance Assessment and Improvement in the Region of the Americas.* Washington, D.C.: PAHO/WHO, 2001.

management decision-making by the health system and should not be conceived as a simple academic exercise. Additionally, it should be linked to the definition of desired changes included in current programs of health sector reform, as well as to the real possibility of putting these changes into practice.

At both the national and international levels, the criteria for evaluating the performance of health systems as well as the indicators used should be established by consensus. Otherwise, polemics on criteria and indicators will tend to cloud the assessment results and limit their possible use by policy makers and other interested actors.

Similarly, performance assessment should be seen as a "quantitative and qualitative appraisal that shows the degree of achievement of the objectives and the goals."

Better health is the ultimate goal that societies seek to achieve with their health systems, but the delivery of individual and collective services, along with intersectoral actions, is only one way of improving the health of the population. Factors linked to socioeconomic conditions, the environment, genetics, and collective and individual behavior also have a powerful influence on health. Accordingly, it is necessary to improve our understanding of how these factors interact, how they influence the health status of individuals and populations, and how they contribute to achieving the ultimate goal of the health system, over and above the performance of the system itself.

All of the above also emphasizes the importance of paying particular attention to the intermediate objectives of health systems, that is, to what the systems are actually doing and what they could do better, rather than focusing performance assessment only on some distant final objectives, that is, what should be done. However, operational and performance assessment of intermediate objectives should always be related to the final objectives of the system—that is, to improvement of the health and quality of life of individuals and societies, the ultimate reason for the existence and operation of the health system. This also raises the debate about the relationship between the boundaries of the health system and accountability of health authorities for its performance.

Unlike the comparison of health system performance over time in the same country, the comparison of health system performance among different countries is seen as something desirable but difficult to carry out for technical and political reasons. For such a comparison

to serve as a stimulus to the formulation of health policies in the participating countries, the terms of the comparison—the conceptual framework, the variables that operationalize it, and the measurement indicators—must be subject to consensus among the countries to be compared.

In this regard, as part of rethinking and improving health systems performance assessment, it was considered appropriate to advance a framework that takes into account four dimensions: inputs and resources, functions, results or intermediate objectives, and final objectives of the system.

Performance evaluation should incorporate the different levels of analysis, that is, national, intermediate, and local, as well as the different functions of the systems. It should also consider several potential audiences: political decision makers, other interested actors, the public, etc.

Accordingly, it was agreed in the consultations that health systems performance assessment should include a broad range of areas and levels of intervention, rather than simply equating the concept of performance with that of efficiency. This will allow users of the performance assessment to consider whether progress is being made toward specific goals and whether appropriate activities are being undertaken to promote the achievement of these goals.

The value of this would be in the capacity to identify problem areas that may need special attention, as well as best practices that can serve as models. Thus, performance assessment can also be a tool for regulation and for resource allocation.

Furthermore, it was considered important to define procedures to measure the performance by health authorities of their steering role, taking into account the functions assumed in the majority of the countries by the central, intermediate, and local levels of government.

Therefore, performance measurement of the essential public health functions, as carried out in the Region of the Americas, illustrates the potential of a tool for evaluating the institutional capacities of health authorities. In the first place, it measures a specific aspect of their steering role. It can also be used for continuous improvement of public health practice and for reorienting resource allocation toward specific public health interventions. It does this through a participatory and transparent process within each country involving a self-evaluation of the performance of the health authority in relation to the 11 essential public health functions. Finally, it should be noted that the results are not reduced to a global indicator, nor are they aimed at development of a summary measure for comparing different countries.

2. Purpose of measuring the EPHF in the countries of the Region of the Americas

Health sector reforms face the challenge of strengthening the steering role of the health authorities, and an important part of that role consists of monitoring the fulfillment of the EPHF that are the responsibility of the State at its central, intermediate, and local levels. It is therefore critical to improve public health practice and the instruments for assessing its current status and identifying areas that should be strengthened.

Measuring the degree to which the EPHF are fulfilled by the health authorities in the countries of the Region should enable the ministries or secretariats of health to identify critical factors to be considered when developing plans or strategies to strengthen public health infrastructure, understood as the ensemble of human resources, management practices, and material resources that are needed to enable the health authorities at different levels to carry out their responsibilities optimally.

This measurement is even more relevant in periods such as the current one, marked by determination to reform health systems to enable them to better respond to current health needs. Public health plays a fundamental role in these reform processes, since the potential to achieve greater equity of access to better health conditions lies within its arena of activity.

Given that the majority of the countries in the Region now make decisions on how to allocate the resources aimed at supporting their reform processes, having an accurate diagnosis of the areas with the greatest needs in relation to public health development will be very valuable when it comes to mobilizing and directing the resources for strengthening these areas, as the World Bank recognizes.[2]

As indicated earlier, strengthening public health is of fundamental importance

to support the implementation role of the health authority. This is essential for defining health policies in a manner consistent with the underlying principles of the health systems (equity, efficiency, and responsiveness to citizens' expectations, for example), as well as for ensuring implementation and development of the policies in line with those same principles. Thus, precise measurement of current deficiencies is very important for governments as well as for technical and financial cooperation agencies involved in health.

An emphasis present today in all reform processes is the introduction of a culture of outcomes assessment, looking at the outcomes derived from use of the ever-increasing resources allocated to health care for the population. The measurement instrument proposed by the "Public Health in the Americas" initiative is geared fundamentally to measuring the performance of the health authorities in regard to public health. Its application should result in a diagnosis that does not just present a static image of the current situation but permits a dynamic analysis of the results being achieved currently and those that would be possible in the future if investments are made to close the identified gaps in resources, capacities, procedures, and results.

The heterogeneity of the responsibilities that come under the rubric of public health make it a social practice that, often, can be equated with the full range of functions and activities of a health system.

In conclusion, the purpose of performance measurement is to identify strengths and weaknesses in how the health authorities perform essential and necessary

functions for developing public health practice, leading to an operational diagnosis of the areas of institutional practice that require greater support and development. The development of the proposed measurement is aimed at strengthening public health infrastructure, understood in its broadest sense to include the human, material, and organizational capacities necessary for good performance, as analyzed in chapter 8.

In order to move forward in the achievement of this objective, it is important that the decision to measure performance be followed by the development of a measurement instrument that can be used to analyze the situation of each country, as well as of the subregions and the entire Region of the Americas. This instrument will undoubtedly require continuous enhancement until it reaches a reasonably optimal level that permits its systematic utilization at the different levels of public health practice in the Region.

The set of indicators, variables, and measures defined in the instrument is subject to error and, obviously, cannot pretend to satisfy every possible viewpoint on the subject among public health specialists. Decisions to include, for example, empowerment or stimulus of an intersectoral approach in the functions of health promotion or social participation imply a certain degree of arbitrary agreement. This means that it is not possible to avoid repetition of areas that are included, with different emphases, in more than one function. It is obvious that the reality of daily public health practice does not allow for drawing clear distinctions between the times when the work is fulfilling one or another function, not even in the practice of a single individual.

---

[2] The World Bank. *Public Health and World Bank Operations.* Washington, D.C.: The Human Development Network: Health, Nutrition, and Population Series; 2002.

It is important to mention here the frequent confusion between the State's role in health, normally exercised by the ministry of health or an equivalent health authority, and the responsibility of the State in overseeing and guaranteeing proper performance of the EPHF. Although the State has a non delegable role in the direct delivery or guarantee of the EPHF, this still represents only a fraction of its responsibilities in health. It is a very important fraction, of course, and proper fulfillment of these responsibilities is not only fundamental for improving the health status and quality of life of the population, but is also needed to give greater legitimacy to the State's execution of its steering role and its responsibilities for regulation, financial control, supervision, and expansion of social security coverage in health and other areas. To clarify the point with an example, a public health agency that does not have a minimally comprehensive and reliable health surveillance system can hardly expect to be credible when it decides or acts to allocate financial capital to the different components or sectors of the health system.

One should also mention the difficulty in drawing a clear distinction between the responsibilities of public health for the management of disease prevention and health promotion services for defined population groups and those functions related to the organization of services for individual curative care.

The emphases here are undoubtedly different. The first of these functions is part of the basic heritage of public health, since the public health authority is the only one that performs it. As for the second function, the essential responsibilities of public health focus mainly on ensuring equitable access to services, guaranteeing the quality of service, and incorporating public health perspectives in national health policies. This does not prevent public health professionals from undertaking to manage health services for individuals. On the contrary, it is desirable that they do so, especially in order to incorporate the public health vision in the operation of such organizations. The latter activity, however, utilizes disciplines that go beyond the social practice that has come to be known as public health.

The common concept of public health as embracing all work carried out in the health field contributes to a dilution of responsibilities among areas distinct from public health and can lead to inefficient use of health resources. Measuring the degree to which essential public health functions are being fulfilled and evaluating the performance of ministries and public health agencies should help to avoid this risk.

With a view to strengthening the institutional capacity of the national health authority with respect to public health, it is important that the decision to measure performance of the EPHF be supported by the development of programs to ensure continuous improvements in infrastructure and practice at the different levels of public health in the Region of the Americas.

Defining and measuring the EPHF are conceived as a way of contributing to the institutional development of public health practice and improving the dialogue between public health and other health-related disciplines. Moreover, better definition of what is essential should help to improve the quality of services and lead to more precise definitions of institutional responsibilities in the delivery of these interventions. Public health's accountability to citizens for its performance should start with the areas for which it is exclusively responsible, that is, the EPHF. Furthermore, public health's legitimacy and its capacity to call on the cooperation of other health-related sectors will be heightened by a more precise measurement of the essential components of its work.

In no case is measurement intended to serve as a method of external evaluation of the work of ministries or ministers, nor is its purpose to rank countries on their commitment to public health. Nonetheless, in accordance with the mandate of the Directing Council, PAHO has taken responsibility for facilitating application of the instrument in all the countries of the Region of the Americas. This has permitted a diagnosis of areas of weakness and strength in the participating countries as a group, which is presented in the following chapter.

The purpose of this measurement, then, is to present a self-evaluation of countries at different points in time, allowing for internal comparisons within an overall analysis of the evolution of public health in the Americas. As noted by the Executive Committee of PAHO,[3] this instrument will not achieve its objective unless measurement is carried out periodically and the instrument is used on a continuing basis. For this reason, both this measurement exercise and those to be carried out in the future will require

---

[3] 126th Session of the Executive Committee of PAHO, June 2000.

close collaboration among the participating countries and PAHO.

The instrument provides a common framework for measuring performance with respect to the EPHF, applicable to all countries, that respects the organizational structure of the health system of each country. In countries with a federal structure, for example, it will be necessary to orient the measurement process in accordance with the decentralized exercise of authority by each of the agencies involved.

Finally, defining the EPHF and measuring their level of performance in the Region are fundamental for strengthening public health education in the Americas, an activity whose current crisis has much to do with the lack of a more precise definition of its task. This measurement effort also contributes to honing such a definition, although its purpose is not really to define the scope of public health as an academic discipline or interdisciplinary field. In this regard, recent agreements of the Latin American and Caribbean Association for Public Health Education (ALAESP) support the development of this initiative, which they consider an important contribution to the development of public health teaching and research.

Measurement of the EPHF, understood as the capacities and competencies of the national health authority (NHA) necessary for improving public health practice, is intended to:

1. Help improve the quality of public health practice by strengthening critical performance areas in the NHA.

2. Promote accountability in public health practice, bolstering the commitment of the NHA to carry out public programs aimed at strengthening the EPHF.

3. Promote the development of public health relevant to the current situation, improving the quality and content of information available to those who make decisions about health policies.

4. Strengthen public health infrastructure in its broadest sense by investing in development of the institutional capacities of the NHA, including infrastructure, technology, human resources, financial resources, inputs, etc.

As can be seen, each country made a very substantial effort and there was a broad range of actors involved in the measurement effort, including officials at different levels of the NHA (both national and subnational), as well as representatives of other sectors, of nongovernmental organizations, and of the general public. This broad and representative participation made it possible to achieve a comprehensive evaluation of the performance of the EPHF by the NHA.

Given the difficulties involved in carrying out the measurement exercise in all the countries of the Region, it is important to note the short time period in which this entire process was completed, which again confirms the countries' interest and commitment to meeting this challenge.

Development of the Measurement Instrument

The development of instruments to measure the performance of the EPHF entailed a long process aimed at defining the functions to be measured, as noted in chapter 6, as well as to define the performance indicators, variables, and measures that would serve to verify performance.

1. Definition of the EPHF for the Region of the Americas

The EPHF were defined operationally, in accordance with the conceptual framework set forth in chapter 6, as the conditions that allow better public health practice.

The ministers of health in attendance at the 2000 meeting of the Directing Council of PAHO unanimously adopted a resolution that, in essence, recommended[1] urging the Member States to:

[1] Resolution CD42.R14. Essential Public Health Functions. 42nd Directing Council of PAHO. Washington, D.C.; 25–29 September 2000.

1. Participate in a regional exercise, sponsored by PAHO, to measure performance with regard to the essential public health functions to permit an analysis of the state of public health in the Americas;

2. Use performance measurement with regard to the essential public health functions to improve public health practice, develop the necessary infrastructure for this purpose, and strengthen the steering role of the health authority at all levels of the State.

In the same resolution, the ministers urged the Director General of PAHO to:

1. Disseminate widely in the countries of the region the conceptual and methodological documentation on the definition and measurement of the essential public health functions;

2. Carry out, in close coordination with the national authorities of each country, an exercise in performance measurement with respect to the essential public health functions, making use of the methodology designed;

3. Conduct a regional analysis of the state of public health in the Americas, based on a performance measurement exercise targeting the essential public health functions in each country;

4. Promote the reorientation of public health education in the Region of the Americas in line with the development of the essential public health functions;

5. Incorporate the line of work on the essential public health functions into cooperation activities linked with sectoral reform and the strengthening of the steering role of the health authority.

Furthermore, the XVI Special Meeting of the Health Sector of Central America and the Dominican Republic (RESS-CAD) agreed to support the proposal to carry out the measurement of the EPHF and strengthen the steering role of the ministries of health in the countries of the subregion, as part of the process of PAHO/WHO technical cooperation for institutional and sectoral strengthening of public health.[2]

Based on these normative precedents, one of the most important decisions adopted in the course of developing the Public Health in the Americas initiative, related specifically to design of the measurement instrument, had to do with the need to adopt definitions of indicators and standards for performance measurement of the EPHF. The intention was to make it possible to guide the strengthening of public health practice by building up the institutional capacities of the health authority.

The list of the EPHF that are defined in the instrument is based on an exhaustive process of collective analysis and reflection, as described in chapter 7. However, all the definitions are, obviously, subject to improvement and are not intended to represent all the views on this subject in the field of public health.

Nevertheless, there have been efforts to minimize disagreements and to incorporate the most important aspects as laid out by experts and actors involved in health policy decisions, whenever they have offered their opinions. It should be noted that this instrument represents the first effort on performance measurement of public health in the countries of the Region of the Americas, an endeavour

that can undoubtedly be improved on in the future, especially if the countries take responsibility for the instrument.

2. Definition of performance standards for the EPHF

The information obtained with measurement instruments of this type, which are intended to help the NHA more effectively define and evaluate the function of public health in the health sector, should reflect a vision of the objective to be achieved.

As in other performance measurement processes, a choice had to be made between acceptable and optimum standards. Defining acceptable levels was difficult and necessarily arbitrary, since it implied either choosing a level comparable to the hypothetical average currently existing in the Region or defining the minimum requirements for performing a function based on the judgment of a group of experts. The choice of optimal standards was considered more appropriate whenever, obviously, this fit the general situation of the Region, since such a definition identifies gaps in the current situation with respect to an optimal level. This should lead to continuous improvement, which is precisely what is to be promoted.

Given the heterogeneous practice of the EPHF in the Region, the optimum standards were defined to reflect the best conditions that could be attained in all the countries of the Region within reasonable time periods; this implied the need to rely on expert opinion to determine what those conditions are. Aside from this, opting for these reasonable optimum standards seemed more appropriate and consistent with the ob-

jective of upgrading the public health services infrastructure within the shortest possible time frame.

Based on the selection of the EPHF, the next step was to determine the optimum standard for their general performance in order to facilitate the elaboration of that objective by the evaluation group as regards the expected performance of each function.

Next, the identification and allocation of priorities for the indicators was one of the most complex and difficult steps in the design of the instrument. The indicators, used as summary performance measures of each function, are the most important component of the instrument and determine its quality and usefulness. Ultimately, they constitute the heart of the measurement.

For determining the indicators, one proceeded with the identification of variables that should be measured and the description of the measures and submeasures, in the form of questions, which made it possible to characterize the performance of the functions. For the purpose of enhancing measurement objectivity, the measurements included were, insofar as possible, those that served to verify proper performance.

The objective of this task is to obtain, through the country's response to several measures and submeasures, as complete a profile as possible of the state of public health practice from the national perspective with respect to structure, institutional capacities, processes, and specific outcomes. When the indicators and the associated variables are evaluated through the measurements, it is important to take into account the source of information on which the re-

---

[2] Agreement 14 of the XVI Special Meeting of the Health Sector of Central America and the Dominican Republic. Tegucigalpa, Honduras; 12–13 September 2000.

sponse is based. This information should come from the core group of people interviewed and selected to carry out the evaluation, as well as from available and easily accessible information sources for both quantitative and qualitative data.

In the final analysis, the key indicators are capable of relating the results to the decision-making processes of the system. Thus, the validity of the indicators will make it possible to ensure continued use of the instrument and future improvements in quality assurance in public health practice.

A first draft of the instrument, including definitions of the functions to be measured and definitions of the optimum standards for indicators, was disseminated by the interinstitutional team in charge of elaborating the instrument with various groups of public health professionals and experts, a process that culminated formally in a meeting of a network of institutions and experts convened by PAHO for this purpose.[3]

Subsequently, the instrument, containing the indicators, variables and measurements for each indicator, was validated in four countries of the Region: Bolivia, Colombia, Jamaica, and Chile. The validation was carried out with groups of key informants who included managers at different levels of the health authority (central, intermediate, and local), researchers, and representatives of public health associations or other institutions concerned with pub-

lic health. Those exercises made it possible to enhance the measurement instrument based on the experiences and opinions of the participants.

3. The instrument for measuring the EPHF in the Region of the Americas

The performance measurement instrument for the EPHF in the Region (see Annex I) is organized as follows:

- A brief introduction explaining the basics of the Initiative and describing the instrument.

- The 11 essential public health functions, each with its corresponding definition, are presented in a table containing the practices that identify the work associated with each EPHF, with three to five indicators for each function. Each indicator consists of :

  - A standard that describes the optimal level of performance for the indicator.

  - A set of variables that identify the operational characteristics of the indicator that are the object of the measurement, and are expressed as the percentage of accomplishment of the function, based on the answers given to the measurements.

  - A set of measures and submeasures that serve to verify performance for each variable within each indicator, and that allow for a dichotomous "yes" or "no" response. Based on the methodology of response by consensus of the evaluation group, it was suggested that the country respond in the negative when opin-

ions are not unanimous, in order to facilitate a more exhaustive analysis later to identify gaps with respect to the expected optimal level.

3.1 Sections of the instrument

The instrument is divided into 11 sections, one for each essential public health function. Each function is preceded by a definition of a selected set of capacities necessary for performing that function, from which the indicators and related variables and measurements are derived.

Utilizing this definition, indicators for each function have been constructed and are used to measure the infrastructure, institutional capacities, key processes, and related results, as well as the decentralized exercise of the function. In general, all functions begin with intermediate result indicators, such as:

- EPHF 1: The indicator "Guidelines and processes for monitoring health status".

- EPHF 2: The indicator "Surveillance system to identify threats to public health".

- EPHF 3: The indicators "Building sectoral and extrasectoral partnerships for health promotion" and "Reorientation of health services toward health promotion".

- EPHF 4: The indicators "Empowering civil society for decision-making in public health" and "Strengthening of social participation in health".

Below are indicators for processes considered critical for good performance of each essential function, such as:

---

[3] Expert Consultation. Essential Public Health Functions and Performance Measurement in Public Health Practice. 9–10 September 1999. Washington, D.C.

- EPHF 1: The indicator "Evaluation of the quality of information".

- EPHF 2: The indicator "Capacity of public health laboratories".

- EPHF 3: The indicator "Support for health promotion activities, development of norms and interventions to promote healthy behaviors and environments".

- EPHF 5: The indicator "Development, monitoring and evaluation of public health policies".

All the functions include indicators that measure institutional capacity for the performance of the EPHF, as well as those that measure technical support to the subnational levels. These make it possible to evaluate efforts to strengthen decentralization, and are usually the last indicators for each function. Examples of indicators designed to evaluate institutional capacity are:

EPHF 5: The indicators "Development of institutional capacity for the management of public health" and "Management of international cooperation in public health".

EPHF 6: The indicator "Knowledge, skills, and mechanisms for reviewing, improving, and enforcing regulations".

EPHF 7: The indicator "Knowledge, skills, and mechanisms to improve access to necessary health services by the population".

As a general rule, indicators for each function were established such that they would cover the five areas that would determine performance: 1) the results of the application of the function; 2) the

principal processes for achieving these results; 3) the institutional capacities to carry out the processes; 4) the necessary basic infrastructure, and 5) the competencies delegated to subnational levels for the decentralized exercise of the function. For some functions it was not considered relevant or easy to identify sensitive indicators within each of these five areas; but for all the functions, the measurements cover at least outcomes and processes, capacities and infrastructure, and also decentralized competencies.

Each indicator has, in turn, a standard model that describes in detail the parameters for optimum performance of the function.

Finally, for each of the indicators, variables to be measured have been identified and measures and submeasures designed in the form of questions that further detail the specific capacities described in the standard for each measurement. Those measurements ultimately reveal the degree of development or the degree to which performance approaches the expected optimum level.

As described in previous paragraphs and illustrated below, the format of the instrument is as follows:

The example below shows this with greater clarity:

Essential function 7: Evaluation and promotion of equitable access to necessary health services

Definition

This function includes:

- The promotion of equity in the effective access of all citizens to necessary health services.

- The development of actions designed to overcome barriers when accessing public health interventions and help link vulnerable groups to necessary health services (does not include the financing of health care).

- The monitoring and evaluation of access to necessary health services offered by public and/or private providers, using a multisectoral, multiethnic, and multicultural approach to facilitate working with diverse agencies and institutions to reduce inequities in access to necessary health services.

- Close collaboration with governmental and nongovernmental agencies to promote equitable access to necessary health services.

Indicator

7.1 **Monitoring and evaluation of access to necessary health services**

Standard of the indicator

The NHA:

- Monitors and evaluates access to personal and public health services by the inhabitants of a territorial jurisdiction at least once every two years.

- Conducts the evaluation in collaboration with subnational levels in public health, clinical care delivery systems, and other points of entry into the health system.

- Determines the causes and effects of barriers to access, gathering information on the individuals affected by these barriers, and identifies best practices to reduce those barriers and increase equity of access to necessary health services

Figure 1 Format for the Performance Measurement Instrument

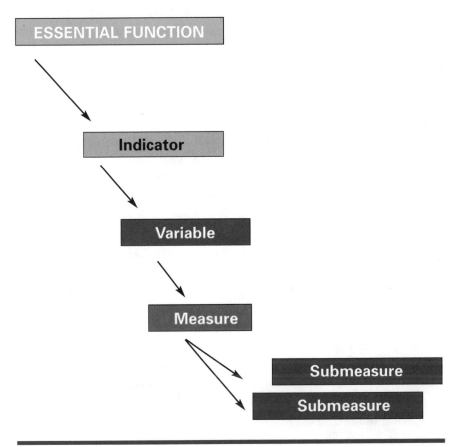

- Uses the results of this evaluation to promote equitable access to necessary health services for the population of the country

- Collaborates with other agencies to ensure the monitoring of access to necessary health services by vulnerable or underserved population groups

Variable

7.1.1 **The NHA conducts a national evaluation of access to necessary population-based health services.**

Measures

Evaluation

7.1.1.1 Do indicators exist to evaluate access?

7.1.1.2 Is the national evaluation based on a collection of population-based services accessible to the entire population?

7.1.1.3 Is information available from the subnational levels to implement the national evaluation?

7.1.1.4 Is the evaluation conducted in collaboration with the subnational levels and different entities of the NHA?

Submeasures

If so,

7.1.1.4.1 Is the national evaluation conducted in collaboration with the intermediate levels?

7.1.1.4.2 Is the national evaluation conducted in collaboration with the local levels?

7.1.1.4.3 Is the national evaluation conducted in collaboration with other governmental entities?

7.1.1.4.4 Is the national evaluation conducted in collaboration with non-governmental entities?

3.2 Limitations of the instrument

The task of developing a common instrument for performance measurement of the EPHF faces a set of self-imposed limits in the design and selection of indicators and variables. While representative of the work of the NHA, these variables cannot possibly reflect the full scope of the functions and activities of the NHA with regard to public health.

In order to design a viable measurement process, a choice was made to concentrate on a small set of indicators that would adequately characterize performance of the 11 essential functions and guide efforts to strengthen infrastructure and significant public health processes in relation to the role of the NHA. The selection of indicators took into account significant aspects concerned with the direct results or key processes related to each EPHF, the institutional capacity or infrastructure needed for proper performance of each EPHF, and the degree of support to subnational levels for strengthening the decentralized exercise of each EPHF.

In addition, for each indicator, a limited subset of variables to be measured was defined; these are also representative of performance, but under no circumstances do they provide a detailed picture of everything needed for good fulfillment of public health objectives.

Moreover, it is important to take into account restrictions imposed by the methodology used for measurement, based on the consensus opinion of a group of key experts that represented adequately the reality of national public health, and who were selected by the NHA to participate in the evaluation process. The selection of national evaluation groups was not exempt from the problems that contributed to the current political and institutional environment, nor from the cultural dynamics related to the performance evaluation of government work in general. In this regard, distortions due to selection of the evaluation groups can be identified, and it is also quite possible that the level of success achieved by each country—not the trends shown in the global profile—may differ depending on when the evaluation was carried out, whether at the beginning, middle, or end of a government's term. It can also vary depending on the breadth and complementarity of the perspectives of the participants, who are mainly representatives of the central levels of the NHA and, to a greater or lesser extent, of subnational levels and of some entities outside the NHA.

It is therefore important to regard the measurement results as reflecting the set of capacities currently characterizing public health in each of the countries involved, based on the consensus of the expert group selected by the government health authority at the time of measurement. Although these results might differ from those that would have been obtained by a different group of national experts, it is clear that they do faithfully reflect the national reality as

the national authorities understand it, and offer the most accurate reflection of a self-evaluation of performance of the EPHF as recommended by the ministers of health in the Governing Bodies of PAHO. Beyond the specific score obtained on each EPHF and each indicator, what is important is that significant trends were identified within critical areas for each country and, accordingly, provide an acceptable basis for efforts toward improvement.

Furthermore, the instrument design and the evaluation methodology are not intended to have validity in the strict scientific sense of the term, given the possibility of error in specific responses if they are contrasted with the reality as depicted by another observer or by independent arbitration. The responses reflect the opinion of the participants with respect to the exercise in which they took part, which means that other readers of the results, who believe they know the national situation, could make different judgments.

However, despite these limitations with respect to validity, the instrument presents a reasonably credible panorama of critical areas. Although it is possible that specific responses would vary if another group of participants were constituted, it is likely that the critical areas would be the same, which confirms the validity of the overall diagnosis put forward.

The design of the instrument for measuring the EPHF, the methodology for which is eminently qualitative, is aimed at constructing a picture of the state of the EPHF within each country. The great advantage of this measurement lies precisely in its capacity to retain the peculiar characteristics of each country and, potentially, to initiate a deeper

analysis of the performance of the NHA with respect to the EPHF. The measurement exercise and subsequent initiatives by the countries to develop actions aimed at addressing the major critical areas encountered demonstrate that these objectives were fully achieved.

These problems could have been solved through external evaluation carried out by a single evaluation agency in all the countries of the Region of the Americas. However, the value of the self-evaluation processes, especially in terms of the commitment of national authorities to strengthening the critical areas diagnosed, reinforces the methodological design chosen.

Moreover, it was decided not to prepare a composite indicator encompassing all the EPHF, given that each function has value in itself and includes significant capacities necessary for the development of public health in the participating countries. It would not be particularly appropriate to calculate a unified score for all the EPHF and present this as an expression of the reality of public health as a whole within each country or in the entire Region.

The scores achieved by the countries are qualitative and cannot be compared quantitatively among themselves, since they depend on a great variety of factors linked to the reality of each country, as noted above. In addition, it is desirable to stimulate cooperation among different countries to improve public health performance. For these reasons, no attempt was made to classify countries according to their level of commitment to public health. Rather, the presentation of results illuminates areas of greatest weakness, providing evidence to support policies and plans for developing public health in national and regional contexts.

Notwithstanding these considerations, presentation of the overall panorama also makes it possible for decision makers to compare their national situation with those of other countries, as well as to define areas of collaboration for the improvement of public health in their areas of responsibility.

4. Analysis of results of the measurement

For presentation and analysis of the results of the measurement, a scoring system was devised that makes it possible to quantify the qualitative responses from the measures and submeasures. At the same time, criteria were developed for classification of the scores obtained from the indicators as either strengths or weaknesses, and, finally, for identification of priority areas for attention and intervention in subsequent efforts to strengthen institutional capacity in order to improve performance of the EPHF.

4.1 Scoring of the measurement

This section describes the methodology that was used to prepare the scoring system based on the responses, and that constitutes the quantitative basis for the analysis of results of the measurement.

The scoring of each indicator that is part of the measurement of each function is based on the scores obtained for the different variables. The value of these variables can range between 0.00 and 1.00, given that they are prepared on the basis of the average value of positive responses on the measures and submeasures that are detailed under each function.

The questions for the measures and submeasures permit only "yes" or "no" responses. If the consensus response was "yes," a value of "1" was assigned for the measure or submeasure in question; if the response was "no," a value of "0" was assigned. Partial responses were not accepted. For this reason, how to obtain the collective response for each measure and submeasure was a significant issue. As a methodological guide for this measurement exercise, it was proposed to the countries that in cases where a consensus of the entire group could not be achieved, at least 60% of the participants should be in favor of the "yes" option in order to count the collective response to the question as positive.

The score for each indicator and its variables has been calculated using the percentage of positive responses to the measures and submeasures. This score is assigned to each indicator and, finally, is used to calculate the average performance level of each essential public health function.

In order to facilitate measurement, the instrument was supported by a computer program that performs direct calculation of the final score for each variable based on the responses to its measures and submeasures. This facilitates automatic calculation of the scores for indicators and functions, and their graphic representation. Utilization of the same computer program in all the measurement exercises made it possible to compile the information instantaneously and using the same criteria.

For this first measurement exercise in the countries of the Region of the Americas, a method of scoring was chosen in which all the functions, indicators, variables, and measures have the same rela-

tive weight, although this can be modified in the future. This decision was based on the difficulty of determining a priori different relative weights for each function or for different indicators and variables. It is more logical to attempt this in the context of the situation in each country, once the measurement has been carried out without differentiating the relative weights of the questions.

In the first stage, the analysis of the results for each country that undertook the measurement was carried out by the country team, which had the support of the instruments that were made available to the country and that are attached in an annex.

The following scale was proposed as a conventional guide for overall interpretation of the performance of each country:

- 76–100% (0.76 to 1.0) Quartile of optimal performance

- 51–75% (0.51 to 0.75) Quartile of above average performance

- 26–50% (0.26 to 0.50) Quartile of below average performance

- 0–25% (0.0 to 0.25) Quartile of minimum performance

Although it is recognized that the scoring mechanism is not yet fully refined, it is sufficient for identifying strengths and weaknesses of the system, as well as for SWOT (strengths, weaknesses, opportunities, and threats) analysis of the public health systems of the countries, especially from the perspective of a systematic and continuous development process. Moreover, application of the instrument in successive measurement exercises will help to identify the evolution of weaknesses in the public health system infrastructure, making it possible to improve the orientation of interventions recommended for strengthening institutional capacity.

4.2 Identification of intervention areas

In preparing plans to develop the institutional capacity of the health authorities in order to improve the exercise of the EPHF pertaining to them, which is the immediate objective of this exercise in performance measurement, two basic premises have been observed:

a) Development efforts should be institutional in nature. This implies a comprehensive approach, rather than isolated interventions targeting the actors and areas of each function. To this end, all the functions have been merged into strategic intervention areas.

b) Interventions for institutional development must seek to overcome weaknesses by taking advantage of strengths. In order to rate performance in the different indicators as strengths or weaknesses, a reference value is needed; this needs to be identified for each country at different points in the process, as a function of the level of performance and development goals. The basic criteria for establishing the reference values are: a) that the weaknesses diagnosed not be accepted or consolidated, and b) that they represent an achievable challenge and a reasonable incentive for continuing efforts at improvement.

Based on the characteristics of the indicators used for measurement of the EPHF in the five aspects that determine the performance level, that is, outcomes, processes, capacities, infrastructure, and decentralization, it was possible to identify three large groups of indicators that represent strategic intervention areas that can be included in programs for strengthening public health. These strategic areas are the following:

1) *Intervention for final achievement of outcomes and key processes,* the fundamental component of the work of the health authority in public health and, thus, the primary goal of interventions to improve performance. It is related to effectiveness, that is to results, and also to the efficiency—or the processes—with which the health authority carries out the public health functions that pertain to it. Accordingly, proper performance of the key processes will lead to success in terms of expected results of the work of the NHA in public health. To this end, this area concentrates mainly on critical areas that require managerial interventions and monitoring to improve performance of the EPHF in the countries, such as:

- Articulating public health with public policies through definition of health objectives and through understanding, analysis, promotion, contribution, and negotiation of policies, as well as their translation into laws and regulations.

- Facilitating the role of the population not only as object—the health of the population—but also as active subject of public health, that is, health for the population. This includes development and strengthening of health promotion, construction of healthy spaces free from threats or harm to public health, and development of citizenship and of the capacity for participation and social control.

- Ensuring equitable access and quality of necessary health services for the entire population, and improving user satisfaction.

- Promoting recognition of the intersectoral character of health services and building partnerships to increase the success of public health initiatives.

2) *Intervention for development of institutional capacities and infrastructure,* understood as the qualitative and quantitative sufficiency of human, technological, knowledge, and resource capacities necessary for optimal performance of the public health functions that are the responsibility of the health authority. Adequate provision and development of such capacities and resources condition performance of the functions and achievement of desired results within the public health work carried out by the NHA. In addition, this type of intervention is basically investment, in its broader sense, and includes aspects such as:

- Strengthening of institutional organization.

- Strengthening of management capacity.

- Human resources development.

- Budget allocation and organization based on performance of the EPHF.

- Strengthening of institutional infrastructure capacity.

Table 1 Indicators for each EPHF according to area of strategic intervention

EPHF	Achievement of results and key processes	Development of capacities and infrastructure	Development of decentralized competencies
1. Monitoring, evaluation, and analysis of health status	1.1 Guidelines and processes for monitoring health status 1.2 Evaluation of the quality of information	1.3 Expert support and resources for monitoring health status 1.4 Technical support for monitoring and evaluating health status	1.5 Technical assistance and support to the subnational levels of public health in monitoring, evaluating, and analysis of health status
2. Public health surveillance, research, and control of risks and threats to public health	2.1 Surveillance system to identify threats to public health 2.4. Capacity for timely and effective response to control public health problems	2.2 Capacities and expertise in public health surveillance 2.3 Capacity of public health laboratories	2.5 Technical assistance and support for the subnational levels in public health surveillance, research, and control of risks and threats to public health
3. Health promotion	3.1 Support for health promotion activities, development of norms, and interventions to promote healthy behaviors and environments 3.2 Building sectoral and extrasectoral partnerships for health promotion 3.3 National planning and coordination of information, education, and social communication strategies for health promotion 3.4 Reorientation of the health services toward health promotion		3.5 Technical assistance and support to the subnational levels to strengthen health promotion activities
4. Social participation in health	4.1 Empowering civil society for decision-making in public health 4.2 Strengthening of social participation in health		4.3 Technical assistance and support to the subnational levels to strengthen social participation in health
5. Development of policies and institutional capacity for planning and management in public health	5.1 Definition of national and subnational health objectives 5.2 Development, monitoring, and evaluation of public health policies	5.3 Development of institutional capacity for the management of public health systems 5.4 Managment of international cooperation in public health	5.5 Technical assistance and support to the subnational levels for policy development, planning, and management in public health

(continued)

Table 1 *(continued)*

EPHF	Achievement of results and key processes	Development of capacities and infrastructure	Development of decentralized competencies
6. Strengthening of institutional capacity for regulation and enforcement in public health	6.1 Periodic monitoring, evaluation, and revision of the regulatory framework 6.2 Enforcement of laws and regulations	6.3 Knowledge, skills, and mechanisms for reviewing, improving, and enforcing regulations	6.4 Support and technical assistance to the subnational levels of public health in developing and enforcing laws and regulations
7. Evaluation and promotion of equitable access to necessary health services	7.1 Monitoring and evaluation of access to necessary health services 7.3 Advocacy and action to improve access to necessary health services	7.2 Knowledge, skills, and mechanisms to improve access to necessary health services by the population	7.4 Support and technical assistance to the subnational levels of public health to promote equitable access to necessary health services
8. Human resources development and training in public health	8.2 Improving the quality of the workforce 8.4 Improving the workforce to ensure culturally appropriate delivery of services	8.1 Description of the public health workforce profile 8.3 Continuing education and graduate training in public health	8.5 Technical assistance and support to the subnational levels in human resources development
9. Quality assurance in personal and population-based health services	9.1 Definition of standards and evaluation of the quality of population-based and personal health services 9.2 Improving user satisfaction with health services	9.3 Systems for technology management and health technology assessment that support decision-making in public health	9.4 Technical assistance and support to the subnational levels to ensure quality improvement in personal and population-based health services
10. Research in public health	10.1 Development of a public health research agenda	10.2 Development of institutional research capacity	10.3 Technical assistance and support to the subnational levels for research in public health
11. Reducing the impact of emergencies and disasters on health	11.1 Emergency preparedness and disaster management in health 11.2 Development of standards and guidelines that support emergency preparedness and disaster management in health 11.3 Coordination and partnerships with other agencies and/or institutions in emergencies and disasters		11.4 Technical assistance and support to the subnational levels to reduce the impact of emergencies and disasters on health

- Development and technological upgrading of information, management, and operational systems.

3) *Intervention for development of decentralized competencies,* related to actions aimed at transferring faculties, competencies, capacities, and resources to the subnational levels, and supporting them so as to strengthen the decentralized exercise of the health authority with regard to public health, consistent with the requirements of State and health sector modernization. This requires, principally, interventions aimed at reorganization of the authority in conjunction with national decentralization policy.

Table 1 details the indicators selected for each area of strategic intervention.

In order to classify strengths or weaknesses based on the measurements obtained in these first evaluations, and with a view to consolidating the results of the different evaluations in the countries of the Region of the Americas so that a regional action plan can be prepared, a choice was made to use as the conventional reference the median of the global results in the 11 functions, so that half the indicators are classified as weaknesses to be overcome. However, despite the uniform use of this criterion for the regional evaluation, it was possible for national authorities to set a different reference level that could be more or less exacting for the purpose of guiding national efforts to improve performance of the EPHF.

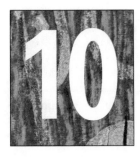

Measurement Process

It must be emphasized that the measurement instrument was designed by groups of experts from different countries of the Region and by staff of the Pan American Health Organization (PAHO), the U.S. Centers for Disease Control and Prevention (CDC), and the Latin American Center for Health Systems Research (CLAISS) to be utilized by key national actors. By developing consensus-based responses to the measurement instrument, actors would be able to report on the EPHF performance profile in their respective countries.

It should be noted that throughout the process, the backing and support of each of the aforementioned participating institutions was provided, in addition to the input and guidance given by the national health authorities, which have been invaluable to the achievement of the measurement objectives. It was through the collaboration among multiple institutions that the measurement of the EPHF could be carried out in each country, utilizing a practical guide to standardize the measurement process.

Consideration must be given to the fact that in this first exercise the main purpose of measuring the EPHF has been self-evaluation of the performance of the NHA. Such institution is responsible for the steering role, which implies, as mentioned in Part I of the book, responsibility for fulfilling other major functions, such as the definition of health policies, financing arrangements, insurance for health care, and regulation of the health sector. As pointed out earlier, in most of the countries of the Region that institution is the Ministry of Health.

Since the work of the NHA in public health implies the collaboration of a broad range of governmental and non-governmental institutions—considering, naturally, universities, health research centers, and public and private service providers, not to mention the government sectors devoted to other areas of collaboration, such as education and the environment—measurement of the performance of the EPHF has been carried out by a group of key actors that represent as faithfully as possible the broad, diverse picture of public health in each national context.

Due to the complexity involved in self-evaluation and the building of consensus for measuring the performance of the EPHF, it was necessary to begin by sensitizing the ministries of health to the importance of the subject and introduce them to the methodology. This was followed by the training of a group of facilitators that would have the knowledge and capacity to support the national measurement exercise to ensure proper implementation and greater control over the process, thus making it possible to obtain reliable results.

In general, the steps followed in the application of the instrument in each country were as follows:

a) Upholding a political agreement between PAHO and the government for the implementation of the exercise.

b) Formalization of an agreement between PAHO and the Ministry of Health to carry out the exercise.

c) Identification of the Ministry of Health personnel who would assume responsibility for the preparation and execution of the exercise.

d) Holding of a cycle of meetings between the two counterparts in which the following was discussed:

- The underlying philosophy of the "Public Health in the Americas Initiative".

- The characteristics and details of the development of the measurement instrument.

- The need to stay on top of problems to control potential risks that might be incurred during the preparation and execution of the exercise, such as:

  – Unfounded fear of what might be implied by a supposedly "external evaluation" of the upper levels of health management and of each person responsible for the areas addressed specifically by the instrument.

  – Apprehension that the "evaluation" would lead to a classification of the countries of the Region according to their degree of support for public health.

e) Selection of participants in the exercise as an exclusive domain of the national health authority. The participant profile that was suggested indicated that the Ministry could select the group, making it as representative and interdisciplinary as possible, ensuring the broad-based origin of its members in accordance with their relevance to the central or subnational level of the NHA or their affiliation with nongovernmental or academic institutions.

f) Preparation of the managerial aspects of the exercise. These included activities such as selecting the place and dates, convening the participants, financing travel and lodging for participants who lived far from the meetings, provision of secretarial support, supplies, and a computer infrastructure.

g) Execution of the measurement exercise. Using the workshop methodology and the application guide, all the participants met to respond to the measurement instrument in an exclusive and intensive fashion. Thus, once the teams were formed, for three days on average, the participants focused on the measurement exercise, structuring a consensus-based response to each of the questions contained in the indicators of the 11 essential functions.

1. Description of the Preparation Process and EPHF Performance Measurement in the Countries of the Region

The responsibility for organizing support for the measurement exercise in the Region of the Americas fell within the realm of the Division of Health Systems and Services Development (HSP) of PAHO, whose main functions were:

a) To promote application of the instrument in all the countries of the Region, in close collaboration with the national health authorities;

b) To support the national measurement processes through the PAHO delegations in each country;

c) To collaborate in training the group of facilitators who would participate in the application of the instrument;

d) To compile the evaluations from each country; and, finally

e) To systematize and analyze the information received, as well as prepare the reports on the results of the EPHF performance measurement in the Region of the Americas.

It should be emphasized that the process has implied an effort to communicate in different languages. This involved an exercise involving much interaction to obtain linguistic and conceptual consistency in English, French, Portuguese, and Dutch for the formulation and application of the measurement instrument, as well as for the execution of the computer program, the analysis of results, and the preparation of the final report.

Thus, using the agreements of the Directing Council of PAHO as the basis, after developing and validating the measurement instrument, the self-evaluation was carried out in each country of the Region. It consisted of the following stages:

1.1 Training of facilitators
1.2 Formation of the group of participants
1.3 Organization and implementation of the measurement exercises

1.1 Training of Facilitators

The first step comprised the selection and training of facilitators who exhibited the leadership and appropriate knowledge to support the application of the instrument. To that end, account was taken of the fact that the work would be carried out in the context of an innovative measurement process. This would involve highly complex deliberations because of the need to arrive at consensus. In addition, the groups of informants were heterogeneous, since their members were trained in different disciplines and had various levels of knowledge, experience, responsibility, and interest, all of which would result in their being sufficiently representative of the realities of the public health service in each country.

Under these premises subregional workshops were held in Argentina, Costa Rica, Haiti, and Jamaica, resulting in the formation of a team of at least three experts from the ministries of health of each country, who had the distinction of being named by the corresponding minister or secretary of health. (Table 1). It should be pointed out that this work and the entire measurement process up through the conclusion of the reports was supported by the staff of the PAHO Representative Offices in the countries that were part of the principal nucleus in charge of formulating the work program and carrying out the

Table 1 Workshops for Training Facilitators in the Application of the Instrument

Subregion	Workshop date	Participants
Central America/Costa Rica	6–8 March 2001	57 professionals
South America/Argentina	29–31 May 2001	59 professionals
English-speaking Caribbean/Jamaica	16–20 October 2001	24 professionals
French-speaking Caribbean/Haiti	29–31 May 2002	14 professionals
Total number of trained facilitators		154 professionals

Table 2 Additional Workshops for Training Facilitators in the Application of the Instrument

Country	Workshop date	Participants
Puerto Rico	1–4 August 2001	15 professionals
Brazil	9–12 January 2002	15 professionals
Paraguay	3–7 October 2001	50 professionals
Curaçao	14–16 November 2001	7 professionals

preparations for the measurement of the EPHF.

To expand this central group of facilitators, other national staff members were subsequently added. They were trained at new workshops in Brazil, Puerto Rico, and Paraguay, as detailed in the following table 2.

1.2 Formation of the Group of Participants

Taking into consideration the mandate of the Directing Council of the Pan American Health Organization (PAHO), which stressed the importance of this measurement as a self-evaluation exercise, it is necessary to emphasize the meticulous care given to safeguarding the autonomy of the NHA in terms of selecting the participants, formulating

the recommendation submitted,[1] and the technical and political considerations that were their exclusive responsibility. With this, the task aimed at achieving effective appropriation of the instrument and the measurement process by each NHA, and consequently the results obtained, take on greater dimensions, making it possible to ensure subsequent implementation of strategies and actions designed to attend to the critical areas revealed in the performance profile.

Consequently, the participating ministries of health in each country of the Region selected technical and professional staff from a variety of institu-

---

[1] The team responsible for the initiative developed a participant profile, which was recommended to each NHA.

tions representative of the public health-related sectors, establishing working groups that assumed responsibility for answering the questions contained in the measurement instrument, with a view to honest collaboration within a process of active, orderly participation.

In each of the 41 countries special attention was given to ensuring the balanced participation of NHA professionals from the national and subnational levels. There was emphasis on the need for informants representative of the intermediate levels—that is, departmental, state, or provincial—and even, at times, from the local level. Efforts were made to include representatives from the academic sector and research groups, as well as from the public and private organizations that provide health care and administer social security, including nongovernmental organizations and other actors in national public health.

With the assistance and coordination of the PAHO delegations, the participation of a representative set of key actors in the application of the instrument, which covered the 11 functions, was achieved. This effort made by the countries of the Region to ensure the intended results is revealed in the following list. The numbers and the profile may at first glance appear inconsistent, but this is due to the unique features of each country and the exclusive decisions of the ministries to carry out the exercise.

Complementing the above description with respect to representativeness, the table below summarizes the types of participants in the EPHF performance measurement. Although the nature of the participants varied among the different countries, it should be noted that in all cases there was a broad range of professionals capable of responding appropriately concerning the performance of the different public health functions.

In addition, it should be recalled that the goal was broad representation from the various disciplines linked to public health: epidemiologists, public health professionals, health economists, lawyers, and specialists in health promotion, social participation, health information systems, public health laboratories, human resources, communications and public relations, environmental health, emergencies and disasters, planning, and others. At the same time, an effort was made to ensure intersectoral representativeness in accordance with the structure and organizaton of each country.

Table 3 National Workshops and Participants in the EPHF Performance Measurement

Country	Dates	Number of participants
Anguilla	29–31 January 2002	19
Antigua and Bermuda	20–22 February 2002	30
Argentina	13–15 November 2001	35
Aruba	20–21 March 2002	25
Bahamas	23 May 2002	71
Barbados	25–27 March 2002	36
Belize	25–27 July 2001	31
Bolivia	15–16 November 2001	54
Brazil	15–17 April 2002	60
Colombia	19–21 September 2001	66
Costa Rica	25–26 April 2001	48
Cuba	19–22 November 2001	56
Curaçao	12–14 November 2001	16
Chile	13–15 December 2000	40
Dominica	10–12 December 2001	25
Ecuador	10–11 October 2001	56
El Salvador	21–23 May 2001	55
Grenada	18–20 February 2002	35
Guatemala	17–21 May 2001	30
Guyana	6–7 December 2001	24
Haiti	24–26 June 2002	29
Honduras	6–8 June 2001	24
Virgin Islands	5–7 March 2002	27
Cayman Islands	11–13 December 2001	27
Jamaica	10–11 December 2001	31
Mexico	19–20 February 2002	40
Montserrat	5–7 February 2002	25
Nicaragua	28–29 May 2001	46
Panama	27–29 June 2001	93
Paraguay	13–15 February 2002	108
Peru	28–29 November 2001	155
Puerto Rico	17–19 October 2001	154
Dominican Republic	7–10 June 2001	102
Saint Kitts and Nevis	12–14 February 2002	41
Saint Lucia	13–15 February 2002	27
Saint Vincent and the Grenadines	28 January–1 February 2002	28
Suriname	24–26 April 2002	36
Trinidad and Tobago	27 February–1 March 2002	42
Turks and Caicos Islands	31 April–1 May 2002	23
Uruguay	24–25 May 2002	45
Venezuela	6–8 February 2002	83
Total Number of Participants in the Measurement of the Region		**1,998**

Table 4 Profile of Participants who Evaluated EPHF Performance in the Countries of the Region

Category	Type of participants
NHA: representatives from the national level 54% of the participants from the NHA	Ministers or Secretaries of Health Advisers to Ministers Health Policy Secretary Secretary of Health Investment Management National Health Council Members Members of National Boards of Municipal Health Secretariats Directors of Administrative Departments Directors-General Of Health and Environment Programs Directors of Promotion Directors of Health Services Development Directors of National Health Surveillance Programs Directors of Human Resources Development Directors of Planning and Institutional Development Directors of National Epidemiology Centers Mass Communication Unit Members
NHA: representatives from the subnational levels 46% of the participants from the NHA	Provincial or state ministries of health Directors of Health Regions Subregional Delegates Regional or Provincial Coordinators PHC Directors Municipal Health Directors National Hospital Directors Provincial Hospital Directors Clinical Unit Heads
Other institutions 15% of all participants	Ministry of Social Action Ministry of Labor Ministry of Agriculture And Livestock Ministry of Finance Or Its Equivalent Social Welfare Secretaries Unions Representatives of professional associations (physicians, other health professionals, lawyers, etc.) Nongovernmental organizations Red Cross, UNICEF German Agency for Technical Cooperation (GTZ) Governors Mayors Representatives of Indigenous Peoples Schools of Public Health Representatives of Universities In The Country Representatives of Institutes of Vital Statistics Institutes of Science and Technology Churches National Nursing Schools Social Insurance, Social Insurance Institutes Offices of People's or Citizens' Advocates Army, Navy, and Air Force Medical Centers National Institutes of Diabetes, Cardiology, Aids, Drug and Addiction Control, etc.

Organization and Development of the Measurement Exercises

Between April 2001 and June 2002—that is, during 15 months of continuous work—a total of 41 national workshops to measure the performance of the EPHF were held. In all of them there was broad participation from the group selected for the exercise. It is worth clarifying that in some cases, when the groups were very large, they were divided into subgroups to ensure that the groups as a whole were able to respond to the different sections of the measurement instrument, identified by the 11 essential functions. In general, the responding groups had similar configurations, with each of them having representation from the various sectors and disciplines that are part of or related to public health, and were convened on a timely basis.

It is necessary to point out that the Ministers of Health, who were totally supportive, strongly backed the initiative. It should be noted that a team of two or three experts from the institutions participating in the design of the measurement instrument served as external facilitators to provide support to each exercise.

To begin the process, the Ministers of Health of the countries convened a working meeting to obtain responses to the questions contained in the measurement instrument. Because of the nature of self-measurement of the performance of the essential public health functions, and in order to familiarize the participants with the instruments, the basic documents for the exercise were annexed to the notice of the meeting. In addition, an effort was made to select a site with the suitable characteristics and environment so that the self-evaluation group could concentrate exclusively on the measurement of the EPHF during the course of the workshop, which lasted from two to three days.

For the measurement process a coordinating group was established in each country to prepare the response to the general and specific aspects of the instrument. Furthermore, as mentioned earlier, key actors and experts or specialists in the area and in the process were able to participate and provided complementary information of both a general and specific nature that was of special value in the measurement of each function. A salient aspect of the measurement was the effort to reach a consensus among the different actors, to ensure that the in-

strument would not become a tool directed exclusively toward the experts of each of the EPHF, but instead yielded a picture that was as representative as possible of the different national and subnational areas and that provided a comprehensive view of national performance.

It is important to emphasize the achievement of one of the main objectives of this measurement, to have each country claim the instrument as its own and to improve it, if it deems that necessary, for later monitoring exercises in its territory. For that purpose the designation and training of national facilitators that could subsequently make use of the instrument for follow-up was basic. To this end, in several countries a series of meetings was held to enable the local facilitators to take charge of the initiative and be responsible for carrying out the measurement.

It is important to note that, in most applications, the participants brought information to the meeting that they considered supportive of their responses to the questions in the instrument. This information could be made available to the team responsible for measuring the EPHF, especially whatever was related to the specific questions aimed at verification.

As a general rule, given the limited time available for the application of the entire instrument, whenever a majority was not obtained an effort was made to achieve consensus through a couple of rounds of voting and presentations. If, at the end of the group discussion, there was still no majority agreement, the response was considered to be negative; when there were doubts about the performance, it was considered preferable to assume it as a deficiency that had to be overcome.

The development of consensus made it possible for those with different opinions on the degree of public health development in their country to make their contribution and inform those who were not familiar with a specific function. However, it should be noted that all the participants were able to contribute to a collective response to the entire instrument and had the opportunity to contribute their knowledge to the contents and aspects implicated in the process.

As a result, it was recognized in all cases that the greatest effort had been made so that the measurement exercise made it possible to obtain the most realistic representation of public health function performance in each country and identify the areas of weakness that required strengthening.

To record and process the responses of the evaluation group, computer software was used that permitted direct instantaneous calculation of the final scoring for each variable, using the responses to the questions and subquestions, and the display of the results in tabular form. To utilize this instrument the only requirement was working knowledge of Microsoft Excel.

After completion of the exhaustive measurement of each function in each country, the workshop continued with a presentation of the summary of results obtained and an analysis of the deficient areas in public health, with the purpose of drawing preliminary conclusions from the measurements. Thus, based on the presentation and the analysis of the performance profiles for each function and to counteract the shortcomings detected, the participants made comments and suggestions for possible future action; these were compiled for the preparation of the final reports from the respective countries. This was the most significant moment of the exercise because, based on the presentation of the weaknesses and the strengths, progress was made toward the development of a common vision of the state of public health in each country. Very significant elements contributed to the development of a plan for the interventions required to improve the institutional performance of the EPHF.

At the end of the exercise, each country summarized the results of the measurement in a document with standard characteristics and format, like the one prepared by the national coordinators and outside experts who supported each exercise. This report contained a description of the measurement process and the results of the application of the instrument, based on the scores obtained for the EPHF and the values of the indicators considered. It also included possible interpretations of the results and identification of priority areas for intervention. Some of those reports have been published by the national authorities. Several countries have already made a commitment to measure the performance of the EPHF again within two or three years and identify the concrete progress, general and specific, that has been made (see example in Annex B).

During the workshop, all the participants were given an opportunity to provide feedback in writing to the team in charge of the project on the content, methodology, and other aspects of the measurement process that they felt could be improved. The evaluation forms used were subsequently analyzed and the results can be found later on in this chapter. Finally, it is important to summarize the principal lines of continuity

and, as appropriate, the resolution defined by the countries, both specific and subregional.

Despite the difficulties involved in completing the measurement in all the countries of the Region, the entire process was carried out within a brief period, which demonstrates the interest and commitment of the countries in the face of this challenge.

It is worth noting that various countries in the Region have begun to plan the development of institutional capabilities to overcome identified deficiencies and consolidate the progress and achievements obtained. Others are in the process of adapting the instrument for use in the measurement of the EPHF at subnational levels, which confirms the motivation generated by the measurement exercise.

Meriting special mention is the fact that in the subregion, made up of the countries participating in the Special Meeting of the Health Sector of Central America and the Dominican Republic (RESSCAD), adopted a resolution[2] designed to formulate a subregional project to support the countries with joint interventions in those functions whose performance received a lower score (Functions 8, 9, and 10). To this end a meeting specifically for building subregional consensus[3] was held, and the project was formulated with a high degree of participation.

[2] Agreement XVII, RESSCAD-NIC-6. Managua, Nicaragua; 29 and 30 August 2001.
[3] Subregional meeting on functions essential to public health as a continuation of Agreement No. 6, XVII RESSCAD. Santo Domingo, Dominican Republic; 15–17 April 2002.

2. Participant Evaluation of the Application of the Performance Measurement Instrument

To enrich this section in which each stage of the measurement process has been described, reference will finally be made to a very important component, namely, evaluation of the entire exercise by the participants from the different countries. For this purpose, the Centers for Disease Control and Prevention (CDC) and the Pan American Health Organization (PAHO) developed a questionnaire to evaluate the application of the methodology and instrument used to measure performance. This questionnaire was used to compile the data on the measurement process carried out through the aforementioned workshops. Accordingly, the evaluation questionnaire was distributed the last day of the workshop in order to:

- Obtain feedback from the participants concerning their impressions of the experience.

- Receive suggestions for improving the measurement process as well as the content of the instrument.

- Ask the participants to provide ratings on a scale analogous to that in the instrument, from the perspective of the national health authority.

In order to begin this evaluation process, all participants were asked to answer the questionnaire anonymously and return it before leaving the session. This survey was administered to practically all the participants with the exception of two countries. A total of 891 adequately answered questionnaires were returned and of these 882, which correspond to 45% of the 1,998 participants, that could be processed and analyzed. The results presented below refer to that universe.

Results

Return rate

The evaluation forms were obtained in time to complete the analysis of the data for 30 countries; evaluation data from the other countries is not available since they did not complete the exercise. Furthermore, it was possible to calculate the return rates for only 23 countries (see Table 5). Data from seven countries could not be calculated because there was insufficient information on the number of registered participants. In many cases a list of the invited participants, divided into groups, was available, but it could not be used as a list of those who actually registered (actual participants). In addition, there was the possibility that, in the dynamic of the workshops, people may have been moved from one group to another to respond to specific functions, so that using this list would not yield the exact number of participants.

Based on the available data from the countries that conducted a strict registration process, the following information was obtained on the number of registered participants and the rates of return. The average return rate was 66%.

Affiliation with the National Health Authority

Of the 882 forms returned, only 768 (93%) contained general information on the type of institution to which the participants belonged and the level of their work; this was because the page requesting this data had not been included in some forms, while in other cases the participants decided not to

Table 5 Countries with Return Rates that Could be Calculated

Country	Return rate	No. of participants registered
Grenada	95%	22
Jamaica	89%	27
Honduras	88%	27
Antigua and Barbuda	81%	32
Belize	80%	20
Saint Lucia	77%	27
Nicaragua	72%	40
Ecuador	70%	39
Venezuela	69%	93
Barbados	67%	36
Saint Vincent and the Grenadines	65%	29
Dominican Republic	64%	81
Saint Kitts and Nevis	64%	30
Guyana	63%	19
Dominica	61%	18
Cayman Islands	58%	31
Brazil	54%	55
Montserrat	52%	21
Anguilla	50%	18
British Virgin Islands	50%	27
Guatemala	48%	31
Colombia	42%	64
Trinidad and Tobago	41%	41

Note: These are the countries that responded completely and in a timely manner to the questionnaire. The rate of return could not be calculated for Argentina, Bolivia, Cuba, El Salvador, Paraguay, Peru, and Puerto Rico.

provide this information. Some participants believed, without sound reasons, that revealing that information would make it possible to determine their identity; however, they were simply asked if they were affiliated with the national health authority, to what level they were assigned, and if their primary specialty was health or something else. Of the forms containing this information, 54% indicated the national level and 46%, the subnational level. Of the 768 forms that included such information, 84% indicated "health" as their primary specialty; the rest, who indicated "other," were from the national health authority, the army medical corps, international agencies, universities, churches, and human rights organizations, as well as health service providers from the private sector.

In addition to their primary responsibilities to the health authority, a limited number of participants (1%) also had responsibilities in other public health organizations, including schools of public health and environmental protection.

Perception of the respondents about the level of their training for participation in the process

In general terms, 37% of the respondents reported that they did not feel well-prepared; 40% felt reasonably well-prepared; and 23%, well-prepared. Although "adequately prepared" and "well-prepared" represented 63% of the responses, the observations of the respondents that did not feel well-prepared were significant. The principal concern expressed was the lack of standardized instructions and the inability of facilita-

116

tors to explain concisely the objective and methodology of the application. They indicated that the instructions varied with the occasion and the process appear inconsistent. These observations were even repeated by respondents who said that they felt sufficiently prepared. It should be noted that at the beginning of the application process there were a large number of such observations. However, as greater experience was gained and the list of more frequently asked questions was expanded, the expressions of skepticism and negative attitudes became less frequent and, at the same time, the presentations in the workshops were better directed, the strategies improved, and the participants understood the process better.

Ninety percent of the respondents indicated that they received adequate directions from the facilitators on how to answer the questions.

Clarity of the instructions
Some 94% of the respondents reported that the instructions were adequate or sufficiently clear; 6% indicated that the instructions were not clear, because:

- The facilitators had not presented the methodology clearly.

- There had been a change in the instructions.

Again, these observations related more to the initial applications.

Distribution of course materials
Fifty-four percent of the participants stated that it was necessary to improve this aspect of the process by allowing more time between the circulation of the materials and the holding of the workshop so that they could be read before-

hand and understood better. The following factors contributed to this delay:

- Little preparation time before the workshops were held.

- Insufficient notice to the participants of the dates and contents of the workshops.

- Late distribution of the materials.

Clarity of the instrument format
The results were very encouraging: 89% of participants considered the format understandable or easy to understand; only 11% found it difficult. The most common reason given for the lack of clarity was related to the way in which the questions were formulated, including the language utilized. This was true for both the Spanish and the English versions. In both cases people felt that some questions were ambiguous and would have preferred the use of clearer, more concise language.

In the Spanish-speaking countries, differences in the meanings of words played a decisive role in determining whether the instrument would be appropriate for local use. A small percentage also indicated that it would be useful to have other options, rather than just yes or no: perhaps a partial or analog scale for the response so that works in process, plans, or signaled changes could be included. This proposal would, of course, eliminate the instrument's capacity to measure conditions as they were at the time. It was not accepted, since the purpose of the exercise was to take a snapshot of the current situation, with no concern for what it might be with the partial option. It should be noted that once it was explained to the participants that the instrument had

been designed to measure what already existed in fact and not what was potential or planned, the lack of an option of an intermediate or partial response was not considered to be so significant.

Number of questions
Sixty-two percent of the respondents indicated that the number of questions was sufficient, while 34% considered that it was too high. It should be noted that certain areas of redundancy were identified and, accordingly, an examination of the instrument is being planned with a view to simplifying and eliminating the possible duplications.

Clarity of the standards for the indicators
The results in this regard were also very encouraging. Some 56% of the respondents thought that the standards were appropriate but needed further clarification; 42% thought that they were well-written, clear, and understandable; and only 2% felt that they were inadequate. The last group were generally from the very small island nations. The participants from those countries suggested that the standards be reviewed and made more applicable to small countries. In view of these responses, the standards and their drafting will be examined. This should be done in cooperation with the smaller countries themselves in order to better respond to local needs.

Difficulty in responding to questions on functions and measurements
Seventy-six percent of the respondents indicated that they had difficulty answering some questions and subquestions. Of this group, 63% gave as their reason the fact that the subject was outside their area of specialization, while 37% of those experiencing the difficulty when the subject was not outside their specialty indicated that they did

not understand the questions because they were ambiguous or unclear, sometimes due to the type of language utilized. Although the evaluation form allowed the participants to make unrestricted observations on the content of the instrument, the participants preferred to do that during the workshop itself. The observations were recorded for use in the iterative development of the instrument.

Linkage of this instrument for use with other national quality improvement or evaluation activities
In regard to this point the respondents offered three options:

a) Validate other, existing national and subnational efforts.

b) Provide data that can be used in conjunction with those from other activities to improve planning at the national and subnational levels.

c) Both a and b.

Of the 825 respondents, 767 (93%) answered this question; 71% selected Option a; 87.5%, Option b; and 59%, Option c. Those selecting Option c felt that the data derived from this instrument played a broader, more significant role, since they could be used to validate existing data and also could be combined with the existing data from other activities to improve planning at the national and subnational levels. Some participants pointed out the need for a mechanism to objectively validate the recorded data. With respect to the request for other areas of possible linkage, the respondents answered:

• Provide data to lawmakers to improve the redefinition and formulation of policies and laws.

• Promote self-evaluation in other areas, for quality analysis.

• Work with other sections of government, especially in the formulation of interinstitutional agreements.

• Strengthen organizational and managerial capacity at every level.

• Continuously improve quality.

• Seek to develop a better fit between human resources and system needs.

• Provide training in leadership and management.

• Use the data to train personnel at all levels of the system.

• Link the data to the standards and accreditation of the organizations in the public health system.

Types of reports that would be of greater usefulness to the respondents
The options presented were:

a) Graphs that indicate the degree of success achieved, by function or indicator.

b) Analyses of strengths, weaknesses, opportunities, and threats (SWOT).

c) Recommendations and interventions to improve system performance, based on the results of the process.

d) All the above options.

Option c was selected in 73% of the cases and Option b in 70%. Only 61% felt that Option a by itself would be useful, while 61% felt that a report that included the three options would be

useful. This indicates very clearly that the type of report that most countries would consider useful would include a graphic analysis of the strong and weak points of the system, together with appropriate recommendations of interventions that would improve system performance.

Use of the results: reports generated based on this activity
The options presented in the questionnaire were:

a) Use the results to improve development of the public health work force.

b) Improve the accountability of the system.

c) Determine and strengthen the weak areas in the system.

d) General strategic planning to improve the system at all levels.

e) Policy evaluation.

f) Capacity development.

g) Use the results to strengthen the capacity to manage the organization.

h) Use the results to promote change within the system, eliminating processes that no longer work.

i) Promote greater adherence to the standards by the national health authority.

j) Modify existing programs and curricula in public health to make them better adapted to the needs of the health sector.

k) Use the results to better define what the public health products should be, depending on the situation in the country.

l) Evaluate the national health authority's capacity for effective leadership.

m) All of the options above.

The respondents could select one or all the options that they considered appropriate. The options most commonly selected were a, c, d, and h: in more than 75% of the responses. Options a and c were the most common, which indicates that the respondents considered the instrument and the methodology useful for the analysis of gaps in the evaluation of the system. It was significant that Option l was selected in only 54% of the responses, which means that the participants did not seem to link the process and the instrument with evaluation of the national health authority's capacity for effective leadership. Only 33% of the respondents recognized the usefulness of reports applicable to all areas. This indicates the need for guaranteeing that the presentations offered beforehand provide pertinent information that allows the participants to establish a connection between the type of report generated and the work of the national health authority. Making the linkage more evident will make it possible for the participants to better understand the relevance and suitability of applying the instruments to their own work.

Use of the instrument for evaluating national health authority performance
Seventy-seven percent of the respondents indicated that they thought the instrument could accurately measure the performance of the NHA. There was no significant difference in this percentage between the participants who came from the national and subnational

levels (chi square = 0.025, P = 0.8). The 23% of the participants who did not believe the instrument would measure the performance of the national health authority indicated that:

- The opinions expressed by the participants were not consistent with reality and expressed only an imprecise idea of the system.

- There was no way of validating the responses. The questions were too subjective.

- The indicators were not applicable to certain countries.

- Lack of participants with experience to answer the questions, inappropriate composition of the groups, not representative of the system.

- Only certain areas of activity were measured.

- The national health authorities in some countries did not use the EPHF framework.

Classification of the usefulness of the instrument in daily practice
The analog scale used by the respondents to classify the usefulness of the instrument in daily practice was as follows: 0 = of no use, 1 = of little use, 2 = of some use, 3 = of average use, 4 = very useful, 5 = highly useful.

The lack of scatter in the responses indicated that most of the participants assigned a high value to the use of the instrument for evaluating the public health service: 70% thought that the instrument was "very useful" or "highly useful." Fewer than the 10% of the participants judged the instrument to be of little use. Figure 1 illustrates the distribution of the responses.

Frequency of application
Seventy-three percent of the participants said that the instrument and the measurement process should be used every one or two years, with 48% opting for annual application. The results can be observed in the following table.

Figure 1 Classification of the Usefulness of the Instrument

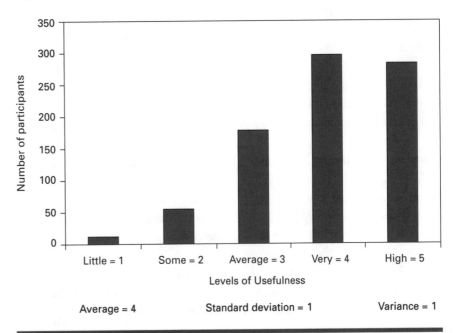

Table 6 Recommended Frequency of Application

Frequency of application	Number of responses	Percentage of responses
Annually = A	288	35
2 years = B	313	38
3–5 years = C	190	23
5–10 years = D	33	4

Suggestions from the respondents
to improve future workshops

This open-ended question solicited observations from the participants, based on their experience in responding to the instrument and participating in the workshop. The observations are very insightful and should be taken into account to help make future workshops more effective and efficient.

- Guarantee diversity in the composition of the group and appropriate representation of all levels for each function.

- Have the support documents in hand to validate the responses.

- Hold preliminary workshops in the country to explain the objectives and methodology, so that the participants can be well-prepared.

- Make sure that the practical guide is concise and the glossary broad enough to cover all the terminology used.

- Improve orientation and standards.

Discussion, conclusions, and lessons
derived from the evaluation

From the perspective of the participants, the instrument and the methodology have proven to be very useful. This is observed in the high rating given to usefulness and the desire to repeat the process

every year or two. The main concerns were focused on the need for reformulating the questions, using more concise language to avoid ambiguities or misinterpretations. Instruments of this type constantly evolve as they go through an iterative refining process. Despite a rigorous phase of pilot studies, certain problems did not become evident until the instrument was used in the field. For these reasons, the drafting and content of the standards, questions, and subquestions are currently undergoing intensive examination before the next version of the instrument is produced.

A stricter approach must be integrated into the application process, so that the facilitators can carry out the evaluation (especially the collection of the completed forms) and guarantee that an exact list of all the participants registered is available from the start. This way, the return rate can be calculated. This component of the application process should be emphasized. Even though return rates are not available for all the countries, information from 825 participants was obtained. The qualitative information obtained by feedback from the participants was very useful, as it contributed data on their perception of the instrument and the application process.

It was clear that it would have been useful to have better strategies "at the country level" to prepare the participants so

that they better understood the objectives of the exercise and the methodology. In most of the countries, the local facilitators held a series of meetings prior to the workshop to familiarize them with the workshop methodology and guarantee that the workshops were held without problems. Unfortunately, this was not done in all the countries. The selection and training of the facilitators is of the utmost importance, and it is essential to select people with the profile, experience, and responsibility required to being a facilitator. As principal factors in the preparation and planning of the countries that wish to use this instrument and this methodology, the following should be emphasized:

a) Be sure that the political will exists and that those in charge will accept and adopt key "in-country" decisions through preliminary meetings and workshops

b) Make sure that effective strategies are in place that guarantee timely receipt of the documents prior to the workshops and data collection exercises.

c) Educate facilitators and promote more effective distribution of the materials by them and by the focal points prior to the workshop.

d) Support the holding of introductory workshops in each country to promote a better understanding of the concept, goals, and objectives of the evaluation. This will also encourage better acceptance by the participants.

Emphasis must be placed on the importance of assigning the participants so that the groups are well-balanced, representative of the issue under analysis, and foster harmony and collaboration among the attendees. Although all participants were not experts in all measurements, that was positive, for it caused the groups to coalesce, with each participant having a specific area of specialization and making significant contributions in that area. Although it is necessary to guarantee that the respondents selected match the function measured, it also is important to avoid introducing biases by having too many "experts" in a particular group.

As can be observed in the information obtained, there is no doubt about the need for some type of objective validation of the responses, to ensure that the data collected are scientifically valid. The application form used in some countries did not give participants access to the instrument as a whole but only to the sections or functions for which their group was responsible. Thus, the participants did not have an overview of the instrument. A balanced mixture of participants from the different levels of the system sometimes acted as a control on the responses themselves and avoided the introduction of excessive bias from dominant individuals in the group. In light of the situations in which there was a lack of objective validation, the balance—or "self-validation"—introduced by the composition of the group made a difference. It also is useful to ask the participants to study the instrument beforehand and to bring to the workshop any document that would help validate their responses to the questions.

Although the participants recognized some deficiencies in the last version of the instrument and methodology, they were able to use the instrument and the data to analyze gaps. This underscores

the success of the exercise and, as stated earlier in this chapter, some countries have already analyzed this information and used it to prepare their own country reports and plans of action. It must be reiterated that regional meetings have already been held to explore the development of regional plans of action and interregional cooperation plans for the formulation of strategic interventions; all of them were geared to boost the institutional capacity of the infrastructure, which will give rise to an improvement in the delivery of public health services at the regional level.

3. General Lessons derived from the Measurement

For the group of Member States, the results presented in Chapter 11, as well as the individual country reports, provide a significant quantity of information that they can use to define their own plans for strengthening public health.

The identification of common areas of weakness and strength can serve as a very useful supporting argument when ministries of health in the Region attempt to pressure those responsible for decision-making in their governments to provide the help needed to develop their health capacities.

However, although there may be continued emphasis on the importance of the measurement process and interest in the results obtained as a faithful representation of the overall situation at the national, subregional, and regional levels, the limitations of the methodology and measurement instrument indicated in the previous chapter should not be overlooked.

Thus, the relativity of the results of specific measurements should not lead to hasty conclusions, but to a more in-depth diagnosis, through the use of more objective instruments and more detailed analysis of the critical areas identified. Only in this manner will it be possible to guarantee the development of programs to improve public health that effectively meet the needs of each country.

Similarly, given the differences in the selection of the national evaluation groups and the asymmetry of the information available to the participants, it is likely that the evaluation of some functions or indicators will not be entirely acceptable to them or to other national experts. In that case, complementary mechanisms should be activated to improve the diagnosis to ensure reliable responses that will assist in the recognition and acceptance of the national challenges to public health. Here, this diagnostic measurement can also serve as a frame of reference for all institutions interested in cooperating in the improvement of public health in the Americas.

For this reason, based on the first measurement exercise at the regional level, it can be concluded that the instrument and its application are in need of improvement. The number of questions and subquestions can be reduced significantly depending on their explanatory power, a conclusion that could not be reached prior to the completion of this first iteration in each country. Similarly, it is also possible to balance the order and the number of questions and subquestions for each indicator. However, even though the instrument does not pretend to have the validity required in a typical diagnosis, it is important to recognize the possibility of improving the questions to ensure greater reliability and, consequently, greater reproducibility of the national responses, thus providing greater value and more objectivity to the measurements, regardless of who the evaluator is.

Furthermore, in response to requests from the countries of the Region, progress is now possible in improving the design of instruments used to measure the EPHF at the subnational levels or in specific spheres of public health activity, allowing greater utilization of the conclusions obtained.

The development of this measurement instrument is thus the starting point of an evaluation process that will allow the countries to better direct their efforts to the improvement of the public health service. Thus, that improvement and evolution will be determined by the national health authorities and by the international cooperation institutions that make this instrument a tool for change and adapt it to their particular needs. Since this first evaluation, initiatives directed toward adapting the instrument for subnational measurements have already appeared, along with proposals designed to require stricter standards, all of which confirm the recognition that this is, in fact, a useful instrument and that it is undergoing continuous improvement.

From the perspective of the institutions in charge of the measurement process in the Region, the exercise has elicited very significant contributions. The main satisfaction lies in the verification that the instrument and measurement methodology developed are useful and meaningful to those responsible for public health services in each country. The exercise has also revealed areas in which the measurement can be improved, a process to which participants in the exercise have contributed with an enthusiasm that makes future improvements imperative. However, perhaps the most important aspect of the whole experience has been witnessing the adoption of the measurement instrument and the methodology for its application by the participating countries.

Finally, the EPHF performance measurement contributes to the development of a baseline for the analysis of the state of public health in the Region of the Americas and provides a point of departure for future evaluation of the progress made by the countries in improving their performance. It also underscores the strategic value of self-evaluation as it applies to the institutional performance of the NHA.

Results of the Measurement of the Essential Public Health Functions in the Americas

Introduction

The following chapter presents the results of the performance measurement of the Essential Public Health Functions. To facilitate the presentation and allow for analysis, the results are explained in detail for the Region as a whole and for each of the subregions. In this manner the reader has at his disposal a summary of what has been an enormous effort of professional and highly participatory work, where as was observed in the previous chapter, the efforts of 1,997 qualified public health workers that participated in the measurement exercise that took place in 41 countries and territories in the Region, are gathered.

First, the average results for the 11 Essential Public Health Functions for the countries of the Region that participated in the exercise are examined; secondly the results of the performance of the EPHF are presented by subregions in the following order: Central Amer-

ica, the Caribbean, the Andean subregion and the Southern Cone and Mexico. Finally, the chapter closes with a section on conclusions, that far from being a final discussion and analysis—product of many work sessions with the groups of participants and experts in the field, both from the countries and the participating institutions—represent an open door for communication and continued discussion to advance in the purpose of promoting the development of the EPHF, starting from the foundation of the self-evaluations of the countries which has always had the intention of being objective and integral.

1. Regional Analysis

1.1 General results of the measurement

As an example of the results obtained in the Region concerning the performance of the EPHF, the following chart provides the median values for this group of countries (Figure 1). This type of

summary was chosen because the results in each country do not make it possible to dispense with the normal distribution as an explanatory model of the country's performance for any of the EPHF.

In general, a low-intermediate performance profile was observed for the group of 11 EPHF. The best relative performance was observed in the functions of reducing the impact of emergencies and disasters (EPHF 11) and in public health surveillance (EPHF 2), although neither of these exceeded a 70% fulfillment rate with respect to the standard used for this assessment.

The functions of human resources development and training in public health (EPHF 8), quality assurance in health services (EPHF 9), and research in public health (EPHF 10) performed more poorly.

High-intermediate performance was observed in the functions of monitor-

Figure 1 Performance of EPHF Regional of the Americas[1]

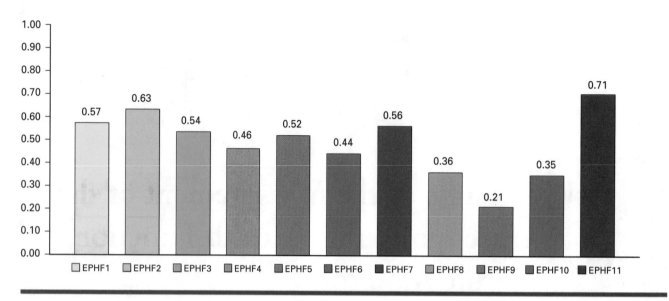

ing, evaluation, and analysis of health status (EPHF 1), evaluation and promotion of equitable access to necessary health services (EPHF 7), development of policies and institutional capacity for planning and management in public health (EPHF 5), and health promotion (EPHF 3). Finally, low-intermediate performance was observed in social participation in health (EPHF 4) and the strengthening of the institutional capacity for regulation and enforcement in public health (EPHF 6).

In general, this EPHF profile shows that functions that can be considered part of the "tradition" of public health development (EPHF 2 and 11) performed better, while more recent functions, such as quality assurance (EPHF 9), performed more poorly. This requires the Region to undertake a profound review of its public health activities, particularly with a view toward developing its institutional

capacity in order to address new health and management challenges.

An important area of concern is the low performance observed in the function of human resources development (EPHF 8). This fact must be taken into account, given that an essential part of the future strengthening of public health is developing the abilities of the human resources on which the institutional strength of the NHA depend.

An analysis of the dispersion of the results obtained for the Region (Figure 2) indicates that function 1 (monitoring, evaluation, and analysis of health status), function 2 (public health surveillance), function 6 (regarding regulation and enforcement), and function 9 (quality assurance in the health services) are more homogeneous in the various countries.

On the other hand, functions 7 (promotion of equitable access to necessary health services), 10 (research in public health), and 4 (participation in public health) show the greatest degree of variability, indicating the possibility of con-

solidating the experiences of a number of countries which, within the Region, are performing better.

An average dispersion is observed for the remaining functions. Generally speaking, this also indicates that there are groups of countries with relative strengths that could contribute to improving the situations of other countries in the Region that are performing at an insufficient level and need to improve. This indicates that, except for several exceptional cases in which a country is showing generally better performance for the set of EPHF, the vast majority of the Region's countries have areas in which they are performing well and others that are more critical.

The results in terms of the median value, the first standard deviation (representing 66% of the countries), and the maximum and minimum values[2] for each function are provided in the

---

[1] For more details on the overall results with regard to each of the EPHF, all of the summary measurements—median, standard deviation, 25th and 75th percentiles—are given at the end of the chapter.

[2] In this analysis, several results that were identified as outliers in the statistical analysis were excluded.

Figure 2 Distribution of the performance of each EPHF in the Countries of the Region

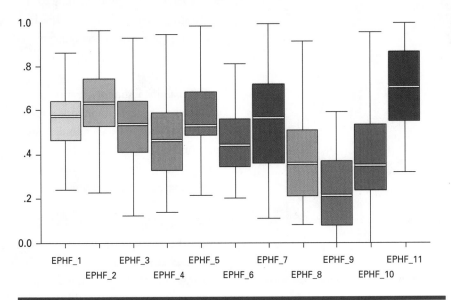

following table. As can be seen, most countries fall within in a similar performance range. A wider range of variability can only be seen for EPHF 7.

1.2 Results of the measurement by function

An analysis of the performance of each EPHF is presented below.

EPHF 1: *Monitoring, Evaluation, and Analysis of Health Status*

Although high-intermediate performance was demonstrated with respect to this function in the Region, it continues to be an area in need of strengthening in some countries. A frequency histogram of the performance of the countries studied is shown below (see Figure 3), showing a median for the Region of 0.58 and a range from 0.24 to 0.97.

The greatest strength was found in the institutional capacity of the NHA to perform this function (Indicator 3). Moderate strength was demonstrated

with respect to the technical support needed to discharge this function (Indicator 4) and NHA assistance to subnational levels (Indicator 5). The most critical areas with those concerning the existence of guidelines for monitoring

and evaluating health status in the countries of the Region (Indicator 1) and evaluating the quality of the data (Indicator 2) with which the profile of health status is drafted, as shown in the following table (Figure 4).

Indicators:

1. Guidelines and processes for monitoring health status

2. Evaluation of the quality of information

3. Expert support and resources for monitoring health status

4. Technical support for monitoring and evaluating health status

5. Technical assistance and support to the subnational levels of public health

Upon analyzing the dispersion of the performance of these indicators for the Region of the Americas, it can be con-

Figure 3 Distribution of the performance level of EPHF 1 in the Countries of the Region

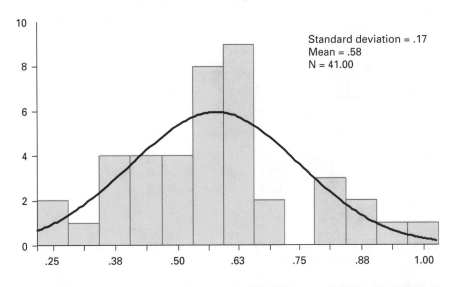

Figure 4 Performance of the Indicators for EPHF 1

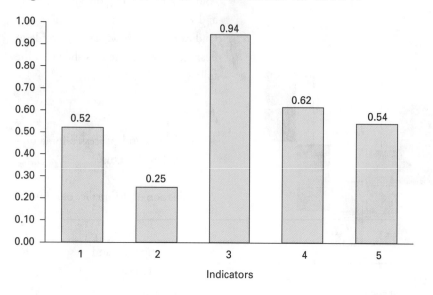

cluded that there is a high degree of variability between the countries of the Region, particularly with respect to the indicator for which the poorest performance was shown (evaluation of the quality of information). However, despite the fact that the majority of the countries showed weaknesses in this area, others demonstrated adequate performance. A similar situation was found with respect to the variability of Indicator 5. In contrast to the previous case, Indicator 5 was a strength for the majority of the countries, although it continued to be an important weakness for others.

Figure 5 Distribution of the performance of the Indicators of EPHF 1 in the Countries of the Region

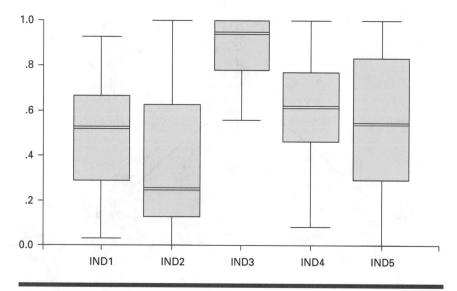

Indicator 3, with respect to which the strongest performance was shown, had a low level of variability, leading to the conclusion that institutional capacities and competencies are a strength for performance of this function.

The remaining indicators, that is, guidelines and processes for monitoring health status (indicator 1) and technical support (indicator 4), should be reviewed by each country, given that they constitute significant weaknesses for some.

The results in terms of the median value, the first standard deviation (representing 66% of the countries), and the maximum and minimum values[3] for each indicator are provided in the following table (Figure 5).

The primary factors determining performance of this function, which were common to all or the majority of the countries are as follows:

- Roughly 70% of the participating countries have guidelines for measuring health status on the national and intermediate levels, and a somewhat higher percentage have guidelines for the local level.

- In the majority of the countries, the health status profile is updated every year and provides information about the use of health services by individuals and groups. It is also used to monitor trends and formulate national goals and objectives. However, the profiles still display shortcomings with regard to using the data to reveal inequalities in access to health services,

[3] In this analysis, several results that were identified as outliers in the statistical analysis were excluded.

guiding activities aimed at improving the effectiveness of the services, and providing information on changes in risk factor profiles and the determinants of health status.

- The primary data used to measure health status are mortality, socioeconomic indicators, and use of health services. In general, barriers to accessing health services are not monitored, less than 30% of the countries monitor risk factors for the most important pathologies, and data on morbidity are inconsistently recorded.

- With regard to the quality of the data, only 16% of the countries have an oversight agency that is independent of the ministry of health. Roughly 30% of the countries replied that they had carried out audits in order to evaluate the quality of the data. A common critical area is the lack of procedures for continually improving information systems. It was also acknowledged that there are no procedures for distributing information concerning the health status of the population to the communications media and to the general public (half of the countries permit public access to the information). Finally, very few countries periodically evaluate how the distributed health status information is used by the recipients of that information.

- Although national bodies responsible for coordinating health statistics exist, fewer than a third meet at least once a year to analyze and evaluate their performance and coordinating activities.

- In human resources education, 80% of the countries have qualified public health professionals at the intermediate level, and half of the countries

Figure 6 Distribution of the performance level of EPHF 2 in the Countries of the Region

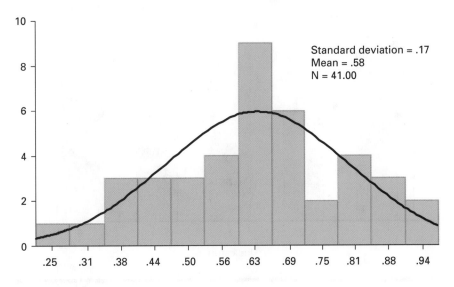

have at least one professional with the title of doctor at the central level.

- The majority of the countries have staff trained in designing plans for sampling and collecting general and specific data on health status. These professionals can consolidate data from various sources, perform integrated data analyses, interpret results, formulate valid conclusions, and communicate pertinent information on the country's health status and related trends to decision-makers.

- Approximately 76% of the countries use computer resources is order to carry out this function at the intermediate level, while only 27% of the countries use them at the local level. Approximately 43% of the countries use electronic communication systems to disseminate data to subnational levels. A common critical area is the lack of fast access to specialized computer systems and equipment maintenance.

- In general, it was acknowledged that the NHA advises subnational levels with respect to data collection, however, the NHA exhibited greater weaknesses with respect to providing support for the interpretation of results.

EPHF 2: *Public Health Surveillance, Research, and Control of Risks and Threats to Public Health*

This is one of the better performing functions for the countries of the Region, with a median of 0.63. A consistent profile was exhibited by the majority of the countries studied,[4] as shown in Figure 6 which provides the median distribution histogram of the countries for this function.

As can be seen, the performance of the majority of the indicators was higher than 50%. The primary areas of strength

[4] Fewer than 25% of the countries performed at less than 50%, according to the standards determined for this function.

127

Figure 7   Performance of the Indicators for EPHF 2

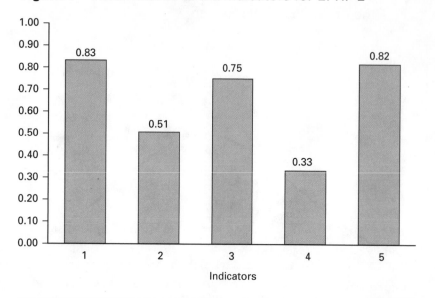

Indicators

Indicators:

1. Surveillance system to identify threats and harm to public health

2. Capacities and expertise in public health surveillance

3. Capacity of public health laboratories

4. Capacity for timely and effective response to control public health problems

5. Technical assistance and technical support for the subnational levels of public health.

were adequate surveillance systems for identifying public health threats, the capacities of public health laboratories, and support for subnational levels. The primary weakness was an insufficient capacity to provide a timely and effective response to control public health problems, as it shown in the following Figure (Figure 7).

Of the results obtained from the countries, the indicator concerning the capacity for timely and effective response exhibited the greatest dispersion. However, although this was a critical area for the Region of the Americas as a whole, it was a strength for some countries. The least variability in the countries' performance was demonstrated by the

results for indicator 1 (public health surveillance system), which can be identified as a strength in the Region.

The results for the remaining indicators exhibited an intermediate dispersion, as shown in Figure 8.

The primary factors determining performance of this function are as follows:

- The surveillance systems make it possible to identify the magnitude and the nature of the threats, to follow adverse circumstances and risks over time, to identify threats requiring a response, and to study trends in diseases determined to be national priorities. The surveillance systems are made up of the subnational levels and are also integrated into supranational surveillance systems. However, they do not integrate information generated by other actors (private health providers, NGOs, etc.)

- The majority of the countries have established the functions and respon-

Figure 8   Distribution of the performance of the Indicators for EPHF 2 in the Countries of the Region

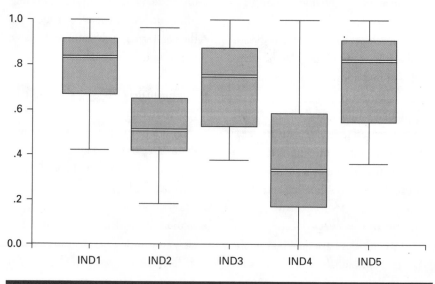

sibilities of the various levels, particularly at the local level.

- Again, weaknesses are manifested in evaluating the quality of the data produced by the surveillance systems, and few countries have established, formal mechanisms for providing feedback on how the surveillance systems are operating.

- The majority of the countries have developed protocols for purposes of identifying the primary public health threats in each country.

- The majority of the countries have qualified personnel to monitor basic sanitation and infectious diseases, as well as to handle evaluation and fast screening techniques. They are also in a position to design new surveillance systems for potential problems. A smaller number of countries (24%) support surveillance with **geofigureic** information systems. The greatest weaknesses are personnel knowledge and experience is epidemiological research on chronic diseases, accidents, and occupational mental health. These constitute the primary health challenges for the Region of the Americas.

- One critical area is the lack of incentive mechanisms or recognition in order to promote good performance by public health monitoring teams.

- Although the vast majority of the countries can give examples of threats to public health that were detected in a timely fashion in the last two years, only a third of the countries evaluate the response capacity of the surveillance system, communicate results, and supervise the implementation of corrective measures.

- The countries maintain up-to-date registries of public health laboratories, have formal coordination and reference mechanisms, and periodically evaluate the quality of diagnoses using international laboratories as reference parameters. However, weaknesses in evaluating the public health laboratories were acknowledged with respect to how the coordination and reference procedures function, and the majority of the countries do not comply with regulations directed toward guaranteeing the quality of their laboratories.

- In all of the countries, the NHA advises and supports the subnational levels in order to help them develop and strengthen their surveillance capacity to an optimal degree.

EPHF 3: *Health Promotion*

This function exhibited high-intermediate performance, with a median for the Region of 0.53. Although the majority of the countries fell near the intermediate values, one can see that several deviated from the average performance of the Region and exhibited better or worse performance, as shown in Figure 9.

A fundamental objective of health promotion is to improve access to available protective factors, such as social support, safe communities, job opportunities, and better education, which can help reduce some of the health inequalities associated with low or disadvantaged socioeconomic level. To this end, the countries of the Region must take necessary actions to improve the critical weaknesses that the performance of this function revealed.

Very similar, intermediate performance was observed for all of the indicators of this function (see Figure 10).

Indicators:

1. Support for health promotion activities, the development of norms, and interventions to promote healthy behaviors and environments.

Figure 9 Distribution of the performance level of EPHF 3 in the Countries of the Region

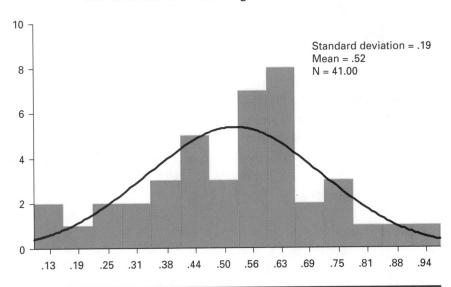

Standard deviation = .19
Mean = .52
N = 41.00

129

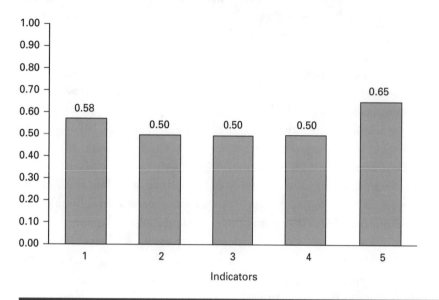

Figure 10   Performance of the Indicators for EPHF 3

2. Building of sectoral and extrasectoral partnerships for health promotion.

3. National planning and coordination of information, education, and social communication strategies for health promotion.

4. Reorientation of the health services toward health promotion.

5. Technical assistance and support to the subnational levels to strengthen health promotion activities.

The results for Indicators 2, 3 and 5 were less variable. Greater dispersion was observed for the remaining indicators, which confirms that health promotion is a strength for some countries and a weakness for others.

The primary factors determining performance of this function, which were generally shared by all countries, are as follows:

• The majority of the countries are aware of the recommendations of international conferences on health promotion and have incorporated them into their action plans. Roughly 49% of the countries have established

health promotion goals and carry out "healthy municipality"-type actions on the local level.

• One critical area is the poor development of systems for supporting health promotion at subnational levels. Only 23% of the countries have systems for recognizing and rewarding health promotion, 35% have "competition" funds designated for stimulating health promotion, and 76% finance health promotion training activities.

• Although policies and standards aimed at promoting healthy behavior and environments are in place and efforts have been made to advocate for the development of health-sensitive public policies (especially with regard to the environment), only 43% of the countries plan actions in this area each year, which may explain the limited observed results.

• In general, the NHA do not carry out systematic studies of the impact of

Figure 11   Distribution of the performance of the Indicators for EPHF 3 in the Countries of the Region

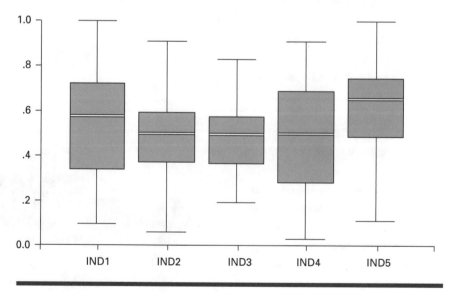

public policies on the health of the population, a practice which would make it possible to proactively support healthy behavior and environments. Only 22% of the countries allocate resources for measuring the impact of public policies on health.

• Approximately 35% of the countries stated that they have specific actions plans for the purpose of establishing partnerships with other actors and sectors, and less than half of them periodically evaluate the results of these actions and correct how they are implemented.

• Throughout the Region, the NHA actively support health promotion activities, particularly local health education. They collaborate with other actors, but do not evaluate the results of this collaboration. The use of television, radio, and the press is common in the majority of the nationally-sponsored campaigns. Only 14% of the countries stated that they have used the Internet to carry out campaigns.

• There are few agencies specifically devoted to providing public health information and education, and the agencies that do exist are not evaluated. Less than a third of the countries use web pages and telephone lines devoted to this purpose.

• Roughly 70% of the countries promote the implementation of models under which the primary strategy for reorienting the health services toward health promotion is the provision of public health services by teams with training in health promotion. However, only 35% of the countries state that they have developed mechanisms for encouraging and fostering the

health promotion approach in primary health care.

• The countries pointed out that obstacles to reorienting health services toward promotion include the fact that only 5% of the countries have established payment mechanisms that support health promotion, that no country has promoted health insurance payment mechanisms that encourage health promotion, and that the majority of the countries do not include activities in support of health promotion in health plans. It was also stated that training in health promotion is not a recognized part of the professional accreditation process.

• The countries stated that they have trained staff in health promotion. Around 59% of the countries encourage training centers to include health promotion in academic training curricula, and 78% have included it in their own human resources training programs.

• The primary critical areas with respect to NHA support for subnational levels are the lack of plans for strengthening health promotion at subnational levels, and the need to improve evaluation and support activities directed toward subnational levels.

EPHF 4: *Social Participation in Health*

This function exhibited intermediate performance for the Region, with a median of 0.49. The performance profile of the countries is quite homogeneous, with the exception of several countries that deviated from the intermediate range, as is shown in Figure 12.

As with the previous function, the indicators measured revealed intermediate performance, although the indicator for strengthening social participation in health was somewhat higher (Figure 13).

Indicators:

1. Empowering citizens for decision-making in public health

Figure 12 Distribution of the performance level of EPHF 4 in the Countries of the Region

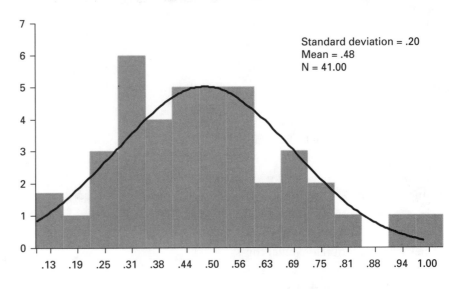

Standard deviation = .20
Mean = .48
N = 41.00

Figure 13 Performance of the Indicators for EPHF 4

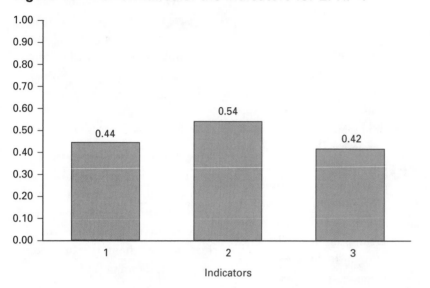

2. Strengthening of social participation in health

3. Technical assistance and support to the subnational levels to strengthen social participation in health.

The Region's results for indicator 2 (strengthening of social participation in health) were less variable, while indicator 3 (support for subnational levels) exhibited the greatest dispersion. The fact that some countries exhibited generally better or worse performance is manifested by the existence of extreme values, as can be seen in Figure 14.

The primary factors determining performance of this function in the Region are as follows:

- Approximately 84% of the countries have formal agencies for receiving public comments on health issues, and 57% have formal forums for consulting with the public on health issues. However, fewer than a third of the countries ensure that comments are answered.

- Half of the countries have an independent "public defense" office, with legal and governmental powers, charged with protecting the public's interest in the area of health.

- Approximately 62% of the countries stated that they issue a public national report on health status at least every

2 years, although only 24% disseminate its results through the communications media. Only a few countries have formal channels for receiving public comments on these reports.

- Procedures and formal channels for receiving and responding to public comments on health issues do not exist.

- Approximately 65% of the countries stated that they have carried out public consultations that were helpful in determining national health goals and objectives and can mention specific examples of citizen contributions in this regard.

- Weaknesses were acknowledged in the development of strategies for informing the public of their rights with respect to health. Only 32% of the countries stated that they had carried out specific actions to this end.

- Personnel trained in promoting community participation in health programs are available, although there are

Figure 14 Distribution of the performance of the Indicators for EPHF 4 in the Countries of the Region

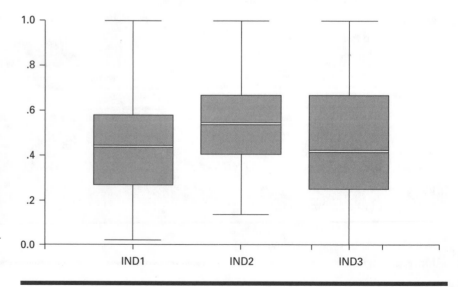

132

weaknesses in the areas of leadership, teamwork, and conflict resolution.

- The countries promote the development of good practices with regard to community participation. Roughly 49% of the countries disseminate these good practices to other countries, and 70% have access to resources (sectoral and extrasectoral) in order to promote community participation activities.

- The majority of the countries have formal mechanisms for promoting social participation in health at the local and intermediate levels, including organization directories and promoting meetings, forums, workshops, and other activities in order to promote participation in health-related subjects.

- In general, the capacity to promote social participation with respect to health and the capacity to use the results of such efforts are not evaluated.

- With regard to support for subnational levels, the primary weaknesses were found in evaluating the results of participation, designing mechanisms for receiving and responding to public comments, designing systems for explaining health status, and designing mechanisms for conflict resolution.

EPHF 5: Development of Policies and Institutional Capacity for Planning and Management in Public Health

This function exhibited intermediate performance, with a median of 0.56 for the Region. In general, it can be observed that the majority of the countries exhibited intermediate performance, and only one country exhibited optimal performance, as shown in Figure 15.

Figure 15   Distribution of the performance level of EPHF 5 in the Countries of the Region

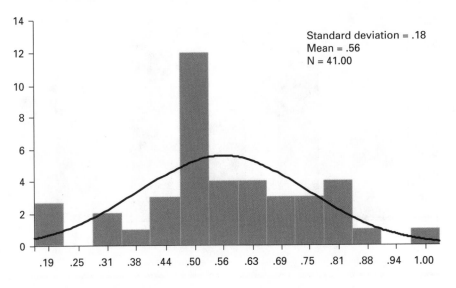

Standard deviation = .18
Mean = .56
N = 41.00

The indicators measured for this function revealed that the areas of lowest performance are the definition of national health objectives (Indicator 1) and NHA support to subnational levels for the performance of this function (Indicator 5). The areas of highest performance are the development of public health policies (Indicator 2) and the capacity for negotiating international cooperation (Indicator 4). Intermediate performance was shown in development of institutional capacity for the management of public health (Indicator 3), as can be observed in Figure 16.

The greatest weaknesses in public health management should alert health authorities to formulate policies, and the NHA in general, on the basis of the current and future challenges facing public health management. In addition, efforts should be made to identify measures that health authorities should take in order to increase institutional capacities, with the ultimate objective of improving public health.

Indicators:

1. Definition of national and subnational health objectives

2. Development, monitoring, and evaluation of public health policies

3. Development of institutional capacity for the management of public health systems

4. Negotiation of international cooperation in public health

5. Technical assistance and support to the subnational levels for policy development, planning, and management in public health.

Of the indicators that revealed the highest performance, the low dispersion of development, monitoring, and evaluation of public health policies (Indicator 2) makes it possible to conclude that this is an area of strength for the Region. This is not the case with regard to

Figure 16   Performance of the Indicators for EPHF 5

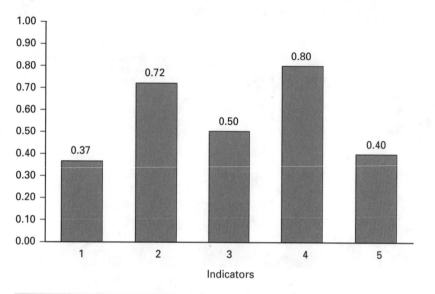

tent (68% of the countries), by the legislative branch. The majority of the countries follow through with legal instruments and needed legislation in order to implement these policies.

• Fewer than half of the countries consult current and potential allies in order to determine the degree of support for developing, implementing, and evaluating the process of improving national health policy. However, the private sector and the public are rarely included in these processes.

• All of the countries have personnel trained in policy development, the preparation of legal documents, and the prioritization of public health policies. In addition, the majority of the countries have qualified personnel and resources for managing international cooperation projects and programs.

• With regard to institutional management capacity, strengths were observed in strategic planning and leadership in the area of health. The

the indicator management of international cooperation (Indicator 4), which exhibited the greatest variability among the countries of the Region; although it generally revealed adequate performance, it continues to be an area of weakness for some countries.

The indicators that presented low and intermediate performance (the definition of public health objectives, the public health management, and support for subnational levels) reveal optimal performance by some countries and weak performance by many others, as shown in Figure 17.

The primary factors determining performance of this function in the Region are as follows:

• In the majority of the countries, the NHA spearheads the process of defining health goals and objectives, which are based on each country's health priorities. However, the countries acknowledged weaknesses in updating health priorities, and 43% stated that health objectives and social policy objectives are directly related. The perti-

nent actors, such as civil society, do not always participate in formulating these objectives. Roughly 51% of the countries stated that indicators had been developed to measure the effective performance of established health objectives.

• By and large, the countries have health policy plans supported by the executive branch and, to a lesser ex-

Figure 17   Distribution of the performance of the indicators of EPHF 5 in the Countries of the Region

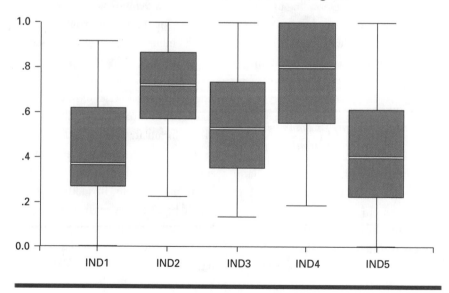

majority of the countries stated that they have skilled and knowledgeable personnel in strategic planning; 64% stated that they have carried out a planning exercise in the last year and that the greatest weakness in this area is evaluating and monitoring the strategic planning process. With regard to leadership, the majority of the countries stated that they have the capacity to generate consensus and promote inter-institutional collaboration with regard to public health, and 65% have used this experience to channel resources toward health. The greatest weaknesses were observed in the areas of conflict resolution and communications skills.

- The countries indicated that adequate financing mechanisms that might help achieve health objectives are unavailable.

- In addition, weaknesses were observed in the development of performance indicators for measuring the achievement of the defined health objectives. Only 51% of the countries have indicators, and 38% develop the evaluation through participatory processes. The majority of the countries do not consult the private sector with regard to this evaluation.

- The NHA has difficulty in establishing alliances in order to implement health policies. In general, they do not work with private sector health services providers, insurers, authorities responsible for health social security, or consumers.

- The primary weaknesses in institutional capacity for public health management are found in the decision making process, based on evidence and organizational development, in order to achieve the desired public health objectives. Some 43% of the countries stated that they did not have a clear organizational vision to guide management; only 32% of the countries learn from changes, and 27% evaluate institutional performance.

- The areas of weakness in support to subnational levels coincide with the areas of weakness in the NHA. It was acknowledged that a widely-shared weakness in the majority of the countries is difficulty in determining necessary actions for supporting management at subnational levels and responding in a timely and appropriate manner.

EPHF 6: Strengthening of Institutional Capacity for Regulation and Enforcement in Public Health

In general, the majority of the countries performed this function at the low-intermediate level, with a median of 0.47 and quite homogeneous results, as shown in Figure 18.

Except for better performance concerning the development of public health regulatory frameworks (Indicator 1), the remaining indicators revealed poor performance, particularly with regard to the enforcement of regulations (Indicator 2), as shown in Figure 19.

Health legislation is regarded as an instrument for the implementation of health policy, taking into account the evolving role of the State and its relationship to civil society. In this regard, the countries' efforts to reformulate existing legal frameworks for the regulation of health-related rights and responsibilities demand that the NHA assist the public, the State, and the private sector in effectively exercising these rights and responsibilities.

Indicators:

1. Periodic monitoring, evaluation, and modification of the regulatory framework

2. Enforcement of laws and regulations

Figure 18   Distribution of the performance level of EPHF 6 in the Countries of the Region

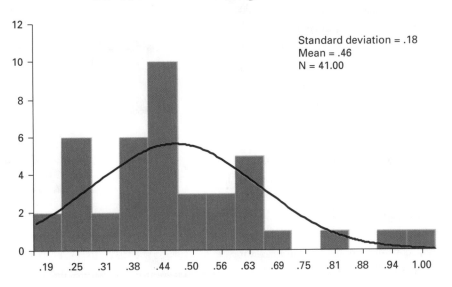

Standard deviation = .18
Mean = .46
N = 41.00

Figure 19 Performance of the Indicators for EPHF 6

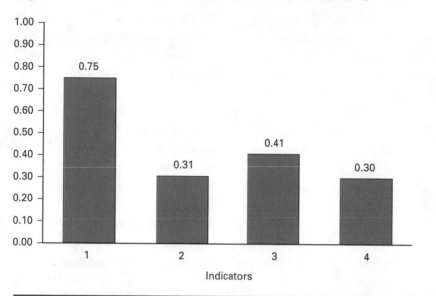

3. Knowledge, skills, and mechanisms for reviewing, improving, and enforcing the regulations

4. Technical assistance and support to the subnational levels of public health in developing and enforcing laws and regulations.

The variability of the results obtained for each country demonstrates lower dispersion with respect to the weaknesses concerning enforcement of regulations (Indicator 2), and lower dispersion with respect to the regulatory framework (indicator 1). The highest variability index was observed in support for subnational levels. This leads to the conclusion that weak enforcement of regulations is common to the majority of the countries. Although institutional competencies and aptitudes, as well as support for decentralized levels, constitute strengths for some countries, they continue to be critical areas for others (see Figure 20).

The primary factors determining performance of this function in the Region are as follows:

• The majority of the countries have competent personnel knowledgeable

in legislative procedures and public health regulations, sufficient health advisory services from international organizations, and sufficient institutional competencies and resources to draft health regulations.

• The countries review existing regulations for purposes of producing and modifying draft legislation. However, only 11% of the participating countries stated that they perform reviews in a timely manner (anticipating problems); 24% perform them periodically. Rather than the above, action is taken in response to pressures external to the NHA, both from the governments and from other actors.

• The NHA leads the process of modifying the regulatory framework, offering technical assistance directly to lawmakers and seeking to persuade the pertinent actors involved in making the suggested legal modifications.

Figure 20 Distribution of the performance of the indicators of EPHF 6 in the Countries of the Region

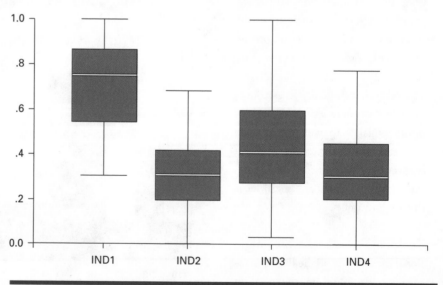

- Although most of the countries identified personnel responsible for enforcement, only 30% stated that they supervise enforcement procedures, while a lower percentage stated that they monitor the timeliness and effectiveness of enforcement efforts. Roughly 80% do not supervise the abuse or misuse of authority by enforcement agencies, and the countries generally do not have systems for promoting the proper use of authority by personnel.

- Approximately 51% of the countries stated that they have mechanisms for educating the public about the importance of following existing regulations, and only 11% have incentives aimed at encouraging the public to comply with regulations.

- Another critical area concerns the promotion of plans and actions aimed at preventing corruption. Although some countries have anti-corruption measures, these are not evaluated, and actions aimed at preventing the influence of power groups are not even considered. Roughly 46% of the countries have warning and punishment systems for illegal practices, and the public is aware of these systems in 35%.

- In general, the countries do not have enough personnel or resources to strengthen enforcement efforts, which is the primary critical area for performance of this function in the Region.

- Although new personnel are trained in enforcement issues and training courses are offered, only 24% of the countries ensure ongoing training in this area. Approximately 40% of the countries stated that they evaluate their training programs.

- In the majority of the countries, subnational levels are provided with support in implementing enforcement procedures and complex enforcement operations. However, the technical assistance that is provided is not periodically evaluated, and subnational levels are not provided with information on the development of local regulations.

EPHF 7: *Evaluation and Promotion of Equitable Access to Necessary Health Services*

This function exhibited intermediate performance for the Region, with a median of 0.55. The performance profile is quite heterogeneous, and some groups of countries were found to have different levels of development for this function, as shown in the Figure 21. Although some countries exhibited lower performance, it is important to point out that a considerable number of countries exhibited performance higher than 70% with respect to the indicators used, which, in some way, reflects the emphasis placed on this health objective.

The lowest performance was for evaluation of access to services (Indicator 1). The remaining indicators—namely, institutional capacities and skills for developing actions to improve access by the population to health services (Indicator 2), advocacy and action to improve access to necessary health services (Indicator 3), and NHA technical assistance and support to subnational levels to promote performance of this function (Indicator 4)—revealed intermediate performance.

Indicators:

1. Monitoring and evaluation of access to necessary health services

2. Knowledge, skills, and mechanisms for improving access by the population to necessary health services

Figure 21   Distribution of the performance level of EPHF 7 in the Countries of the Region

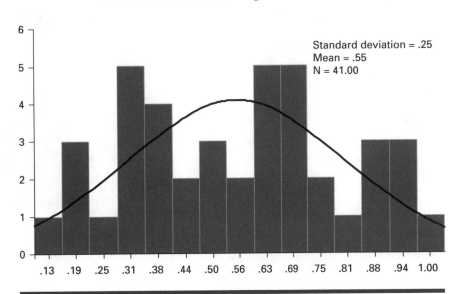

Standard deviation = .25
Mean = .55
N = 41.00

Figure 22   Performance of the Indicators for EPHF 7

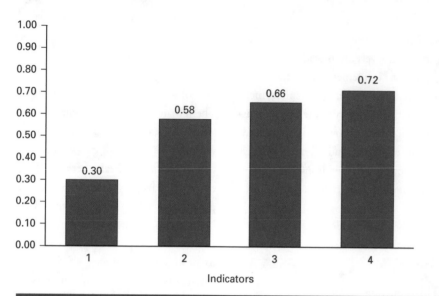

3. Advocacy and action to improve access to necessary health services

4. Technical assistance and support to the subnational levels to promote equitable access to health services.

With regard to the variability of the performance revealed by the indicators in the various countries of the Region, it can be seen that Indicator 7.3 revealed better overall performance and exhibited lower dispersion, essentially confirming that this is an area of strength for the Region. The remaining indicators exhibited maximum dispersion. This implies that there is one group of countries with relatively better performance, and another group of countries for which these indicators are critical areas in need of improvement (see Figure 23).

The primary factors determining performance of this function in all or the majority of the countries are as follows:

• In general, the evaluation of access to population-based health services is better than evaluation of access to personal health services (especially due to the absence of information from private health services and from the social security institutions). Roughly 57% of the countries stated that they have indicators to objectively evaluate access to health services. A critical area common to the entire Region is the failure to identify and disseminate good practices aimed at removing barriers to access. In general, few countries use the results of these evaluations to implement strategies aimed at reducing barriers to access.

• It is noteworthy that a low percentage of the participants identified barriers related to ethnic groups, cultural or religious barriers, or barriers based on sexual orientation. Approximately 46% of the countries stated that they included gender differences as a criterion in this analysis.

• The greatest weaknesses in developing strategies and actions aimed at improving access to health services for people without access to these services are related to the extent to which personnel have knowledge and experience in orienting users when linguistic barriers exist, as well as to designing actions aimed at improving access to services for the most vulner-

Figure 23   Distribution of the performance of the Indicators for EPHF 7 in the Countries of the Region

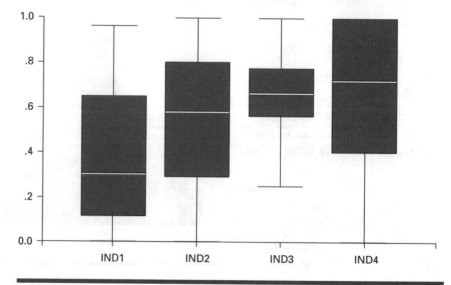

able populations. Another weakness is insufficient systematic evaluations of efforts to reduce barriers to access. On the other hand, the majority of the countries have the institutional capacity to develop early detection programs and to implement innovative methods for improving access (mobile clinics, fairs, etc.)

- The countries performed well with respect to developing laws and regulations aimed at improving access for the neediest and with respect to carrying out actions directed toward reducing barriers to access, especially for vulnerable groups. Half of the countries advocate incorporating this knowledge into human resources education and inform decision-makers of findings concerning barriers to access. In general, the greatest weaknesses of the NHA were in developing actions designed to enable other actors responsible for providing health services to reduce barriers to access (private organizations and social security institutions).

- In terms of actions directed toward reducing existing gaps, all of the countries exhibited strength in their capacity to inform the public of how to access health services.

- Major weaknesses exist in the development of incentive systems for service providers (public and private) aimed at reducing the access gaps that were found. Approximately 46% of the countries indicated that they have local measures for encouraging the development of actions aimed at promoting more equitable access to health services.

- All of the countries provide subnational levels with assistance in deter-

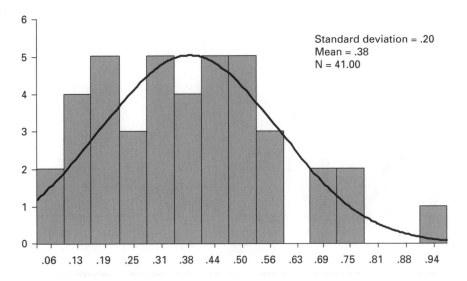

Figure 24 Distribution of the performance level of EPHF 8 in the Countries of the Region

Standard deviation = .20
Mean = .38
N = 41.00

mining a basic package of individual and collective services that should be available to the entire population. However, the performance of those responsible for providing this basic package of pre-established services is not regularly evaluated, particularly with regard to the most vulnerable or underserved populations.

EPHF 8: *Human Resources Development and Training in Public Health*

This function exhibited low performance, with a median of 0.38 for the Region. In general, it can be said that the majority of the countries exhibited low and intermediate performance; however, a limited number exhibited better performance, as shown in Figure 24.

Although all of the indicators revealed low performance, the following areas are critical for the Region: improving quality, promoting continuing education and graduate training in public

health, and increasing concern about educating personnel in issues that promote the culturally appropriate delivery of services to the populations of these countries (see Figure 25).

Indicators:

1. Description of the public health workforce

2. Improving the quality of the workforce

3. Continuing education and graduate training in public health

4. Upgrading human resources to ensure culturally appropriate delivery of services

5. Technical assistance and support to the subnational levels in human resources development.

In general, the results for this function exhibit little variability for Indicators

Figure 25 Performance of the Indicators for EPHF 8

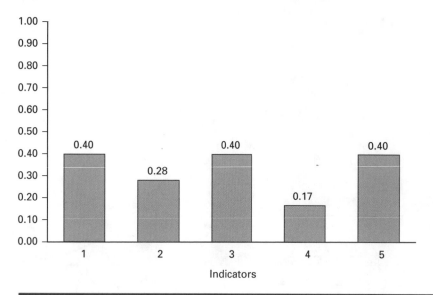

8.3 (continuing education) and 8.2 (Improving the quality of the workforce). The remaining indicators (8.1, 8.4 and 8.5) exhibit greater dispersion, which indicates that some countries exhibit better performance in comparison to the rest of the Region (Figure 26).

The primary factors determining performance of this function in all or the majority of the countries are as follows:

• Although the participating countries evaluate the characteristics of the workforce, only 50% define personnel needs for public health functions, including determining the size, profile, and required competencies of the staff. This hinders NHA efforts to strengthen appropriate human resources development for public health, both with regard to the individuals they train themselves and with regard

to those who graduate from training centers. In addition, one of the greatest weaknesses was found to be criteria for determining needs for future growth.

• As for improving the quality of the workforce, although guidelines for personnel accreditation do exist, adherence to these guidelines in hiring is not evaluated. Strategies for selecting and retaining workers are evaluated in only a few countries. Approximately 19% of the participating countries stated that their training programs include ethics as a pertinent field of study. Incentives for strengthening leadership among public health personnel do not exist, and only 11% of the participating countries promote the retention of leaders. Although half of the countries have performance evaluation systems, only 32% establish measurable results, and few use the results for allocating responsibility and incentives for retaining workers on the basis of demonstrated merits.

• In the majority of the countries, participation in continuing education is encouraged, training for less-experienced personnel is offered, and agreements have been reached with training centers for this purpose. However, none of the countries have clear policies and regulations for ensuring that human resources education is of an appropriate level, none have systems for evaluating the results of human resources education and training, and none have mechanisms for retaining the most qualified personnel, resulting in an ongoing loss of the potential benefits of these education and training activities.

• With regard to support for subnational levels in the performance of this function, less than a third provide sup-

Figure 26 Distribution of the performance of the Indicators for EPHF 8 in the Countries of the Region

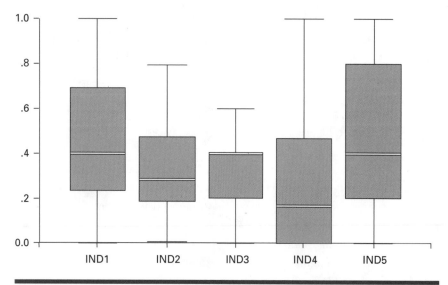

port for the identification of human resources appropriate to the sociocultural and linguistic characteristics of the users, while 51% of the countries do not promote decentralized strategies for improving human resources management in accordance with the needs of local and intermediate levels.

EPHF 9: *Quality Assurance in Personal and Population-based Health Services*

This function exhibited the lowest performance for the Region, with a median of 0.26. The profile of the participating countries reveals similar results; all of the countries exhibiting low-to-intermediate performance, with the exception of one country that exhibited better performance and clearly distanced itself from the group, as shown in Figure 27.

Although all of the indicators revealed very low performance, it is worth noting that there were small advances with regard to health technology assessment to support decision-making in public health (Indicator 3) and the improvement of user satisfaction with health services (Indicator 2). The low support for the subnational levels (Indicator 4) is due to the low development of this function in general (see Figure 28).

Indicators:

1. Definition of standards and evaluation to improve the quality of population-based and personal health services

2. Improving user satisfaction with the health services

3. Systems for technological management and health technology assessment to support decision-making in public health

Figure 27 Distribution of the performance level of EPHF 9 in the Countries of the Region

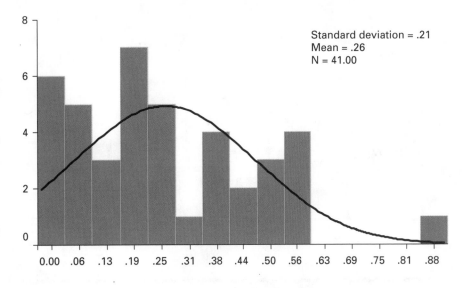

Standard deviation = .21
Mean = .26
N = 41.00

4. Technical assistance and support to the subnational levels to ensure quality improvement in the services.

The greatest variability in the results obtained by the participating countries was found in the definition of standards and evaluation to improve the quality of health services (Indicator 9.1), and in support for the subnational levels (Indicator 9.4), which, despite being a weakness for the Region, is an area in which there was considerable progress in some countries. On the other hand, concern for improving user satisfaction with health services is a critical area for all of

Figure 28 Performance of the Indicators for EPHF 9

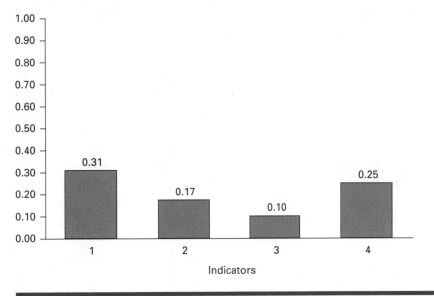

141

Figure 29 Distribution of the performance of the Indicators of EPHF 9 in the Countries of the Region

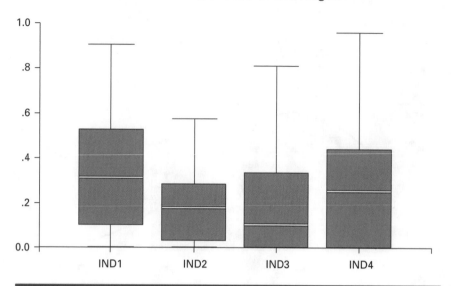

the participating countries and exhibited the least dispersion. It was confirmed that a third of the Region's countries failed to exhibit any progress with respect to Indicator 9.3 (see Figure 29).

The primary factors determining performance of this function in the majority of the countries are as follows:

- Approximately 49% of the countries promote policies aimed at continuously improving the quality of health services. Some 43% apply quality performance standards, and 27% have measured their progress in this area. In general, few countries evaluate the quality of services, and even fewer disseminate results to the public. Only 22% of the countries have autonomous agencies that accredit and evaluate the quality of health services providers.

- By and large, a greater increase was observed in actions aimed at evaluating the quality of personal health services (particularly those aimed at

evaluating processes and, less frequently, results) than in those aimed at evaluating the quality of population-based health services.

- In general, national systematic and periodic strategies for evaluating user satisfaction with health services (both personal and population-based health services) have been developed by very limited degree; however, the participating countries described several isolated experiences at the local and intermediate levels. Approximately 41% of the countries use the results to enhance strategies for improving health services quality, but it was acknowledged that these results are not used to guide decision-making in this area and that the results are not communicated to users. In general, the majority of the countries do not have mechanisms for ensuring the confidentiality of information provided by users.

- Approximately 30% of the countries have an agency responsible for technological management and for sup-

porting decision-making in this area, although no evidence was provided of any major successes related to supporting the health policy decision-making process or delivering recommendations on technology use to health services authorities. Although insufficient, the countries acknowledged some progress in evaluating the safety and effectiveness of technology.

- In keeping with the low level of performance exhibited for this function, it was observed that the NHA provides partial support to subnational levels, particularly with respect to evaluating the quality of personal health services.

EPHF 10: *Research in Public Health*

Public health research is another function exhibiting low performance, with a median of 0.42. Based on the results obtained, the distribution profile of the participating countries indicates that a majority exhibited low-to-intermediate performance, with the exception of several countries that exhibited higher performance, as shown in Figure 30.

With regard to the performance revealed by the indicators used in this measurement, the Region's primary weakness is the lack of national public health research agendas. Better relative performance was exhibited in developing the institutional research capacity of the NHA (Figure 31).

Indicators:

1. Development of a public health research agenda

2. Development of institutional research capacity

3. Technical assistance and support for research in public health at the subnational levels

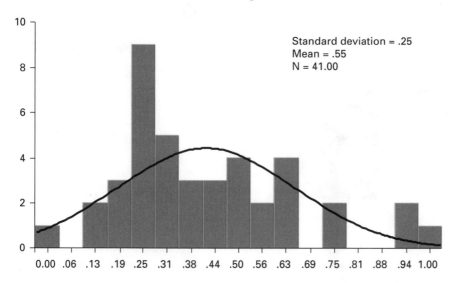

Standard deviation = .25
Mean = .55
N = 41.00

As for dispersion, low variability was generally observed for indicator 10.1, indicating that the lack of national public health research agenda is a weakness for the Region. The other indicators exhibit greater variability; while the majority of the countries did not demonstrate sufficient development in these areas, other countries exhibited strengths (see Figure 32).

The primary factors determining performance of this function in all or the majority of the countries are as follows:

- Although 49% of the countries stated that they have an agency in charge of the national agenda, significant weaknesses were observed in the preparation of these agenda. In general, the

Figure 31 Performance of the Indicators for EPHF 10

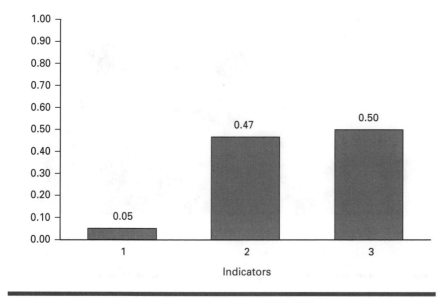

Indicators

countries stated that public health research does not consider the current lack of knowledge with regard to managing health priorities, does not conduct tests in order to improve health services management, does not ensure the economic feasibility and sustainability of innovations in public health, and does not provide support for making important political decisions with regard to public health.

- Progress in fulfilling the public health research agenda is not periodically evaluated; if it is evaluated, the results are not communicated to the parties involved.

- Weakness exists in the relationship with researchers, particularly researchers who come from outside the NHA (e.g., from academia), and the results of NHA research are only partially disseminated to the rest of the scientific community.

- No mechanisms exist for ensuring that public health research corresponds to national priorities. Although half of the countries have procedures for approving research, only 19% evaluate the importance of the subject. Few countries stated that they have formal, transparent mechanisms for assigning research funds.

- The availability of tools and experts for the promotion of public health research, as well as the fact that the NHA tend to use research results, are strengths in all of the countries. The vast majority of the countries can give examples of public health research in the last two years.

- The primary research strengths are epidemiology and food poisoning;

Figure 32 Distribution of the performance level of EPHF 10 in the Countries of the Region

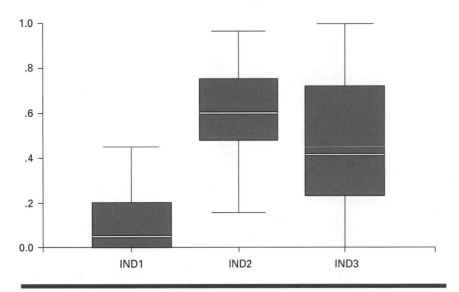

gency and disaster management efforts are insufficient.

Indicators:

1. Reducing the impact of emergencies and disasters

2. Development of standards and guidelines that support emergency preparedness and disaster management in health

3. Coordination and partnerships with other agencies and/or institutions

4. Technical assistance and support to the subnational levels to reduce the impact of emergencies and disasters on health.

The greatest variability among the countries was observed for Indicators 11.1 and 11.2. Several countries acknowledged that they had made no progress in these areas, particularly in the develop-

the primary weaknesses are research on risk factors for chronic diseases and research on collective interventions and community health.

• The countries provide subnational levels with partial support for research, and the majority promotes the participation of subnational level professionals in research. In addition, 32% of the participating countries indicated that they disseminate the results of this research.

EPHF 11: *Reducing the Impact of Emergencies and Disasters on Health*

This is one of the best-performing functions for the Region, with a median of 0.69. The distribution profile indicates low dispersion in the specific results for each country, with the exception of several countries for which this continues to be a critical area, as shown in Figure 33.

Although the majority of the indicators revealed good performance, shortcomings were still observed in the perfor-

mance of the NHA in the area of management for reducing the impact of emergencies and disasters (Indicator 1). This profile of the Region demonstrates that, despite the existence of institutional mechanisms, the results of emer-

Figure 33 Distribution of the performance level of EPHF 11 in the Countries of the Region

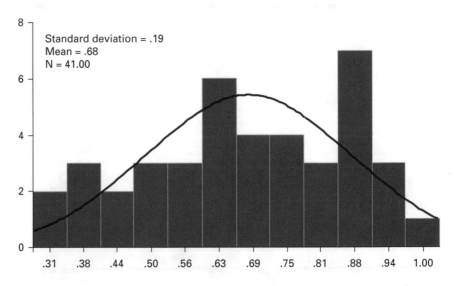

Figure 34 Performance of the Indicators for EPHF 11

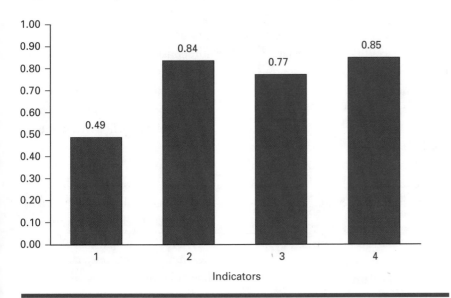

ment of standards and guidelines. This indicates that although this function is, for the most part, performed acceptably well throughout the Region, some countries still exhibit significant weaknesses.

The primary factors determining performance of this function in the Region are as follows:

- Approximately 80% of the countries have sectoral plans integrated into a national emergency program, and 50% have maps of hazards and risks for emergencies and disasters. Approximately 70% of the countries have a specialized body devoted to the subject, and 30% indicated that this body has an allocated budget.

Figure 35 Distribution of the performance level of the Indicators of EPHF 11 in the Countries of the Region

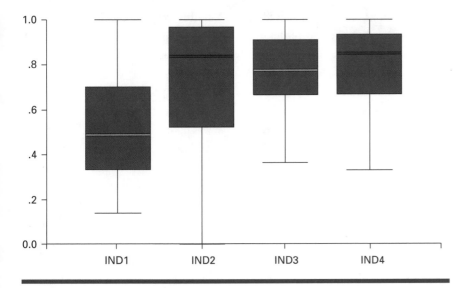

- The countries acknowledged that one of the critical areas concerning NHA management of emergencies and disasters is insufficient coordination within the health sector in the event of emergencies and disasters.

- The health sector's primary weaknesses in the management of emergencies and disasters are in addressing mental health problems, managing health services under these circumstances, and periodically carrying out simulation exercises. However, with regard to human resources education, it was acknowledged that adequate institutional capacity exists to address subjects such as basic sanitation, vectors, and infectious and communicable diseases.

- The greatest weakness in current regulations concerns treatment of mental health problems; 50% of the countries acknowledged weakness with respect to the vulnerability of health infrastructure.

- The countries stated that there is good coordination between the remaining institutions, and between national institutions and international organizations, in these cases. In general, the countries maintain relationships with the vast majority of the organizations concerned with disaster response issues, and they collaborate with neighboring nations and other bodies in the event of emergencies.

- In general, the NHA provide a high level of support and assistance to the subnational levels. Roughly 70% of the participating countries stated that they periodically assess the needs of subnational levels in the event of emergencies and disasters, although this does not necessarily mean that the shortcomings that are uncovered are corrected, given the limited availability of resources for this purpose.

1.3 Identification of priority intervention areas in order to prepare a program for strengthening the EPHF in the Region of the Americas

1.3.1 Profile of all indicators

In order to provide a guide for the preparation of national and Regional plans for developing the institutional capacities of the national health authorities of the participating countries, as well as for structuring a program for strengthening public health in the Region, the indicators have been ordered so as to facilitate an integrated analysis. For the majority of the countries, the analysis will cover indicators representing strengths that must be maintained and strengthened, and other areas of poorer performance that should be strengthened.

The Region exhibited the lowest performance in the development of national public health research programs.

Reflecting the low performance of the function, all of the indicators related to health service quality assurance (definition of standards, monitoring health service quality, improving user satisfaction, health technology assessment) constitute critical areas that should be strengthened.

The development of human resources in public health and, in particular, efforts aimed at improving the quality of human resources, also constitute a major challenge in ensuring the improvement of public health in the countries of the Region.

In addition, the evaluation of the quality of information in order to subsequently evaluate health status, the monitoring of equitable access to necessary health services, and the generation of timely responses to public health threats are all common critical areas in need of improvement.

Finally, a critical issue concerning the role of the NHA and regulation is the low performance exhibited with regard to compliance with existing regulations.

1.3.2 Analysis of the Indicators by Area of Intervention

The profile of all of the indicators determined to be strengths or weaknesses for the Region appears below, organized according to the three intervention areas described in the previous chapter. In order to facilitate the analysis, the indicators for each function have been given a different color.

Based on a level of success equal to or higher than 70% of the established standard, the primary strengths exhibited by the majority of the countries of the Region in performing the essential public health functions, and which should be maintained in the programs of the pertinent countries, are as follows:

- Intervention and action in the most important processes for achieving results; surveillance systems aimed at identifying public health risks and threats; developing, monitoring, evaluating health policies; reviewing, evaluating, and modifying the regulatory framework; developing standards and guidelines for reducing the impact of emergencies and disasters on health; and collaborating and estab-

lishing alliances with other agencies and/or institutions for this purpose.

- The development of public health institutional capacities and infrastructure; monitoring and evaluating health status; the capacities of public health laboratories; and the capacity to manage international cooperation.

- With regard to developing the competencies of decentralized bodies in performing public health functions, subnational levels must continue to be supported in the areas of public health monitoring, research, controlling risks and threats, and reducing damage caused by emergencies and disasters.

Based on a level of success equal to or lower than 40% of the established standard, the primary weaknesses exhibited by the Region, and which should be included in a program for the improvement of public health, are as follows:

- In order to strengthen important processes, progress should be made in: evaluating the quality of information available for monitoring the health status of the population; enforcing health regulations; improving user satisfaction; and developing national public health research programs.

- With respect to investing in institutional capacities and infrastructure, as was pointed out earlier, it is necessary to: improve the quality of human resources; develop actions for promoting continuing education, life-long education, and graduate education in public health; and to train human resources to provide services in ways that take into account the sociocultural backgrounds of the users. Finally,

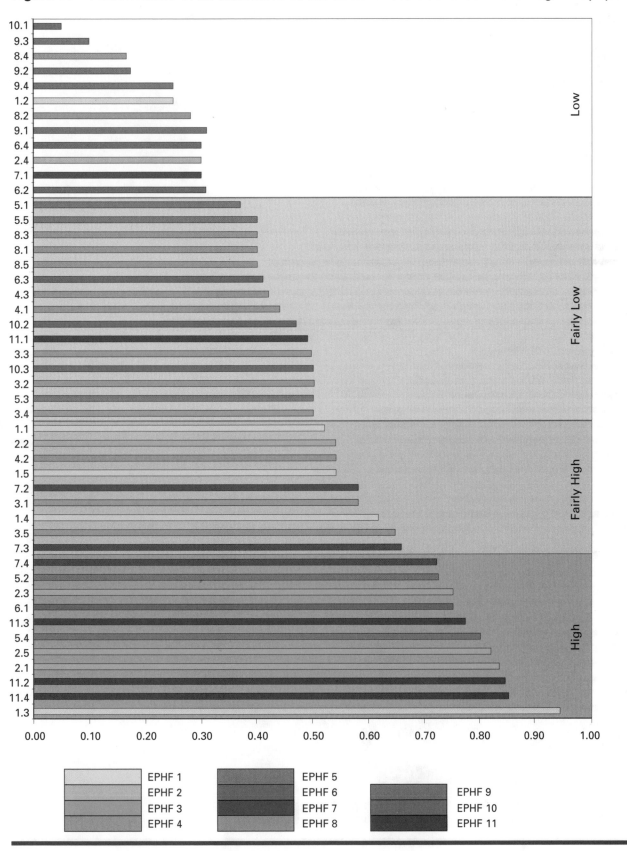

Figure 37 Performance of all the indicators of the EPHF according to priority areas of intervention

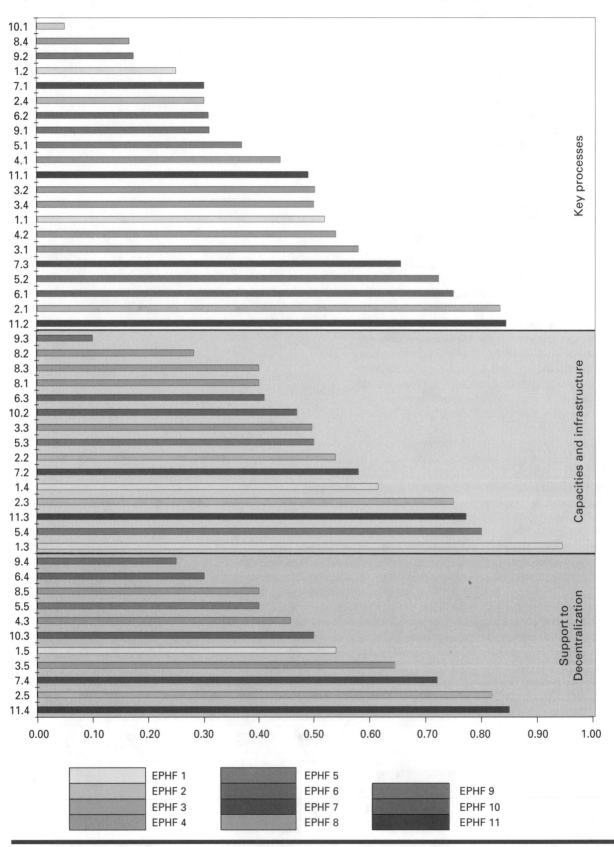

the primary weakness of the Region is the insufficient development of technological management and health technology assessment systems to support decision-making.

- The primary weaknesses with respect to NHA support for subnational levels in the performance of public health functions are enforcement of health laws and regulations, and guaranteeing and improving the quality of personal and population-based health services.

1.3.3 Performance Profile According to the Action Priorities of the World Bank

Finally, the indicators have been regrouped in order to make the results of the measurement useful within the framework of the cooperation strategies of the World Bank. This will make it easier to identify action priorities that correspond to the significant gaps in the public health profiles of the countries in question, as well as to identify investment needs. The proposed categories[5] are:

1. Development of health policies.

2. Collection and dissemination of evidence to guide public health policies, strategies, and actions.

3. Disease prevention and control.

4. Intersectoral intervention to improve health.

5. Human resources development and building public health institutional capacity

[5] The indicators assigned to each of these categories are defined at the end of the chapter.

These categories enable one to give priority to public health actions in the health policy and financing debate, making it possible to define health improvement goals on the basis of the characteristics of the health system, infrastructure, and institutional capacity to respond to public needs, rather than on the basis of the specific health problems.

The level of EPHF performance makes it possible to test the effects of health policies and programs, which helps to determine how and why particular efforts fail to achieve the expected level of performance. As a result, policies and action programs can be adjusted as necessary.

It is also possible to use the results of the EPHF measurement to monitor and evaluate the formulation and implementation of health strategies designed to reduce poverty, particularly those aimed at guaranteeing equitable access and health services quality.

Measuring the EPHF makes it possible to identify the countries' gaps in knowledge, resources, human capital, and institutional capacity to respond to health challenges, making it easier to quantify what resources are needed to ensure an adequate public health infrastructure.

Development of health policies

The areas in need of strengthening must be seen in relation to the ability to define national health objectives in cooperation with the actors involved in improving health; these objectives must also be consistent with decisions concerning the structure of the health system. It is particularly important to point out that one of the most significant weaknesses is the lack of *indicators* for evaluating the achievement of national objectives over

time. Although the countries have the knowledge and institutional capacity to monitor and evaluate health policies, these efforts are still focused on the actions of the public sector, without taking into account the existence and potential policy contributions of other actors (the private sector, social security institutions, and others). A critical area in the Region is the insufficient capacity of the NHA to ensure the quality of both personal and population-based health services; the capacity to define standards in order to subsequently evaluate quality is particularly weak. Another current challenge is the development of strategies aimed at including user satisfaction as key element in actions designed to improve health systems.

Collection and dissemination of evidence to guide public health policies, strategies, and actions

A critical area that must be strengthened is defining a *priority health research agenda* for the countries of the Region and promoting greater *interaction with the scientific community and other actors* capable of providing data that could support the decision-making process. The Region is beginning to develop technological management and health technology assessment strategies and actions that could help to improve public health policies. It should also be noted that many countries have not developed a systematic practice of *evaluating the quality of information* compiled by national health authorities. This weakness must be corrected in light of the fact that changing national priorities make it necessary to continually address the need for new data with respect to damage and risk factors, as well as with respect to the use of, and access to, health services. In many countries, the moni-

Figure 38 Performance of all the indicators of the EPHF according to priority areas of intervention Proposed by the World Bank

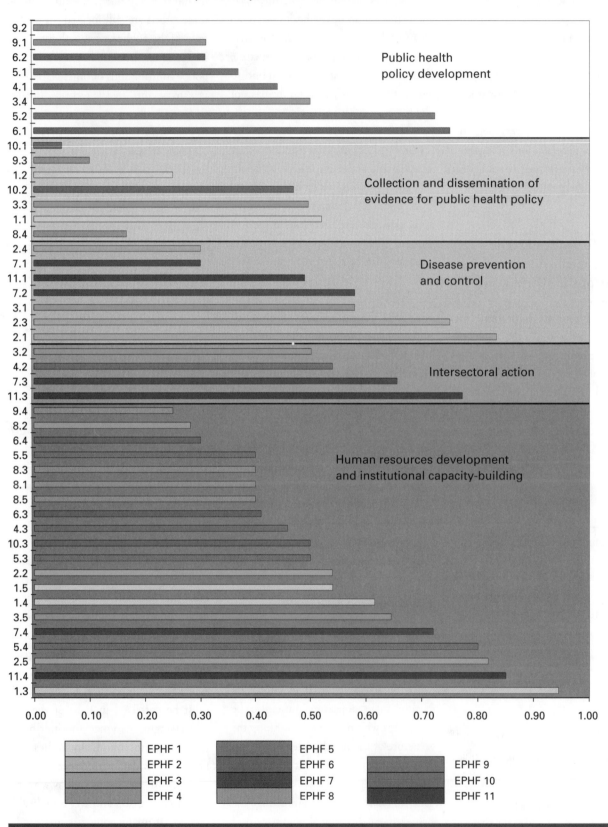

toring and evaluation of health status does not include analysis of risk factors, which are important variables for new diseases and for identifying trends in current priority epidemiological problems. Particular weakness was noted in the areas of mental health, risk factors for chronic diseases, and occupational health, among others.

Disease prevention and control

It is important to point out that shortcomings were observed in more than half of the participating countries in the *integrity of the sources of information for disease prevention and control*. The data continue to focus on the public sector, despite the growing role of the private sector (nonprofit and for-profit) in delivering services and the fact that this information must therefore be included in order to monitor public health threats. With regard to new areas of development, the principal deficiencies were observed in the monitoring of *threats to mental health, threats deriving from the work environment, and chronic disease or risk factors for chronic disease*. With regard to the health services, it is troubling that evaluations of public access to services are *barely used* to correct policies and plans aimed at improving the ability of poorly-served populations to access services. In the majority of the countries, the NHA addresses priorities through direct actions aimed at correcting the gaps in the populations at greatest risk, and less effort is made to encourage other pertinent actors to assume their roles and responsibilities with regard to this problem.

Human resources development and building institutional capacity

In this area, it is necessary to strengthen institutional capacity for performing

"emerging" public health functions, such as quality assurance, developing strategies designed to improve public access to health services, and providing support to subnational levels in order to increase health promotion and social participation in health. As was mentioned earlier, the majority of the countries generally exhibit low performance with regard to developing public health human resources, which constitutes a serious obstacle to improving the EPHF in the Region.

1.4 Initial Exploratory Analysis of the Performance of the EPHF and Their Relationship to Other Indicators

An initial exploratory analysis of the relationship between the performance of the essential public health functions, and some relevant characteristics of the participating countries, are provided below.

Although not the primary purpose of this evaluation, it is interesting to analyze the performance of the EPHF in relation to some of the indicators in order to determine whether differences exist between the EPHF profiles associated with these variables.

It is important to note that this analysis only attempts to show that such relationships exist; it does not attempt to explain the observed relationships, let alone establish cause-and-effect, since such efforts would go beyond the purpose of this evaluation. However, it is hoped that new lines of research based on the results given below will make it possible to achieve advances in this regard.

The chosen indicators are as follows:

DemoFigureic and socioeconomic features of the countries. These variables are understood to be independent of the performance of public health and may be determinants of the results exhibited by the countries in this measurement.

- Population
- Rural population percentage
- Per capita gross domestic product
- Population income equity: 20% higher income/20% lower income
- Total per capita health expenditure

Country organization. This refers particularly to how the governments and health systems are organized.

- Federal states/unitary states
- Type of health system: integrated public, mixed regulated, and segmented.

Health and quality-of-life outcome indicators. These are variables that can be influenced by the performance of the public health functions.

- Infant mortality
- Maternal mortality
- Mortality due to infectious diseases
- Life expectancy at birth
- Human development index

In the analysis presented below, the median performance of the various country groups has been used as a measure of the overall performance of the EPHF for purposes of evaluating performance.[6]

---

[6] The countries of the Region have been grouped by quartiles and terciles in order to analyze groups with more or less indicators.

1.4.1 The EPHF and the demoFigureic and socioeconomic features of the countries

The EPHF and the population

A comparison of the performance of each essential function for groups of countries with smaller populations (fewer than 120,000 inhabitants) and groups of countries with larger populations (more than 10 million inhabitants) reveals a generally similar performance profile. For EPHF 3 (health promotion), EPHF 5 (policies and management in public health), EPHF 8 (HR development), and EPHF 11 (disaster reduction), the smaller countries generally performed slightly better than the larger countries. The opposite situation was observed for the remaining functions, with the exception of EPHF 9 (quality assurance) and EPHF 7 (equitable access), for which performance was very similar.

Upon analyzing the performance of EPHF 8[7] by population quartiles, an inverse relationship is observed between population and EPHF performance, although this is not the case for the third quartile (countries with population between 2 and 10 million inhabitants). Leaving this fact aside, it may be stated that potentially better performance of this function depends upon the size of the country. In general, the most geoFigureically concentrated countries—which, for purposes of this analysis, are the smaller countries of the Caribbean—could achieve better performance in human resources development, because the necessary investment for achieving this end is much smaller than in larger

---

[7] The EPHF for which the two groups exhibit the greatest difference.

Figure 39   Performance of the EPHF according to Population Size of the Countries of the Region

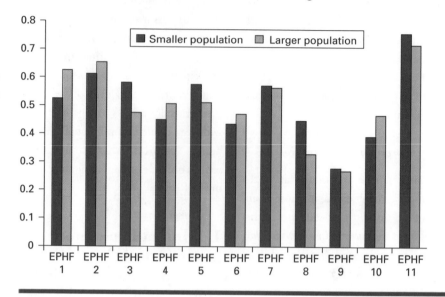

countries. The previous is confirmed by the fact that a positive correlation exists between the performance of this function and the educational level of the population, because the small countries of the Caribbean also have the highest literacy rates.

The EPHF and the rural population percentage

An analysis of performance of the EPHF in the countries grouped according to rural population percentage indicates that, for all of the functions (except EPHF 11), the median score of the group with the smaller rural population (less than 25%) is significantly higher than that of the group with the highest rural population (more than 53%), as shown in Figure 40.

If the performance of the countries is analyzed in terms of rural population percentage quartiles, it can generally be stated that the group of countries with the smallest rural population exhibits a significantly better performance profile

than the remaining groups, as shown below (see Figure 41).

In view of the above, it is important to keep in mind that results are more difficult to achieve in countries with larger rural populations, and that the drop-off point occurs at a rural population of approximately 25% (the last quartile).

The EPHF and per capita gross domestic product

The EPHF performance profile of groups with greater per capita GDP (higher than US$8,400) as compared to groups with lower per capita GDP (up to US$3,800) is heterogeneous. EPHF 7 and, to a lesser extent, EPHF 9 and 11 correlate positively with expenditure; in other words, the group with the highest per capita expenditure level also exhibits better performance of these functions. On the other hand, the opposite is true for EPHF 4 and, with insignificant differences, for EPHF 1, 5, 6, 8 and 10. The two groups exhibit virtually no difference for EPHF 2 and 3.

Figure 40   Performance of the EPHF according to Percentage of Rural Population in the Countries of the Region

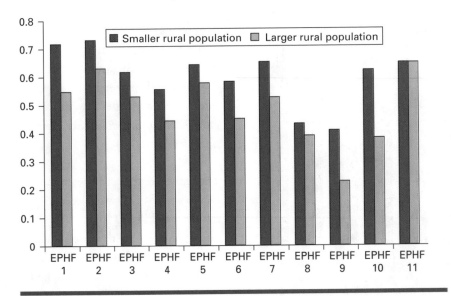

The fact that the poorest group of countries exhibited better performance with regard to social participation in health (EPHF 4) is consistent with the significant efforts and achievements of the governments of these countries. These efforts were aimed at promoting generally greater public participation, particularly in health, and they were often supported by nongovernmental organizations and international cooperation programs.

The following table (Figure 43) shows the EPHF profile of the participating countries, grouped by quartiles. The poorest quartile clearly stands out from the other groups, which indicates that performance of this function improves as per capita gross domestic product increases. This confirms what was indicated earlier, since the international cooperation organizations focus their interventions on the poorest countries of the world.

On the other hand, the opposite holds for equitable access to health services (EPHF 7), with regard to which the richest group exhibits the best performance. This partially reflects the population's generally higher standard of living. As a result, the users are more demanding, probably require the health authority to make a greater commitment to this fundamentally important task, and also have greater resources for health.

The poorest group of countries exhibits a slightly higher average than the quartile that follows it, despite the variability of the results exhibited by this group. This could partially reflect the efforts of multilateral agencies in recent decades, which have invested in projects aimed at improving public access to health services, particularly for the poor.

The EPHF and Income Distribution Equity

The coefficient separating the income of the richest 20% from that of the poorest 20% was used as an indicator for this analysis, both because it is an internationally accepted measure of income equity and because this information was available in the majority of the countries of the Region.

A comparison of the EPHF performance of countries with lower income distribution equity to the EPHF performance of countries with greater in-

Figure 41   Performance of the EPHF according to the Quartiles of Rurality of the Countries of the Region

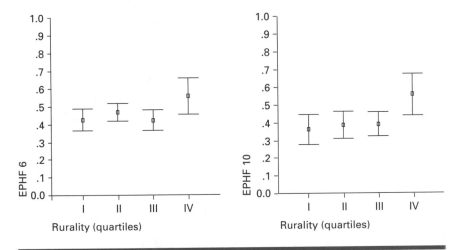

Figure 42 Performance of the EPHF According to GDP Per Capita

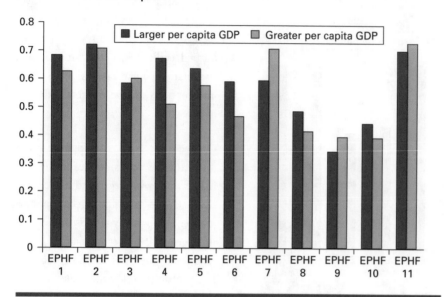

■ Larger per capita GDP ▨ Greater per capita GDP

come distribution equity[8] reveals better performance by the group with lower equity (except for EPHF 11). Considering that the health systems, particularly the public health system, should give first priority to serving groups at greatest health risk, and that poverty as a result of income inequity is an important public health risk factor, it may be concluded that the countries' performance (particularly that of the State) has been heading in the right direction with regard to the public health functions.

An analysis of various EPHF performance profiles for the countries of the Region grouped according to quartiles of income distribution equity always indicates that countries tend to exhibit better performance if they have lower income distribution equity, particularly

in the fourth quartile, which comprises the countries with the lowest equity in the Region.

This finding makes it possible to state (or at least not to discount) that countries with larger at-risk populations have carried out greater efforts in the area of public health.

Figure 43 Performance of the EPHF 4 According to GDP Per Capita

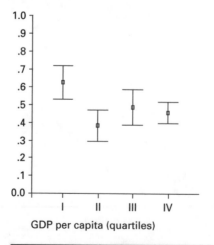

GDP per capita (quartiles)

---

[8] It is important to note that the comparison is of countries within the Region, which means that the description "greater equity" might not apply if the indicator were evaluated with respect to the entire world.

The EPHF and total health expenditure

An analysis of the relationship between performance of the EPHF and total per capita health expenditure reveals that the average performance of the group of countries with higher health expenditures is generally better than that of the group of countries with lower expenditures (see Figure 45).

The greatest difference between the two groups was observed with respect to performance of EPHF 7 (promotion of equitable access to health services). This is reasonable given that countries that invest more in health invest more in health services that meet public demands. It is therefore to be expected that better performance was observed in countries with higher health expenditures. The situation with respect to EPHF 10 (public health research) is similar, probably because countries with greater health resources are also able to invest in research. This does not occur in the countries in which health expenditures are more restricted, where allocation priorities are surely oriented primarily toward attempting to solve basic problems of public access to health services.

In particular, an analysis of the average performance of EPHF 7 by the countries grouped in quartiles according to health expenditure indicates a positive correlation between higher expenditure and better performance in the first three quartiles; the correlation is lower for the group with the most resources for health. These observations coincide with other studies on health variables that have demonstrated that performance increases significantly up to a certain level of expenditure, but that results do not improve beyond this level

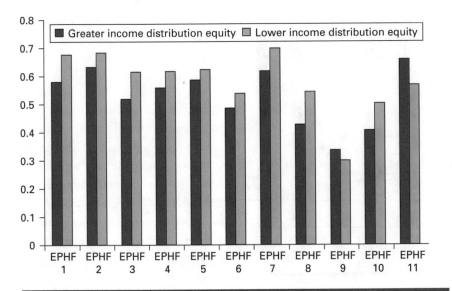

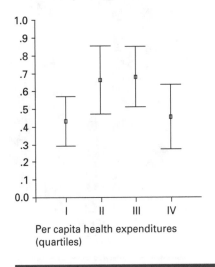

Per capita health expenditures (quartiles)

merely through an increase in expenditures (Figure 46).

The opposite situation was observed with respect to performance of EPHF 4 (social participation in health). This indicates that performance of this function is not necessarily associated with the availability of resources. As a result, countries with fewer health resources could obtain better results in this area if desired. The same is true for the observations for per capita gross domestic product.

1.4.2 The EPHF and country organization

The EPHF and type of government organization

It is interesting to evaluate the differences in the EPHF performance profiles of unitary countries and compare them with those of federal countries, as shown in Figure 47.

In general, the performance profile of the federal countries is higher than that of the unitary countries for all of the functions. The greatest differences were observed with respect to EPHF 1, 2, 3, 4, 5, 6, 7 and 10, the performance of which require significant institutional capacity, both in terms of infrastructure and organizational development. To some extent, these results are in accord with the situation concerning other governmental institutions, which, as a result

Figure 45   Performance of the EPHF According to Total Per Capita Expenditure in Health in the Countries of the Region

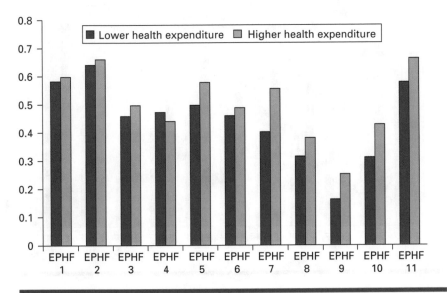

Figure 47   Performance of EPHF in Unitarian and Federal
Countries

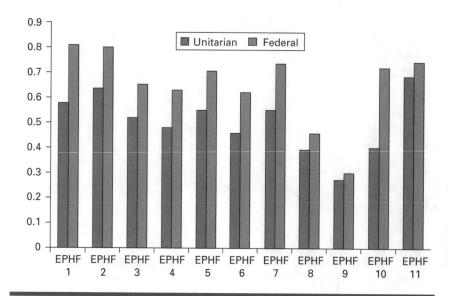

This assertion is consistent with the results exhibited for overall performance of the public health functions, presented previously, which indicated the existence of several more traditional models of public health management that assign a major role to the central health authority.

In light of this evidence, it is necessary to review how public health performance has been affected in greater depth, particularly in connection with health system reforms currently being implemented in the Region emphasizing mixed systems (public-private) under which the State plays a primarily regulatory role.

of federal organization into states, require greater institutional development at the decentralized level in view of insufficient capacities at the central level.

EPHF 8 and EPHF 9 do not show significant differences, which may reflect the generally poor development of this function throughout the Region regardless of this variable. Although federal countries have greater public health institutional capacities, the areas of public health human resources and quality assurance are still in need of development.

The EPHF and the type of health system

The health systems of the countries of the Region have been grouped into the following categories (defined by PAHO) according to their similarity: 1) integrated public system, 2) regulated mixed system, and 3) segmented system.

In general, performance of the EPHF is better (or very similar in the case of

EPHF 2) in countries with integrated public systems than in countries with other health systems. The regulated mixed system exhibits the poorest performance (with the exception of EPHF 11).

It is well known that the separation of the health functions, with the health authority being made responsible for regulating and supervising the good performance of the other actors in the health system (insurance and service

Figure 48   Performance of the EPHF According to Type of
Health System of the Countries

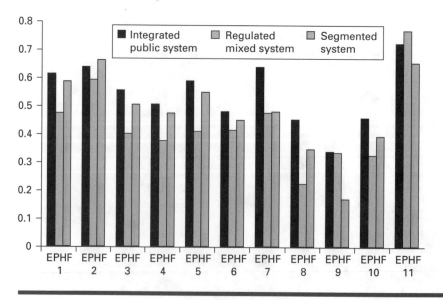

Figure 49 Performance of EPHF 1, 7 and 8 according to type of Health System of the Countries

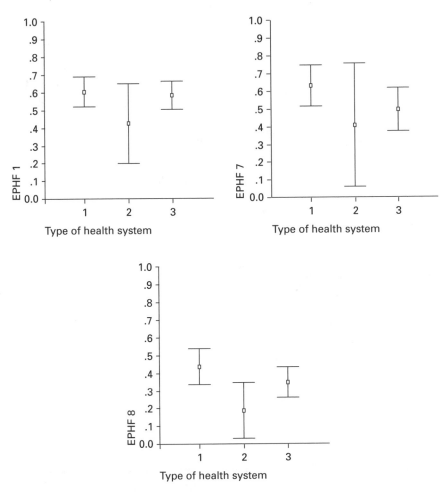

Note: 1) integrated public system, 2) regulated mixed system and 3) segmented system

gion. This may be explained by the greater weakness of the health authority under this type of system, since the health authority is responsible for developing standards, accrediting service providers, and evaluating the quality of services provided. If some of the public health functions for this group had to be prioritized, EPHF 9 should probably be a priority. The greater dispersion in the performance of this function in countries with regulated mixed health systems should be studied in greater depth in order to obtain useful data with respect to the better-performing countries.

The EPHF and the health and quality-of-life outcome indicators

Several health and quality-of-life indicators that are frequently available for all of the countries of the Region have been selected.

Given that health outcomes (specifically any of the indicators used in this analysis) have many causes, it is not our in-

Figure 50 Performance of EPHF 9 According to the Level of Infant Mortality

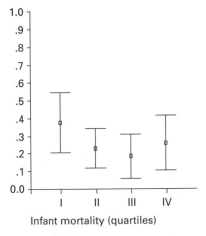

Note: infant mortality is lower in quartile 1 and higher in quartile 4.

providers), has been a difficult process that is still very far from achieving optimal performance, a factor which, in this case, also affects public health performance. This finding applies to both "traditional" functions (such as EPHF 1, monitoring health status) and other functions. The low performance of the regulated mixed group is particularly significant with respect to EPHF 8 (human resources development), a fact that undoubtedly affects—or will affect—the possibility of further developing public

health institutional capacities. In the case of EPHF 7 (promotion of equitable access to health services), great dispersion is exhibited in the performance of the countries with mixed regulated health systems, indicating the variability of an area that has been an emphasis in reform efforts (see Figure 49).

On the other hand, the performance of EPHF 9 (quality assurance) is lower in the group of countries with segmented health systems than in the rest of the Re-

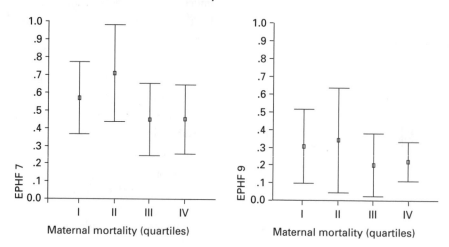

Figure 51 Performance of EPHF 7 and 9 According to Level of Maternal Mortality

Note: maternal mortality is lower in quartile 1 and higher in quartile 4.

tention to state here that better or worse performance of the essential functions necessarily causes a health outcome, although it can indeed influence it. Consequently, this part of the analysis will consider the characteristics of particular functions with respect to these indicators, selecting those EPHF for which significant differences are observed.

The EPHF and infant mortality

The average performance of EPHF 7 (promotion of equitable access) and EPHF 9 (quality assurance) presents an inverse correlation with the countries grouped into quartiles. The countries with lower infant mortality rates (less than 12.8 per 1,000 live births) exhibit better relative performance of both functions than countries with higher infant mortality rates (greater than 23.5 per 1,000 live births), as shown in Figure 51. Although infant mortality is affected by a number of factors, it is possible to state that a relationship exists between the performance of these func-

tions and this indicator. This underlines the importance of improving the performance of these functions, particularly quality assurance in health services, which is performed at an insufficient level throughout the Region.

The EPHF and maternal mortality

The relationship between performance of EPHF 7 and 9 and the maternal mortality rate is found to be very similar to the relationship observed for the previous indicator, although with less significant differences (see Figure 52). This same profile is also exhibited with regard to performance of EPHF 11 (disaster reduction).

The EPHF and mortality due to infectious diseases

An analysis of the EPHF performance profile in relation to mortality due to infectious diseases indicates that performance of the public health functions is generally better (except for EPHF 3 and 10) in the group of countries with a lower mortality rate (less than 41.8 per 100,000 people) than in the group with a higher mortality rate (greater than 82), as shown in the following table (Figure 53).

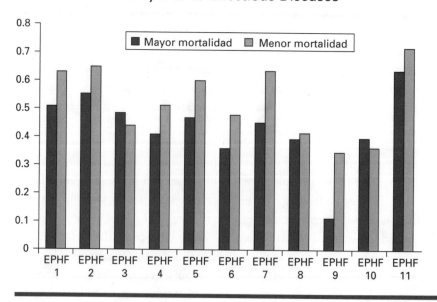

Figure 52 Performance of EPHF According to the Level of Mortality Due to Infectious Diseases

Figure 53   Performance of EPHF 8 and 10 According to the Level of Life Expectancy at Birth in the Countries of the Region

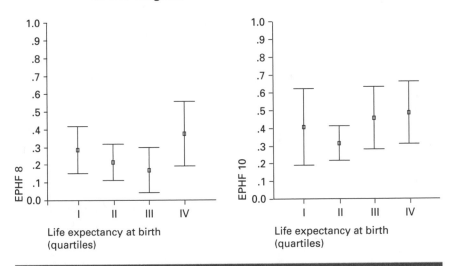

Life expectancy at birth (quartiles)

Again, the greatest differences are observed in the performance of EPHF 7 and 9.

The EPHF and life expectancy at birth

An analysis of the EPHF performance profile in relation to life expectancy at birth reveals a positive correlation in the case of EPHF 7 and 9. This confirms the conclusions already found with respect to infant mortality and infectious diseases, given that life expectancy in the Region is strongly determined by the infant mortality rate, especially for children under one year of age.

A positive correlation is also found with respect to other public health functions, a fact that is more of an expression of the overall development of the countries. Thus, the better performance of EPHF 8 (human resources development) and EPHF 10 (public health research) associated with countries with greater life expectancy rates may be a re-

flection of their overall level of development, because more developed countries generally invest more in these areas of public health, given that they have the infrastructure and institutional ca-

pacity to do so (training centers, human and financial resources for research, etc.). The differences are accentuated in quartile 4, which comprises the countries with the highest life expectancy rates in the Region.

The EPHF and the Human Development Index

The Human Development Index (HDI) is another measure of a country's development. This indicator is derived from the simple average of three indicators of the country's success in securing the health and longevity of its population (measured by life expectancy and infant mortality rates), education (measured by adult educational level), and standard of living (measured by per capita gross domestic product, adjusted for purchasing power parity). This indicator shows how far the countries of the Region are from achieving the following goals: 1) life expectancy of 85 years, 2) 100% adult lit-

Figure 54   Performance of the EPHF in Relation to the Level of Human Development in the Countries of the Region

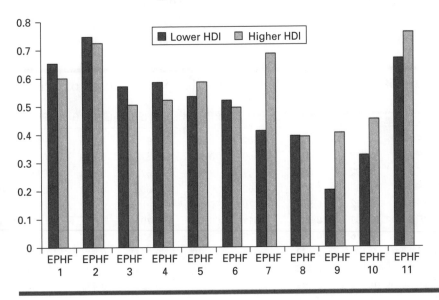

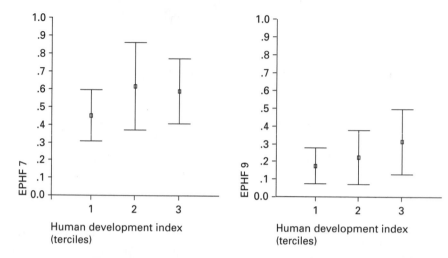

least makes it possible to infer that their performance is affected by other external factors.

However, a positive correlation is observed for EPHF 7, 9 and 10; that is, the higher the HDI, the better the performance of these functions. As shown in the following table (Figure 56), in the case of EPHF 7 (promotion of equitable access to services), the countries in the first tercil, with HDI below 0.72, exhibit the lowest performance; and in the case of EPHF 9 (health quality assurance), each tercil shows sustained improvement in direct proportion to higher HDI.

1.5 Correlations between functions

eracy, and 3) real per capita GDP of US$40,000.

The relationship between the EPHF and the HDI exhibits two phenomena that are difficult to differentiate: a) on the one hand, the inclusion of health outcome indicators (life expectancies) could enable one to state that performance of the EPHF might contribute to better results for these indicators, and 2) the HDI, as a summary measure of a country's development, might in some way affect the level of development of the health authority and, accordingly, the possibility that it will exhibit good performance of the EPHF.

As shown in the table 54, the EPHF performance profile for the majority of the functions is relatively similar for the quartile with the lowest HDI as compared to the group with the highest HDI. For some functions, such as health promotion and social participation, the profile is inverted, which at

Correlations between the performance scores of the different EPHF in the participating countries were also analyzed.[9] This analysis revealed a high correlation between the various functions (Figure 56), with the exception of EPHF 11 (reducing the impact of disasters), whose performance profile exhibits a very low and insignificant correlation

[9] Using the Pearson correlation method, which is briefly explained at the end of the chapter.

Figure 56 Correlations between performance scores of EPHF

	EPHF 1	EPHF 2	EPHF 3	EPHF 4	EPHF 5	EPHF 6	EPHF7	EPHF 8	EPHF 9	EPHF 10	EPHF 11
EPHF 1		0.733	0.502	0.500	0.512	0.609	0.476	0.475	0.496	0.622	0.036
EPHF 2	0.733		0.559	0.608	0.577	0.599	0.360	0.478	0.436	0.350	0.146
EPHF 3	0.502	0.559		0.662	0.670	0.511	0.676	0.668	0.523	0.372	0.049
EPHF4	0.500	0.608	0.662		0.663	0.663	0.640	0.703	0.650	0.367	0.161
EPHF 5	0.512	0.577	0.670	0.663		0.702	0.532	0.611	0.524	0.393	0.169
EPHF 6	0.609	0.599	0.511	0.663	0.702		0.407	0.614	0.637	0.449	0.120
EPHF 7	0.476	0.360	0.676	0.640	0.532	0.407		0.626	0.553	0.430	0.262
EPHF 8	0.475	0.478	0.668	0.703	0.611	0.614	0.626		0.589	0.352	0.194
EPHF 9	0.496	0.436	0.523	0.650	0.524	0.637	0.553	0.589		0.345	0.242
EPHF 10	0.622	0.350	0.372	0.367	0.393	0.449	0.430	0.352	0.345		0.157
EPHF 11	0.036	0.146	0.049	0.161	0.169	0.120	0.262	0.194	0.242	0.157	

Figure 57   Main Summary and Dispersion Measures of the EPHF in the Countries of the Region

	EPHF 1	EPHF 2	EPHF 3	EPHF 4	EPHF 5	EPHF 6	EPHF 7	EPHF 8	EPHF 9	EPHF 10	EPHF 11
Number of countries	41	41	41	41	41	41	41	41	41	41	41
Average	0.58	0.63	0.52	0.48	0.56	0.46	0.55	0.38	0.26	0.42	0.68
Median	0.57	0.63	0.54	0.46	0.53	0.44	0.56	0.36	0.21	0.35	0.71
Standard education	0.17	0.17	0.19	0.20	0.18	0.18	0.25	0.20	0.21	0.23	0.19
25th percentile	0.46	0.52	0.41	0.33	0.49	0.34	0.33	0.21	0.08	0.24	0.54
75th percentile	0.64	0.75	0.64	0.60	0.70	0.56	0.73	0.51	0.39	0.54	0.87

Note: A very high correlation is defined as p < 0.01 (dark blue) and a high correlation as p < 0.05 (light blue)

with the remaining functions. EPHF 10 (public health research) only exhibits a significant correlation with EPHF 1 (monitoring of health status).

The most notable of the observed correlations was the strong correlation between performance of EPHF 5 (policies and management in health) and the vast majority of the other functions, particularly EPHF 3 (health promotion) and EPHF 6 (strengthening of institutional capacity for regulation and enforcement). This confirms the importance of concentrating more efforts on improving the critical areas that pertain to this function throughout the Region.

One fundamental responsibility of the health authority is ensuring access to the health services, particularly for the neediest sectors of the population. The high correlation between performance of this function and other so-called "emerging" functions (health promotion, social participation in health, quality assurance in health services) leads to the conclusion that, at present, strengthening these new public health functions is of fundamental importance in promoting equitable access to health services. Furthermore, the correlation between this function and EPHF 8 (human resources development) obliges the participating countries to continue their efforts to develop these resources as an essential step in im-

proving their performance and promoting greater access to health services.

2. Subregional Analysis

To compliment to the Regional analysis, the following presents the results of the measurement by subregions: Central America, Caribbean, Andean Countries, and Southern Cone and Mexico. The criteria used in these groupings are based on the one hand on facilitating the possibility of future strategies and collaboration among countries; for example, countries that have agreements or previous cooperation activities, such as the Health Services Network of Central America (RESSCAD), The Andean Pact and MERCOSUR. On the other hand the criteria of grouping countries based on traits or common characteristics as in the case of putting Mexico with the Southern Cone countries, Belize with the Caribbean and Cuba with Central America. These criteria were used with the perspective of identifying or developing cooperation strategies between countries.

2.1 Central America, Spanish-speaking Caribbean and Haiti

2.1.1 General results of the measurement

The results of the measurement in the countries of Costa Rica, Cuba, El Salva-

dor, Guatemala, Haiti, Honduras, Nicaragua, Panama, Puerto Rico, and the Dominican Republic are presented below.

The overall performance of the countries of the Region with respect to the EPHF is shown in the following table summarizing the average performance of the Region (Figure 1). This average was chosen as a summary measure in order to eliminate the influence of the extreme scores on the small number of observations for the nine countries.

In general, a relatively good performance profile was observed for the functions of public health surveillance (EPHF 2) and reducing the impact of emergencies and disasters (EPHF 11).

Lower performance was observed for the functions of quality assurance in the health services (EPHF 9) and human resources development in public health (EPHF 8).

High-intermediate performance was exhibited with respect to: monitoring, evaluation, and analysis of health status (EPHF 1); promotion of equitable access to necessary health services (EPHF 7); social participation in health (EPHF 4); development of policies and institutional capacity for planning and management in public health (EPHF 5); and strengthening of institutional ca-

Figure 58   Performance of the EPHF in the subregion of Central America, Spanish-speaking Caribbean and Haiti

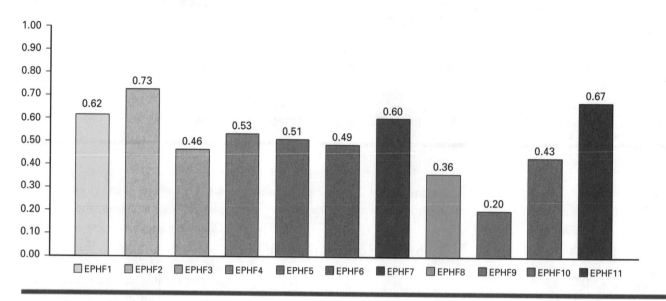

pacity for regulation and enforcement in public health (EPHF 6).

Low-intermediate performance was exhibited with respect to health promotion (EPHF 3) and public health research (EPHF 10).

In general, the profile of the EPHF for Central America reveals relatively better performance of functions that may be considered part of the "tradition" of public health development (EPHF 2 and 11) and poorer performance of emerging functions (EPHF 9).

A noteworthy area of concern is the low performance exhibited with respect to human resources development (EPHF 8). This is very important to take into account, because the future improvement of public health in the Region depends on developing the competencies of human resources, which are the foundation of the institutional strength of the NHA.

If one studies the variability of the results (Figure 58), one can see that EPHF 9 (quality assurance)—exhibits the lowest performance, as well as EPHF 8 (human resources development) reflecting a weakness throughout the countries of the subregion.

On the other hand, while EPHF 10 (public health research) is a weakness for the subregion as a whole, its greater dispersion indicates that it is a strength for several countries. Similarly, some countries exhibited adequate performance with respect to EPHF 5 (policies and management in public health) and EPHF 7 (equitable access to health services), while the performance of other countries indicates that these functions are critical areas that require intervention.

An analysis of the EPHF performance profile for the countries indicates that—with the exception of one country that exhibited generally good performance of

all functions—the countries of the subregion[10] exhibited good performance in some areas and relatively poor performance in other, more critical areas, which vary from country to country.

The results for EPHF 11 (reducing the impact of emergencies and disasters) revealed relatively good performance and low variability, indicating that this is an area of overall strength for the subregion.

On the other hand, the results for EPHF 8 (human resources development) and EPHF 9 (quality assurance in the health services) revealed relatively poor performance and low variability, indicating that this is an area of weakness for all of the countries.

The results for some functions revealed intermediate performance and low variability, such as EPHF 4 (social partici-

---

[10] Hereafter, 'the subregion' refers to Central America and the countries previously mentioned.

162

Figure 59   Distribution of the Performance of each EPHF in the subregion of Central America, Spanish-speaking Caribbean and Haiti.

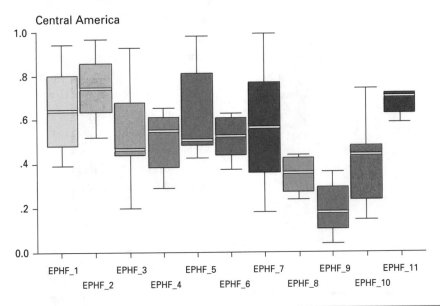

Central America

pation in the health) and EPHF 6 (regulation and enforcement).

Finally, the results for EPHF 5 (policies and management in public health) and EPHF 7 (promotion of equitable access to health services) revealed the highest variability among the countries, suggesting the possibility that countries which have achieved more progress in these areas might cooperate with countries for which these areas are significant weaknesses.

2.1.2 Analysis of the results for each EPHF

The results for each of the essential public health functions in the subregion are analyzed in detail below.

***EPHF 1:** Monitoring, evaluation, and analysis of health status*

The relatively good performance exhibited for EPHF 1, with an average score

of 0.64 for the subregion, is fundamental to enabling the health authorities to make decisions related to national health policy priorities on the basis of solid information. Although the results for this function revealed high-intermediate performance, the countries of the subregion exhibited some common weaknesses.

First of all, it must be pointed out that the countries have not established the practice of systematically evaluating the quality of the information that is gathered by the national health authorities. It is very important that this weakness be corrected, given that changing national priorities make it necessary to continually gather new data on public health threats and risk factors, as well as data on how the health services are used and accessed. However, in view of the fact that reform processes demand an increasingly clear separation between functions related to service delivery and

functions related to health system financing and regulation, it is important to establish clear guidelines with regard to collecting and evaluating the quality of information, and to evaluate the true usefulness of that information in the decision-making process. In the majority of the countries, there are no clear guidelines or criteria requiring that the quality of information be evaluated at the various levels of health authority action or at the level of service providers.

It is also important to point out that, despite the fact that the countries of the Region have indicated that they are deeply concerned about improving equitable access to health services, the greatest weakness of the information systems lies precisely in their ability to systematically evaluate the distribution of access to health services, particularly for the most disadvantaged.

Another weakness that should be addressed is the limited coordination between the management of monitoring systems and the management of national statistics systems, which is essential to measuring health status from an intersectoral perspective.

In addition, in view of the increasingly important role of people in caring for their own health and the increasingly important role of public participation in the health policy decision-making process, it is vital to strengthen the ability to adequately communicate the results of health status monitoring to the various actors in society and the general public.

Generally speaking, significant weaknesses were not observed in the knowledge and skills of human resources that monitor and analyze health status, even

Figure 60 Performance of the Indicators for EPHF 1 in the subregion of Central America, Spanish-speaking Caribbean and Haiti.

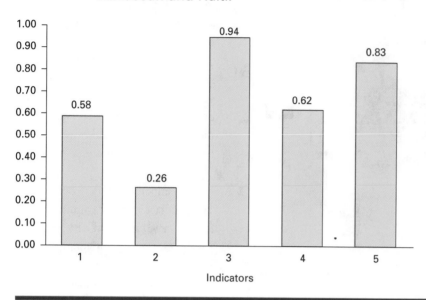

at intermediate levels, which indicates good performance of this indicator (Indicator 3). Although the countries have been addressing the issue of computer support through various initiatives in recent years (Indicator 4), the greatest weaknesses were inadequate computer equipment and information technology at the local level, and deficiencies in equipment maintenance at all levels.

Indicators:

1. Guidelines and processes for monitoring health status

2. Evaluation of the quality of information

3. Expert support and resources for monitoring health status

4. Technical support for monitoring and evaluating health status

5. Technical assistance and support to the sub national levels of public health

EPHF 2: Public health surveillance, research, and control of risks and threats to public health

The countries of the subregion exhibited their best performance with respect to EPHF 2, with a score of 0.74. Nevertheless, it is possible to identify some areas that should be strengthened in order to adapt the good performance of a "traditional" function by the public health systems to the current epidemiological outlook and the future of public health in general.

The greatest dispersion of the results for this EPHF was noted in the indicators designed to evaluate the capacity for timely response to control public health threats. Given the importance of this capacity, without which efforts to gather information and perform research on public health risks and threats would be meaningless, it must be emphasized that efforts to strengthen surveillance must be concentrated in this area.

As with EPHF 1, deficiencies were noted in the evaluation of the quality of information gathered through surveillance programs. This area must be improved in order to ensure that the population is protected against known threats or emerging diseases. It also is important to point out that deficiencies in the integrity of information sources were observed in some countries, information sources that are still centralized in the public health system, despite the increasing role of the private sector, both nonprofit and for-profit service providers, resulting in deficiencies in the information needed to monitor public health threats.

The primary deficiencies with regard to new areas of development were observed in the training of teams responsible for monitoring the collection and analysis of data on mental health threats, threats deriving from work environments and diseases, or risk factors for chronic diseases.

With regard to surveillance system management, it should be noted that deficiencies were observed in the coordination of public health laboratory networks at the national and international levels. Finally, there is a lack of incentive programs aimed at promoting the performance of the teams responsible for public health surveillance and protection, particularly in view of the threats likely to be controlled by these warning systems.

Indicators:

1. Surveillance system to identify threats and harm to public health

2. Capacities and expertise in public health surveillance

3. Capacity of public health laboratories

164

Figure 61 Performance of the Indicators for EPHF 2 in the subregion of Central America, Spanish-speaking Caribbean and Haiti

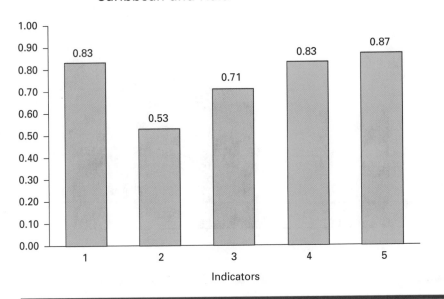

Given the importance of the communications media and public education in improving public health, it is important to note that the measurement revealed weakness in assessing the impact of these sectors on public health, which is essential to decision-making in this area.

Although all of the countries have accepted the recommendations of world conferences with regard to health promotion, one of the Region's major weaknesses is related to one of these recommendations: the importance of orienting personal health services toward health promotion. Virtually none of the countries stated that they have clear incentives aimed at orienting services toward health promotion.

4. Capacity for timely and effective response to control public health problems

5. Technical assistance and support for the subnational levels of public health.

EPHF 3: Health promotion

The results for this EPHF were clearly more heterogeneous, with some countries exhibiting greater development with regard to health promotion than others. In general, weaknesses were observed in the following areas.

First of all, a limited participation of the health authorities in designing public policies that have an acknowledged impact on public health. Although intersectoral commissions aimed at developing health promotion programs do generally exist, systematic efforts on the part of the health sector to influence policy in sectors such as education,

housing, public works, and transportation must be strengthened, particularly with regard to evaluating the health effects of such policies.

Finally, it is important to note that the countries of the Region have not developed plans to encourage health promotion at the subnational levels in which the ministries of health play a central role.

Figure 62 Performance of the Indicators for EPHF 3 in the subregion of Central America, Spanish-speaking Caribbean and Haiti

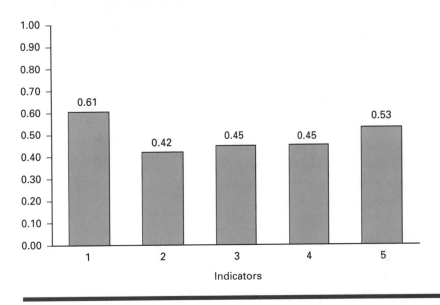

165

1. Support for health promotion activities, the development of norms, and interventions to promote healthy behaviors and environments

2. Building of sectoral and extrasectoral partnerships for health promotion

3. National planning and coordination of information, education, and social communication strategies for health promotion

4. Reorientation of the health services toward health promotion

5. Technical assistance and support to the subnational levels to strengthen health promotion activities.

EPHF 4. *Social participation in health*

The countries of the Region exhibited intermediate performance of this function as well, but significant variations may be observed. All of the countries stated that they have some type of ombudsman's office with the capacity to protect the rights of citizens in health-related matters. However, it should be noted that formal channels of social participation for receiving and responding to public concerns and opinions regarding health policies and the organization of the health services do not exist. In addition, it is difficult to clearly ascertain the extent to which national health authorities are interested in analyzing and channeling public contributions in the process of defining sectoral goals and strategies.

A major deficiency is educating the public about health law. As with other functions, weaknesses were observed in the systematic evaluation of social participation in health.

Figure 63 Performance of the Indicators for EPHF 4 in the subregion of Central America, Spanish-speaking Caribbean and Haiti

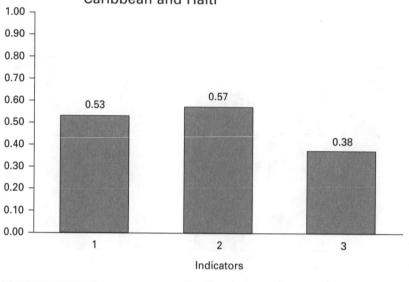

Finally, NHA support to the decentralized levels in the performance of this function is the lowest performing indicator. Given that the best place to establish contact between the public and the health system is at the local level, this deficiency indicates that the system is weak.

Indicators:

1. Empowering citizens for decision-making in public health

2. Strengthening of social participation in health

3. Technical assistance and support to the subnational levels to strengthen social participation in health.

EPHF 5. *Development of policies and institutional capacity for planning and management in public health*

Although three countries of the subregion exhibit greater development with regard to the preparation of public health policies, it is important to evaluate these results keeping in mind that at least two of them are currently involved in health system reform processes marking a milestone in the formulation of new health laws. These reform processes tend to positively evaluate the capacities of the ministries of health in the area of policy development; however, these capacities may be directly influenced by the success of these reforms.

Specific deficiencies were observed in the capacity to define national health objectives in coordination with decisions made about the structure of the health system. It is particularly important to point out that one of the most significant weaknesses in this area is the lack of indicators that would make it possible to evaluate the achievement of national objectives over time.

It is important to note that practically all political efforts in the area of public health concern the development of the public sector. Although it is logical to consider this to be the pertinent sector in evaluating NHA performance of reg-

Figure 64 Performance of the Indicators for EPHF 5 in the subregion of Central America, Spanish-speaking Caribbean and Haiti

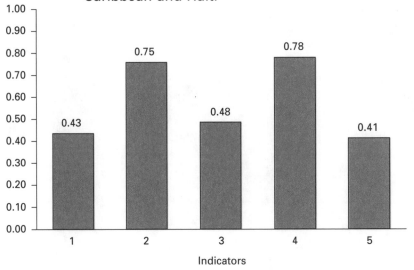

The countries of the subregion exhibited intermediate performance of this function. In general, better performance was observed with respect to personnel expertise in the development of regulatory instruments than with respect to monitoring compliance with existing regulations. Although enforcement teams are properly trained, it was noted that the primary weakness in enforcing the regulatory framework is a lack of human and financial resources.

The countries do not regularly review their guidelines for regulating the health system. These guidelines tend to focus on establishing laws and regulations, rather than on providing incentives for ethical compliance with regulations.

ulatory functions, it is significant that the private sector is generally not taken into account in national public health decisions.

Finally, efforts to base political decisions with regard to public health on data must be significantly strengthened. It should also be noted that the countries acknowledged shortcomings in organizational development; standards are not defined and institutional performance with regard to public health is not evaluated.

Indicators:

1. Definition of national and subnational health objectives

2. Development, monitoring, and evaluation of public health policies

3. Development of institutional capacity for the management of public health systems

4. Management of international cooperation in public health

5. Technical assistance and support to the subnational levels for policy development, planning, and management in public health.

EPHF 6. Strengthening of institutional capacity for regulation and enforcement in public health

There appears to be a lack of specific interest in establishing policies to prevent staff corruption and abuse of authority. This is as a very important deficiency recognized throughout the subregion, given that inspectors are susceptible to these types of administrative and legal transgressions.

Figure 65 Performance of the Indicators for EPHF 6 in the subregion of Central America, Spanish-speaking Caribbean and Haiti

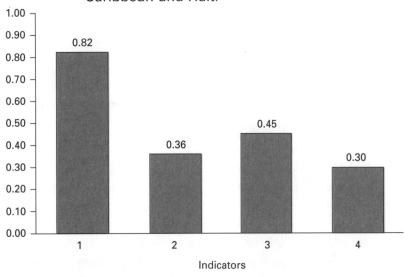

Indicators:

1. Periodic monitoring, evaluation, and modification of the regulatory framework

2. Enforcement of laws and regulations

3. Knowledge, skills, and mechanisms for reviewing, improving, and enforcing the regulations

4. Technical assistance and support to the subnational levels of public health in developing and enforcing laws and regulations.

EPHF 7: Evaluation and promotion of equitable access to necessary health services

Performance of this function in the subregion varied considerably. Generally speaking, better performance was observed in the promotion of equitable access to health services. It should be noted that evaluations of public access to personal health services are under utilized to correct policies and plans aimed at improving access to these services for underserved populations.

The difficulty of the NHA in increasing its role in improving access to health services is of particular concern, given that the steering role is being separated from the role of providing services. It may be inferred that the NHA is still acting as a service provider (primarily for the poorest) and, in this way, is seeking to solve the problem. Insufficient understanding of the cultural issues involved in improving access to services is a weakness that must be addressed, particularly in countries characterized by significant cultural diversity.

The countries acknowledged that a major deficiency is insufficient staff knowledge and technical expertise in

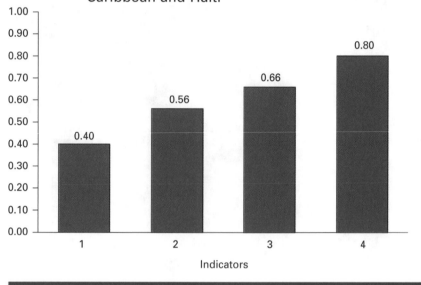

Figure 66 Performance of the Indicators for EPHF 7 in the subregion of Central America, Spanish-speaking Caribbean and Haiti

improving access to adequate health services for underserved populations, particularly competencies for adapting health services to the cultural features of the population.

In addition, the countries stated that difficulties exist in the promotion of equitable access to health services due to other decision-makers with influence in this area. Given that access to health services is a major focus of health sector reform, it is significant that the countries—when faced with a subject that tends to be central to these reforms; namely, establishing guaranteed packages of health benefits—have difficulty evaluating the extent to which these packages have been made accessible in these countries.

Indicators:

1. Monitoring and evaluation of access to necessary health services

2. Knowledge, skills, and mechanisms for improving access by the population to necessary health services

3. Advocacy and action to improve access to necessary health services

4. Technical assistance and support to the subnational levels to promote equitable access to health services.

EPHF 8. Human resources development and training in public health

One of the principle problems that should be addressed by the countries of the subregion is their low performance with regard to the development of human resources in public health. This insufficiency endangers all of the accumulated capital for adequate performance of the EPHF, and therefore endangers many years of investment in this matter. The countries' low performance with regard to human resources development in public health is a warning sign to the NHA of these countries that they could lose their position as leaders in meeting the challenges of sectoral reform.

Virtually none of the countries have made efforts to establish the characteristics of the workforce—in terms of com-

Figure 67 Performance of the Indicators for EPHF 8 in the subregion of Central America, Spanish-speaking Caribbean and Haiti

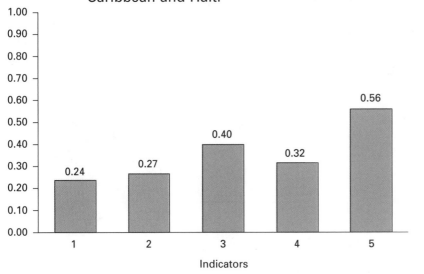

5. Technical assistance and support to the subnational levels in human resources development.

EPHF 9. Quality assurance in personal and population-based health services

A critical weakness throughout the subregion is the capacity of the NHA to ensure the quality of personal and population-based health services.

Deficiencies were observed in the capacity to ensure the quality of personal and population-based health services, particularly the latter.

Fewer than half of the countries reported progress in using technological systems as an basic tool in improving the quality of each type of health service. The capacity of the NHA to perform this function is further weakened by difficulties in defining quality standards for the health services.

petencies and professional training—needed to fulfill current public health responsibilities.

Another significant deficiency is the lack of cooperation between the health authority and human resources education centers in developing plans and programs for training and continuing education.

With regard to retention and development of human resources, it is clear that there are insufficient performance incentives for public health workers.

Finally, it should be noted that deficiencies exist in training health workers to interact with populations of various cultural groups in each country.

Indicators:

1. Description of the public health workforce

2. Improving the quality of the workforce

3. Continuing education and graduate training in public health

4. Upgrading human resources to ensure culturally appropriate delivery of services

One of the subregion's greatest weaknesses is the lack of interest at all levels

Figure 68 Performance of the Indicators for EPHF 9 in the subregion of Central America, Spanish-speaking Caribbean and Haiti

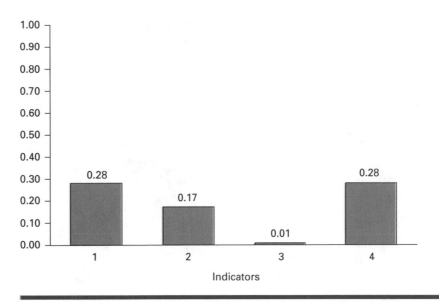

in evaluating and improving user satisfaction with provided services.

Indicators:

1. Definition of standards and evaluation to improve the quality of population-based and personal health services

2. Improving user satisfaction with the health services

3. Systems for technological management and health technology assessment to support decision-making in public health

4. Technical assistance and support to the subnational levels to ensure quality improvement in the services.

EPHF 10. *Research in public health*

As with EPHF 8 and EPHF 9, the countries of the subregion exhibited low performance of this function. Two noteworthy deficiencies are the absence of a priority public health research agenda in each of the countries, and insufficient interaction between the ministries of health and the public health scientific community at both at the national and international level.

The countries acknowledged that very little research has been performed on the impact of public health interventions and current risk factors for chronic diseases. Another area of limited development is research on health systems and services.

Indicators:

1. Development of a public health research agenda

2. Development of institutional research capacity

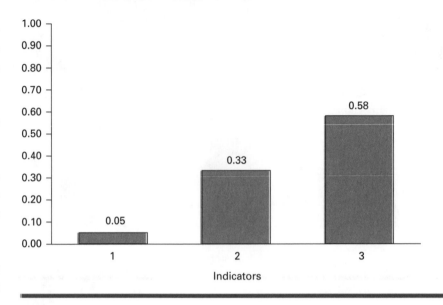

Figure 69   Performance of the Indicators for EPHF 10 in the subregion of Central America, Spanish-speaking Caribbean and Haiti

3. Technical assistance and support for research in public health at the subnational levels

EPHF 11: *Reducing the impact of emergencies and disasters on health*

The countries of the subregion exhibited relatively good performance of this function. Nevertheless, it is important to point out that coordination within the health sector must be improved in order to effectively address emergencies and their impact on health.

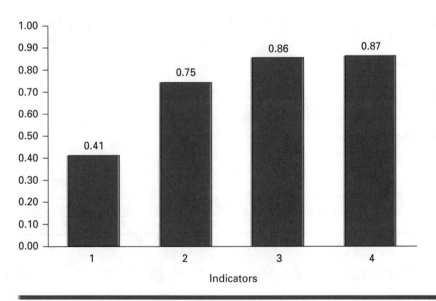

Figure 70   Performance of the Indicators for EPHF 11 in the subregion of Central America, Spanish-speaking Caribbean and Haiti.

One particularly sensitive area in need of attention throughout the subregion is the vulnerability of the hospital infrastructure and the weakness of policies and plans aimed at improving hospital evaluation and correcting deficiencies, making it possible to manage emergencies that may damage the hospital infrastructure or hinder its ability to reduce the overall harm caused by disasters.

Indicators:

1. Reducing the impact of emergencies and disasters

2. Development of standards and guidelines that support emergency preparedness and disaster management in health

3. Coordination and partnerships with other agencies and/or institutions

4. Technical assistance and support to the subnational levels to reduce the impact of emergencies and disasters on health.

2.1.3 Identification of priority areas of intervention to prepare a program for strengthening the EPHF in Central America

2.1.3.1 Performance of all indicators

A profile of all of the indicators, classified as strengths or weaknesses for the subregion, is presented below. In order to facilitate the analysis, the indicators for each function have been given a different color.

The general profile indicates significant weaknesses in all of the indicators for EPHF 9 (quality assurance of the health services); the lack of progress in health technology assessment is particularly noteworthy. The majority of the indicators for EPHF 8 (human resources development) revealed low performance, with the exception of continuing education and graduate training, which registered intermediate performance.

In addition, it was noted that little progress has been made in defining national public health research agendas, and that the capacity of the NHA to directly perform research is insufficient.

Although the countries of the Region exhibited adequate performance with regard to developing the regulatory framework, they exhibited low performance with regard to enforcing existing regulations.

On the other hand, the subregion exhibited clear strengths with regard to emergency and disaster management, development of the public health surveillance system, and the capacity for timely response to public health threats.

2.1.3.2 Performance by intervention area

The primary *strengths* of the majority of the countries of Central America in performing the essential public health functions (with a score equal to or greater than 70% of the established standard), and which should be maintained in the subregional plan, are as follows:

• Intervention in these important processes: surveillance systems to identify risks and threats to public health; capacity for timely and effective response to control public health problems; developing, monitoring, and evaluating public health policies; reviewing, evaluating, and modifying the regulatory framework for public health; developing standards and guidelines aimed at reducing the impact of emergencies and disasters; and coordination and partnerships with other agencies or institutions in emergency and disaster management.

• Intervention with regard to developing institutional capacities and infrastructure: capacity and expert assistance in monitoring and evaluating health status; capacity of public health laboratories; and capacity to negotiate international cooperation.

• The development of decentralized competencies: NHA support to the subnational levels for performance of the functions; monitoring, evaluating, and analyzing health status; public health surveillance, research, and control of risk and threats to public health; evaluating and promoting equitable access to necessary health services; and reducing the impact of the emergencies and disasters.

The primary *weaknesses* of the Region (with a score equal to or less than 40% of the established standard), and which should be included in a public health strengthening program for Central America, are as follows:

• Intervention in these key processes: evaluating the quality of information for monitoring the health status of the population; defining national and subnational public health objectives; monitoring compliance with health regulations; describing the characteristics of the health workforce; continuing education in public health; definition of standards and evaluation to improve the quality of personal and population-based health services; improving user satisfaction; and developing a public health research agenda.

171

Figure 71 Performance of the indicators of the EPHF in the subregion of Central America, Spanish-speaking Caribbean and Haiti

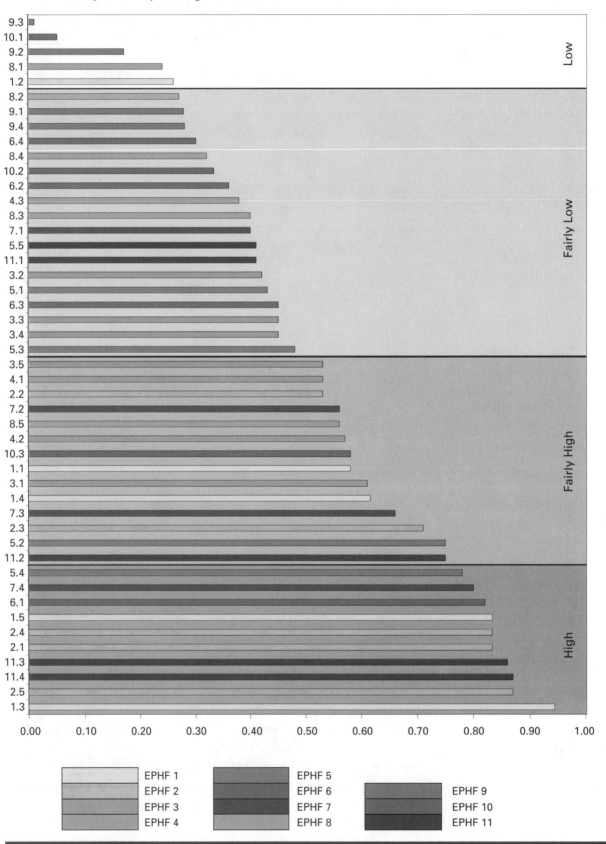

- Intervention to develop institutional capacities and infrastructure: improving the quality of human resources in public health; upgrading human resources to ensure culturally-appropriate delivery of services; developing systems for technology management and health technology assessment to support decision-making in public health; and developing institutional capacity for public health research.

- The development of decentralized competencies: NHA support to the subnational levels for the performance of the functions: technical assistance and support to the subnational levels in the policy development, planning, and management in public health; technical assistance and support to the subnational levels in enforcing laws and regulations; and promoting quality improvement in personal and population-based health services.

2.1.3.3 Performance according to the action priorities of the World Bank

The indicators have been regrouped in order to make the results of the measurement operational within the framework of international financing and cooperation strategies. The objective is to identify action priorities based on: *a*) significant differences in the public health profile of the countries, and *b*) investment needs. The categories that were considered and the results of the analysis are given below.

- Development of health policies

- Data collection and dissemination to orient the public policies, the strategies, and the actions with regard to public health

- Disease prevention and control

- Intersectoral action to improve the level of health

- Human resources development and creation of institutional competencies for public health

a) Development of health policies

Specific deficiencies were observed in the capacity to define national health objectives in coordination with decisions made about the structure of the health system. It is particularly important to point out that one of the most significant weaknesses in this area is the lack of indicators that would make it possible to evaluate the achievement of national objectives over time.

Although the countries of the subregion have the knowledge and institutional capacity to monitor and evaluate health policies, they focus on examining public sector activity, without considering health policies or what other actors (the private sector, social security institutions, etc.) could contribute to these policies. It was also noted that little action has been taken in the Region to involve other actors in the process of defining and designing health policies.

A critical weakness throughout the subregion is the capacity of the NHA to ensure the quality of personal and population-based health services, particularly the capacity to define standards in order to subsequently evaluate these services.

Another challenge is building interest in developing strategies that include user satisfaction as an essential element of improving the health system.

b) Collection and dissemination of information to guide public health policies, strategies, and actions

Notable weaknesses include the absence of a priority public health research agenda in the countries of the subregion and weak interaction between the scientific community and other actors that could provide information to improve the decision-making process.

Strategies and actions for technological management and health technology assessment, which could effectively contribute to the improvement of public health policies, are just beginning to be developed.

It must also be taken into account that many countries have not established the practice of systematically evaluating the quality of the information that is gathered by the national health authorities. It is very important that this weakness be corrected, given that changing national priorities make it necessary to continually gather new data on public health threats and risk factors, as well as data on how the health services are used and accessed.

In many countries, the monitoring and evaluation of health status does not include analysis of risk factors, which are important variables for emerging diseases and for identifying trends in current priority epidemiological problems. Particular weakness was noted in the areas of mental health, risk factors for chronic diseases, and occupational health, among others.

c) Disease prevention and control

It is important to point out that shortcomings were observed in more than half of the countries in the integrity of

Figure 72 Performance of the indicators of the EPHF in the subregion of Central America, Spanish-speaking Caribbean and Haiti, according to Priorities Areas of Intervention

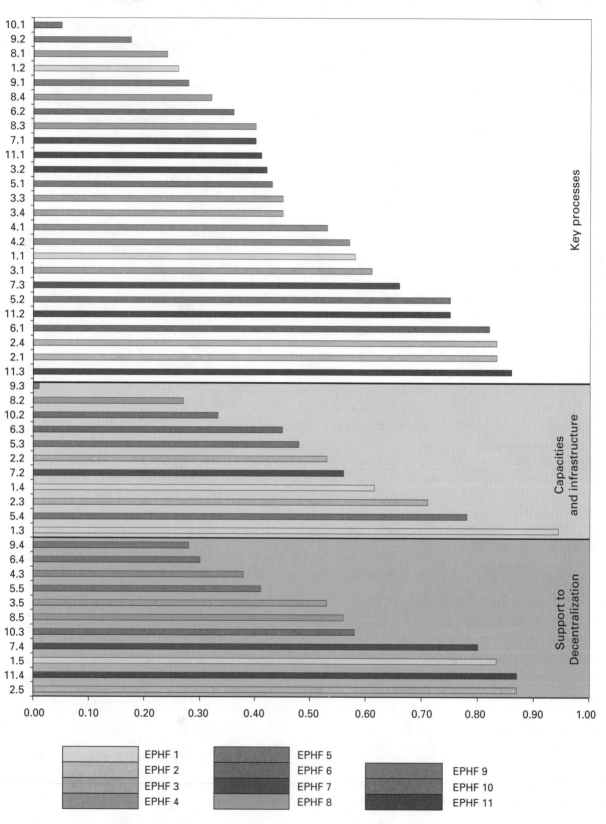

the sources of information, which continue to center on the public sector, despite the growing role assumed by the private sector (nonprofit and for-profit) in delivering services and the fact that this information must therefore be included in order to monitor public health threats.

With regard to new areas of development, the principal deficiencies were observed in the monitoring of threats to mental health, threats deriving from the work environment, and diseases or risk factors for chronic disease.

With regard to the health services, it was observed that evaluations of public access to services are barely used to correct policies and plans aimed at improving the ability of poorly-served populations to access services. In the majority of the countries, the NHA addresses priorities through direct actions aimed at correcting the gaps in the populations at greatest risk, and less effort is made to encourage other pertinent actors to assume their roles and responsibilities with regard to this problem.

d) Intersectoral intervention to improve health

In general, the countries of the subregion exhibited adequate performance in this area. However, one area of critical concern continues to be the establishment of partnerships to encourage health promotion. The countries may be able to learn from the process of establishing partnerships for managing emergencies and disasters and their relatively better performance in that area.

e) Human resources development and building institutional capacity

The primary deficiencies in building institutional capacity are associated with

performing "emerging" public health functions, such as quality assurance, developing strategies designed to improve public access to health services, and providing support to subnational levels in order to increase health promotion and social participation in health.

Most of the countries exhibited low performance with regard to developing human resources in public health, which constitutes a serious obstacle to improving the EPHF in the Region.

2.1.2 Conclusions

The results of this first measurement of the performance of the EPHF in the Region of Central America are primarily descriptive in nature, although they may serve as a basis for analyzing the major trends in the countries' performance of the EPHF.

As a result of this measurement, each country is provided with a detailed analysis of the current performance of the EPHF at the level of the national health authority. This profile of the current status of the health infrastructure may be very useful in making decisions with regard to strengthening the NHA's basic capacity to exercise a steering role in relation to the entire health system. As all of the participating countries have clearly recognized, the value of the instrument does not lie in its perfection as a diagnostic test, but rather in its capacity to promote a *proactive* discussion on the current status of national public health, the reasons for this status, and appropriate formulas for overcoming weaknesses and bolstering strengths.

A transverse analysis of the performance of all of the functions reveals several common critical areas. These critical areas affect a number of essential public

health functions and should be priorities in the effort to strengthen NHA performance.

These critical areas are:

- Strengthening the capacity to periodically evaluate implemented actions and strategies (included feedback from the pertinent actors: decentralized levels in the performance of NHA functions, other actors, and the general public)

- Designing and implementing a system of stimuli and incentives for achieving results in public health, and

- Improving public health information systems, particularly those intended to support data-based decision-making.

From the subregional perspective, this exercise makes it possible to draw a number of conclusions concerning common areas of weakness and strength that may be very useful in supporting the efforts of the ministries of health and in encouraging the decision-making bodies of each government to provide necessary support for developing health capacities. This first diagnostic evaluation should also serve as a frame of reference for institutions interested in cooperating with these national efforts.

In general, it may be concluded that critical areas in the performance of the EPHF in the subregion are: strengthening quality assurance in the health services (particularly with regard to considering user satisfaction as an indicator of quality); human resources development in public health; strengthening the capacity to enforce public health regulations; and developing national public health research agendas. All of these

Figure 73 Performance of the indicators of the EPHF in the subregion of Central America, Spanish-speaking Caribbean and Haiti, according to priority areas of intervention proposed by the World Bank

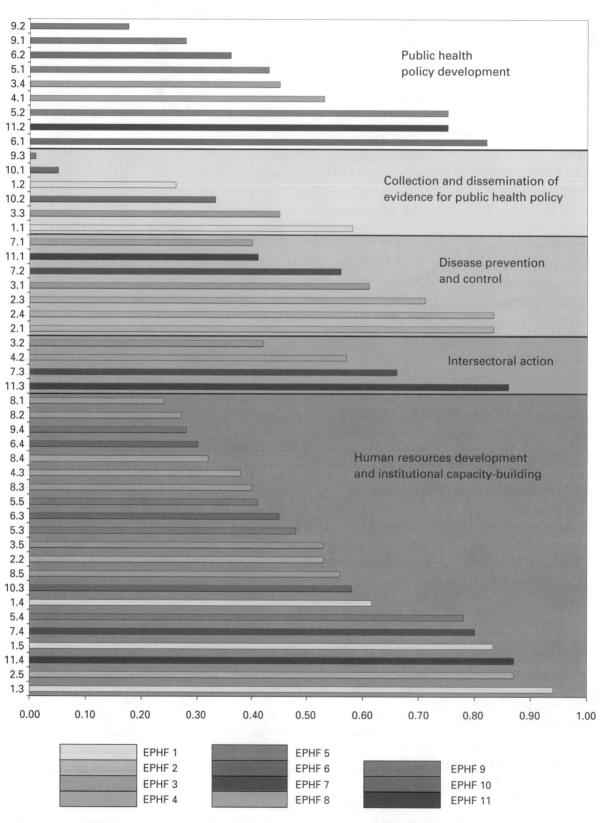

Figure 74 Performance of the EPHF in the subregion of the English-speaking Caribbean and the Netherlands Antilles

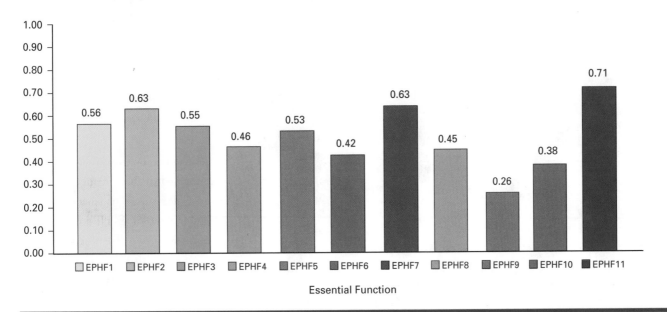

areas could be improved through actions undertaken for Central America as a whole. One area in need of particular attention is health technology management and assessment directed toward providing information to agencies with decision-making power in important areas such as investments, as well as providing information to clinicians on clinical protocols for improving health practice.

The program's priorities with regard to the remaining functions will depend on the analysis carried out by each country with regard to its own performance profile, which will guide each country in determining its national priorities for the improvement of public health.

2.2 English-speaking Caribbean and Netherlands Antilles

The results of the measurement in the twenty countries that comprise the Re-

gion of the Caribbean are presented in this report: Anguilla, Antigua, Aruba, Barbados, Bahamas, British Virgin Islands, Cayman Islands, Curaçao, Dominica, Grenada, Guyana, Jamaica, Montserrat, Saint Kitts and Nevis, Saint Lucia, Saint Vincent, Suriname, Turks and Caicos, and Trinidad and Tobago, with the addition of Belize.[11]

2.2.1 General results of the measurement

The overall performance of the countries of the subregion with respect to each of the evaluated EPHF is shown in Figure 74. Here, the average is used as a summary measure to eliminate the influence of the extreme scores.

---

[11] Although geoFigureically part of Central America, Belize has been included in this group because of its political-sanitary characteristics, that are closer to the profile for a Caribbean country.

The general performance level exhibited varied from low to intermediate. In the subregion adequate performance was exhibited only for the function of reducing the impact of emergencies and disasters in health (EPHF 11).

The countries exhibited a high-intermediate performance in the functions related to evaluation and promotion of equitable access to necessary health services (EPHF 7); public health surveillance, research and control of risks and threats to public health (EPHF 2); monitoring, evaluation, and analysis of health status (EPHF 1); health promotion (EPHF 3); and development of policies and institutional capacity for planning and management in public health (EPHF 5).

The functions for which low-intermediate performance was exhibited are: social participation in health (EPHF 4); human resources development and training in public health (EPHF 8);

Figure 75 Distribution of the Performance of the EPHF in the subregion of the English-speaking Caribbean and the Netherlands Antilles

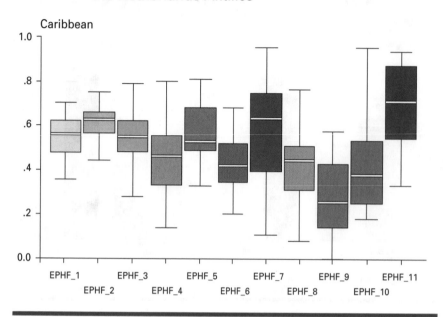

eleven essential public health functions shows a relatively homogeneous pattern among all the countries analyzed (Figure 75). Generally speaking, the countries exhibited performances ranging between 40 and 80% for functions 1 to 6. From there on, a wider dispersion of scores became evident, with a marked trend toward lower scores for EPHF 9.

Although the countries of the Region exhibited their highest performance in reducing the impact of emergencies and disasters in health (EPHF 11), a high degree of dispersion was observed among the countries, making it a weakness in some cases.

The two functions for which the lowest overall performance (EPHF 9 and 10) also manifested high degrees of dispersion, and even the highest scores were insufficient to make them a strength for some countries of the subregion.

The limited dispersion among countries in performing EPHF 2 (public health surveillance, research, and control of risks and threats to public health) and, on the other hand, the high dispersion in the performance of EPHF 7 (evaluation and promotion of equitable access to necessary health services) were noteworthy among the functions in which high-intermediate performance was exhibited. In the latter case, this function represented a strength in some countries of the Region.

2.2.2 Analysis of the results for each EPHF

The performance of each of the essential public health functions in the subregion is analyzed in detail below.

strengthening of institutional capacity for regulation and enforcement in public health (EPHF 6).

The countries of the Region exhibited their lowest performance in public health research (EPHF 10) and quality assurance in personal and population-based health services (EPHF 9).

Generally speaking, this profile indicates that the countries of the Caribbean have not achieved satisfactory levels of performance with respect to the essential public health functions in the areas considered most traditional. However, the processes of reform have allowed progress to be made in other areas of more recent impetus, such as evaluation of equitable access to health services and health promotion, as well as strengthening of the institutional capacity for management in public health.

There is a clear need for strengthening the functions related to the steering role of the health sector, management of resources, and, especially, quality assurance of services offered to the public.

Further exploration of the overall performance requires an analysis of the dispersion in the performance of each EPHF by the countries of the subregion. To this end, Figure 75 shows the average score, the first standard deviation (representing 66% of the countries), and the maximum and minimum scores[12] for each function.

The performance profile of the countries of the Caribbean with regard to the

---

[12] This analysis excludes some results identified in the statistical analysis as "outliers" (external elements).

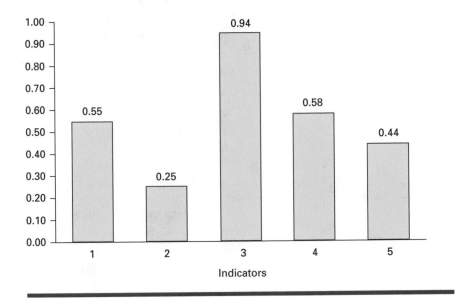

EPHF 1: Monitoring, evaluation, and analysis of health status

In the English-speaking Caribbean and Netherlands Antilles subregion, average performance of this function was 56% of the preestablished optimal standard for this measurement.

Only the institutional capacity to monitor and evaluate health status (Indicator 3) stood out in the performance of this function, thanks to the high levels of training among the human resources.

In the preparation of guidelines and processes for the performance of this function, as well as technical assistance and support to the subnational levels, the index achieved in the subregion was only intermediate.

No country in the subregion has information available on the obstacles in access to health care, and a limited number include monitoring of the relevant risk factors in their epidemiological profile, which prevents the use of the health status profile to solve the problems of inequity and to evaluate the impact of the initiatives aimed at controlling or modifying health risk factors.

Although adequate material exists, its process of dissemination is deficient. The design of these instruments does not take into account their target audience and there are deficiencies in the timeliness with which information is disseminated.

The lowest degree of performance was exhibited in the evaluation of the quality of information. This is due to the fact that the majority of the countries of the subregion do not have an entity at the level of the health authority responsible for carrying out this function, nor are audits performed to evaluate the quality of data. Deficiencies in intersectoral coordination also occur in compiling the relevant information on vital statistics required for monitoring health status. Despite the foregoing, all the countries registered good performance with regard to the medical certification of deaths.

Indicators:

1. Guidelines and processes for monitoring health status

2. Evaluation of the quality of information

3. Expert support and resources for monitoring health status

4. Technical support for monitoring health status

5. Technical assistance and support to the subnational levels of public health

EPHF 2: Public health surveillance, research, and control of risks and threats to public health

The countries of the subregion exhibited intermediate performance in this function, with an average score of 63% with regard to the defined optimal standard.

The capacity for timely and effective response to public health problems (Indicator 4) and the insufficient expert development of public health surveillance at the level of the NHA (Indicator 3) stood out in their limited performance.

Indicators:

1. Surveillance system to identify threats and harm to public health

2. Capacities and expertise in public health surveillance

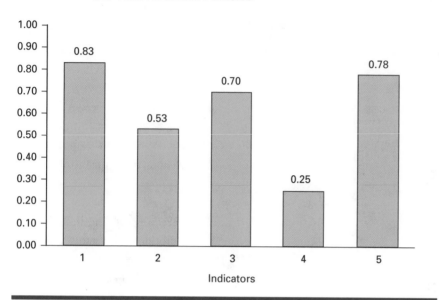

gard to surveillance of accidents and occupational health. Finally, despite the existence of trained staff and action protocols that would enable the health authority to respond effectively to threats and harm to public health, the capacity for timely response is neither stimulated nor evaluated periodically, nor have incentives been defined to improve the performance of personnel responsible for surveillance in public health.

EPHF 3: *Health promotion*

The performance of the subregion with respect to this function was from low to intermediate, with an average score that was 55% of the optimal performance.

3. Capacity of public health laboratories

4. Capacity for timely and effective response to control public health problems

5. Technical assistance and support for the subnational levels of public health

The majority of the countries have an effective surveillance system to identify threats and harm to public health that includes a support laboratory network, but its quality generally is not evaluated on a regular basis.

Even though technical assistance is provided to the subnational levels in the Region is sufficient to support their surveillance capacity, the health authority generally does not have appropriate and timely feedback mechanisms on the information produced at these levels.

With regard to expertise in epidemiology, the subregion has experienced per-

sonnel trained in this area. Its capacity in the area of mental health is particularly strong, and its principal deficiencies are associated with the lack of regular evaluation of the surveillance systems, as well as weaknesses with re-

The English-speaking Caribbean and Netherlands Antilles subregion exhibited intermediate and relatively homogeneous performance for all the indicators, although the indicator related to technical assistance at the subnational levels (Figure 78) was slightly higher.

Figure 78   Performance of the indicators for EPHF 3 in the subregion of the English-speaking Caribbean and the Netherlands Antilles

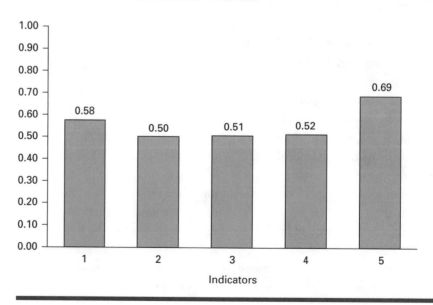

The subregion has various levels of support for promotion activities, although the majority of countries manifest the importance of these activities through written promotion policies.

In general, the levels of participation by other sectors and actors are low. Progress has been achieved in promoting healthy behaviors and environments, although mechanisms to evaluate the impact of social and economic policies are not available.

The health authorities of the countries of the English-speaking Caribbean and Netherlands Antilles subregion are not effective in convening or building partnerships with other sectors, especially due to the low feedback they receive from joint efforts that have been conducted.

Despite the previous, the majority of the countries of the subregion have prepared programs for disseminating information and educating the public on subjects related to health promotion. Some have conducted promotion campaigns, that have not been evaluated, or established entities for the purpose of disseminating information on these subjects among the population.

Health promotion is a topic of frequent discussion in the decision-making bodies of the subregion. Furthermore, primary care is being strengthened and efforts are being made to train human resources in this area. In general, the countries have still not developed actions to reorient health services toward health promotion.

Although the capacity to provide support at the subnational levels is available and the use of tools to improve public access to health promotion has been strengthened, most of the countries of the subregion are unaware of the needs for trained staff.

Indicators:

1. Support for health promotion activities, development of norms, and interventions to promote healthy behaviors and environments

2. Building of sectoral and extrasectoral partnerships for health promotion

3. National planning and coordination of information, education, and social communication strategies for health promotion

4. Reorientation of the health services toward health promotion

5. Technical assistance and support for the subnational levels to strengthen health promotion activities

EPHF 4: *Social participation in health*

The countries of the English-speaking Caribbean and Netherlands Antilles exhibited low to intermediate performance in this function, as reflected by their average score of 46% of the optimal score for this measurement.

The aspect of this function for which an improved, although intermediate, performance was exhibited relates to the strengthening of social participation in health (Figure 79).

With regard to empowering citizens for decision-making in public health, a certain degree of progress has been achieved thanks to the implementation of citizen consultation mechanisms, although these are usually informal in nature and their contributions to health policy design are not monitored.

The establishment of ombudsman's offices and the concept of public account-

Figure 79 Performance of the indicators for EPHF 4 in the subregion of the English-speaking Caribbean and the Netherlands Antilles

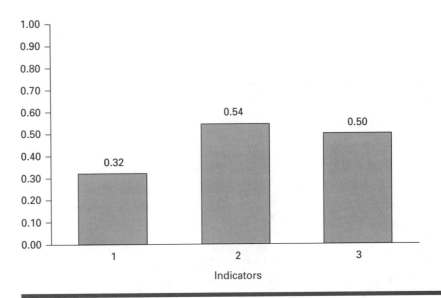

ability are recent occurrences in the subregion.

The strengthening of social participation in health-related matters is an aspect of irregular development across the subregion and, although citizen participation is an element of policy in almost all the countries, it is implemented on an informal basis. In most cases, procedures have not been established for considering public opinion in decision-making, and the information provided to citizens on their rights with regard to health is limited.

Nevertheless, most of the countries have personnel trained to work in these areas and have allocated specific financing for the development of actions in this regard. The evaluation of these aspects is deficient, however.

Finally, although support is provided to the subnational levels with certain regularity, its scope is limited.

Indicators:

1. Empowering citizens for decision-making in public health

2. Strengthening of social participation in health

3. Technical assistance and support for the subnational levels to strengthen social participation in health

EPHF 5: *Development of policies and institutional capacity for planning and management in public health*

The countries of the Region exhibited intermediate performance in this func-

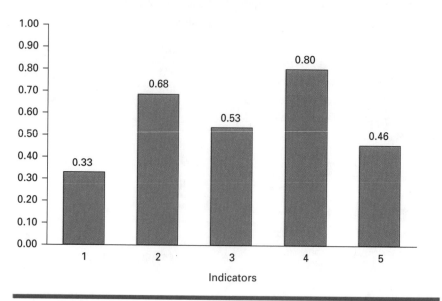

Figure 80 Performance of the indicators for EPHF 5 in the subregion of the English-speaking Caribbean and the Netherlands Antilles

tion, with an average score of 53% of the optimal score for this measurement.

Of particular note was the subregion's high performance with respect to the management of international cooperation in health public, and, on the other hand, its limited ability to define public health objectives, both at the national and subnational levels (Figure 80).

The low performance exhibited in the subregion with regard to the development of plans with goals and objectives that relate to sanitary priorities is attributable to the fact that, although this is a process spearheaded by the health authority, it lacks both a well-defined health system profile to serve as a basis, and financing for the implementation of plans and programs; in addition, neither the indicators to evaluate performance or achievement of the objectives, nor the ability to recognize the partnerships necessary for their fulfillment, have been adequately developed.

The health authority of the countries assumes leadership in the process of developing, monitoring, and evaluating public health policies through a program supported by all State powers, but with limited participation by other sectors. And although the countries have implemented policies that have been translated into laws and have trained personnel in these areas, not all of them have evaluated their impact.

Most of the countries of the subregion have human resources trained in public health management, but they have limited leadership capacity in this area and their supervisory mechanisms are weak. The institutional capacity for information-based decision-making is limited, primarily due to insufficient access to information systems to support and manage this information. The majority of the countries use strategic planning in management but acknowledge that this methodology is not used systematically. Organizational development and the institutional capacity for human resources management are limited, especially with respect to the lack of skilled personnel.

The majority of the countries of the English-speaking Caribbean and Netherlands Antilles have resources, technology, and capacities with regard to the management of international cooperation, and are familiar with the mechanisms and requirements of the various international organizations for allocating resources.

The countries have trained personnel to provide technical assistance to the subnational levels, but the provision of these services is limited for reasons relating to the policy, planning, and management of public health activities, continuous training, and the availability of resources, as well as the inability to determine technical assistance needs at the subnational levels.

Indicators:

1. Definition of national and subnational health objectives

2. Development, monitoring, and evaluation of public health policies

3. Development of institutional capacity for the management of public health

4. Negotiation of international cooperation in public health

5. Technical assistance and support for the subnational levels for policy development, planning, and management in public health

EPHF 6: Strengthening of institutional capacity for regulation and enforcement in public health

The countries of the Region exhibited low performance in this function, with an average score of 46% of the optimal score for this measurement.

In the group of countries that comprise the subregion, only the capacity to establish guidelines for regulating the health system stood out with an intermediate performance level. The other areas exhibited limited development (Figure 8).

Indicators:

1. Periodic monitoring, evaluation, and modification of the regulatory framework

2. Enforcement of the laws and regulations

3. Knowledge, skills, and mechanisms for reviewing, improving, and enforcing the regulations

4. Technical assistance and support to the subnational levels of public health in developing and enforcing laws and regulations

To perform this function, most of the countries of the English-speaking Caribbean and Netherlands Antilles have adequate resources and technical assistance to formulate regulations, but timely and periodic studies of the impact or adverse effects of current regulations are not always performed.

Although the majority of the countries have personnel assigned to enforcement tasks and systematic processes for enforcing regulations, they generally do not have guidelines for the enforcement process. Those who regulate compliance are trained and educated, but there is a lack of incentives for compliance. On the other hand, the implementation of policies and plans aimed at preventing corruption is not a frequent practice.

Figure 81 Performance of the indicators for EPHF 6 in the subregion of the English-speaking Caribbean and the Netherlands Antilles

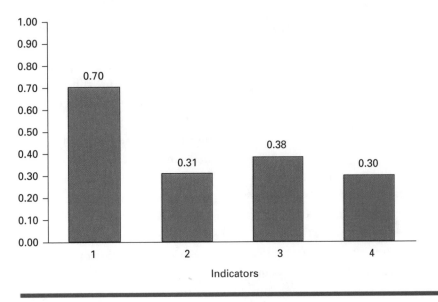

The institutional capacity to perform the regulatory and supervisory function is irregular in the subregion, mainly due to limitations in technical capacity and resources to perform the function and enforce the regulations established by the health authority. Personnel training is incomplete and mechanisms to evaluate training needs generally have not been established.

As a result, assistance to the subnational levels is limited and usually consists of support with regard to enforcement. There is no process available to evaluate the quality of technical assistance or its impact.

EPHF 7: *Evaluation and promotion of equitable access to necessary health services*

The countries of the Region exhibited intermediate performance in this function, with an average score of 63% of the optimal score for this measurement.

In performing this function, the countries of the subregion have demonstrated progress in promoting and taking action to improve access to necessary health services and technical assistance to the subnational levels. Their level of performance in other aspects was lower, especially with regard to the monitoring and evaluation of access to health services (Figure 82).

Indicators:

1. Monitoring and evaluation of access to necessary health services

2. Knowledge, skills, and mechanisms for improving access by the population to necessary health services

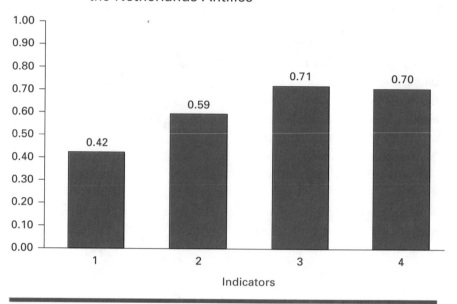

Figure 82 Performance of the indicators for EPHF 7 in the subregion of the English-speaking Caribbean and the Netherlands Antilles

3. Advocacy and action to improve access to necessary health services

4. Technical assistance and support to the subnational levels to promote equitable access to health services

In the majority of countries, the monitoring and evaluation of access to necessary health services is a process that is performed by the respective health authority, in a more or less centralized manner, which translates into an incomplete analysis of levels of public access, especially due to difficulties in identifying the obstacles involved. Consequently, the criteria needed to promote equity in access to essential services is not available.

In the majority of countries, the health authority is familiar with the pattern of health services used by the population, but with limitations due to the weaknesses already mentioned and, as a result, a low capacity for approaching the

community and influencing behavior. In addition, although health personnel receive training in various areas, they are not subject to periodic evaluation, nor is the impact of their actions measured.

The countries of the subregion carry out activities to promote the improvement of public access to health services with varying degrees of success, and accompanied in most cases by concrete actions that are not always evaluated. Furthermore, the establishment of incentives for service providers to promote access to health services is an area of weakness.

Support for the subnational levels is provided unevenly by the different countries of the subregion, with the greatest success in the coordination and dissemination of information and major deficiencies in the capacity to detect obstacles to access, as also occurs at the health authority level.

184

Figure 83 Performance of the indicators for EPHF 8 in the subregion of the English-speaking Caribbean and the Netherlands Antilles

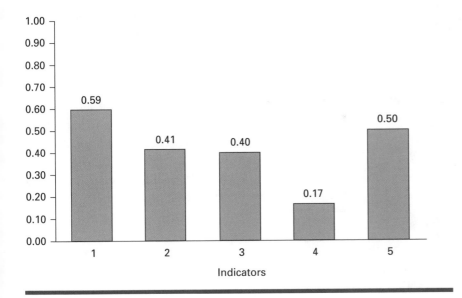

Indicators

EPHF 8: Human resources development and training in public health

The countries of the subregion exhibited low performance in this function, with an average score of 45% of the optimal score for this measurement.

Performance of each aspect of the function was limited in the English-speaking Caribbean and Netherlands Antilles Region, particularly with regard to improving the quality of the workforce for culturally appropriate delivery of services (Figure 83).

The majority of the countries of the subregion have undertaken actions aimed at determining the characteristics of the workforce and defining the skills required for performing the essential functions and population-based public health services, although difficulties occur in identifying the discrepancies between these factors.

The characteristics of the existing public health workforce are not always evaluated with sufficient frequency, nor are steps taken to fulfill future needs. Other types of institutions are also excluded from this process.

Indicators:

1. Description of the public health workforce

2. Improving of the quality of the workforce

3. Continuing education and graduate training in public health

4. Upgrading human resources to ensure culturally appropriate delivery of services

5. Technical assistance and support to the subnational levels in human resources development

The strategies to upgrade the workforce are limited, particularly with regard to the development of service careers, ethical issues, and the strengthening of leadership.

The majority of the countries of the subregion have service performance evaluation systems, but this information is rarely utilized to improve decision-making. Furthermore, there is a marked shortage of continuing education programs.

The most deficient aspect is the process of upgrading the workforce to take into account the sociocultural characteristics of users, at both the health authority and subnational levels. In this area, however, the majority of the countries support the implementation of decentralized human resources development and management plans.

EPHF 9: Quality assurance in personal and population-based health services

The countries of the English-speaking Caribbean and Netherlands Antilles exhibited their lowest performance with respect to this function, with an average score of only 26% of the optimal score for this measurement.

The countries of the subregion exhibited low performance for all aspects of this function, especially with regard to improving the degree of user satisfaction (Figure 84).

Indicators:

1. Definition of standards and evaluation to improve the quality of the population-based and personal health services

2. Improve user satisfaction with the health services

185

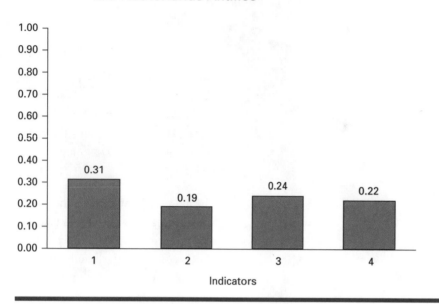

3. Systems for technological management and health technology assessment to support decision-making in public health

4. Technical assistance and support to the subnational levels to ensure quality improvement in the services

In performing the function of the definition of standards and evaluation to improve the quality of population-based and personal health services, the health authorities of only some countries of the subregion apply policies with respect to the continuous improvement of health services quality. The preparation of standards and the periodic evaluation of their fulfillment have not been sufficient, with respect to both population-based and personal services, except in enforcement-related issues.

Efforts to evaluate user satisfaction for services received have been very limited. These evaluations are usually conducted through surveys of the population served and on personal rather than population-based services.

The health authorities in the countries of the subregion seldom promote technological management and health technology assessment; when technology assessment is carried out, it usually has been limited to aspects of safety and effectiveness. Accordingly, decisions made with regard to technology do not tend to be based on the available data. Furthermore, the health authority seldom assesses its capacity in this area.

The subnational levels are provided with limited support for technology development and the evaluation of the quality of both population-based and personal services. This assistance is usually limited to aspects of organizational structure and overall capacity.

EPHF 10: *Public health research*

The English-speaking Caribbean and Netherlands Antilles Region exhibited its second-lowest performance in this function, with an average score of 38% of the optimal score for this measurement.

Of the three aspects, the countries demonstrated the least progress with regard to the development of a public

Figure 85   Performance of the indicators for EPHF 10 in the subregion of the English-speaking Caribbean and the Netherlands Antilles

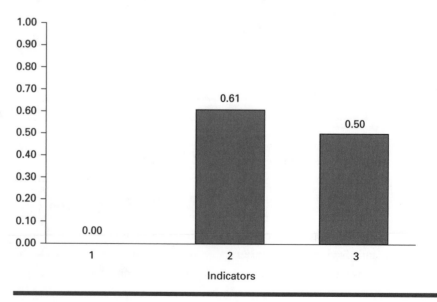

health research agenda. Intermediate performance was exhibited in the aspects concerning institutional capacity and technical assistance at the subnational levels (Figure 85).

Indicators:

1. Development of a public health research agenda

2. Development of institutional research capacity

3. Technical assistance and support for research in public health at the subnational levels

The generalized absence in the subregion of a public health research agenda is the principal weakness in the performance of this function.

Nevertheless, the health authorities have developed a certain level of institutional capacity for autonomous research, thanks to the availability of trained technical teams and computer equipment to provide adequate support for the analysis of information.

Furthermore, certain technical assistance is provided at the subnational levels in operations research methodology and the interpretation of results. Unfortunately, although the professionals at these levels are encouraged to participate in research of national relevance, the results are rarely disseminated among them or to the rest of the scientific community.

***EPHF 11:** Reducing the impact of emergencies and disasters on health*

The countries of the English-speaking Caribbean and Netherlands Antilles exhibited their highest performance in this function, with an average score

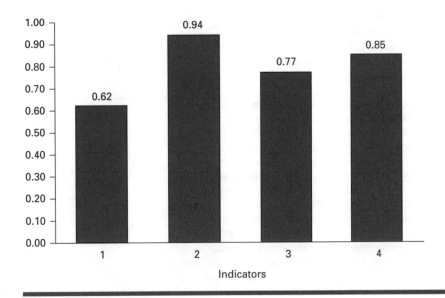

Figure 86 Performance of the indicators for EPHF 11 in the subregion of the English-speaking Caribbean and the Netherlands Antilles

of 71% of the optimal score for this measurement.

Of all the aspects of this function, the one in which the highest level of performance was exhibited is the development of standards and guidelines, while the lowest performance was exhibited with regard to management. In general, intermediate to high performance levels were achieved in the remaining aspects (Figure 86).

Indicators:

1. Reducing the impact of emergencies and disasters

2. Development of standards and guidelines that support emergency preparedness and disaster management in health

3. Coordination and partnerships with other agencies and/or institutions

4. Technical assistance and support to the subnational levels to reduce the impact of emergencies and disasters on health

Management to reduce the impact of emergencies and disasters in the subregion is limited, since not all the countries have an institutionalized national plan to confront these situations, a fact that generally is associated with the lack of a specific health authority unit that is also funded with a designated budget allocation.

Health personnel receive a relatively high level of training in performing this function, but it is not usually included in professional education programs.

The establishment of regulations and standards for dealing with the impact and aftermaths of emergencies and disasters is clearly a strength of the

187

Figure 87 Performance of all the Indicators of the EPHF in the English-speaking Caribbean and Netherlands Antilles

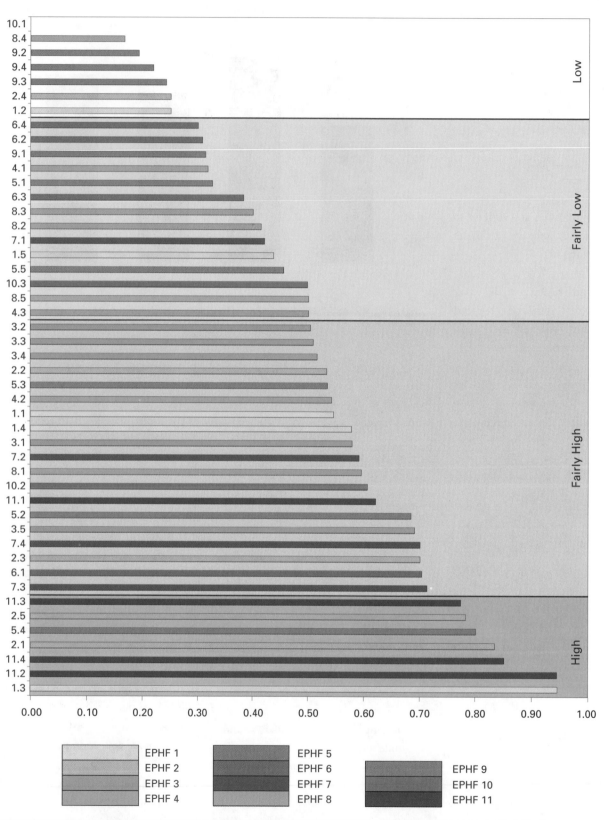

English-speaking Caribbean and Netherlands Antilles Region and encompasses all aspects, except for the impact on mental health.

Coordination between the health authority and other agencies or institutions to confront this type of situation frequently occurs in the countries of the English-speaking Caribbean and Netherlands Antilles, both at the national and international levels. This is supported by the existence of protocols for the dissemination of relevant information through the communications media.

Assistance to the subnational levels in this area is widely developed in the subregion, especially with respect to the strengthening of technical capacity and management of resources, thanks to a needs assessment performed at these levels.

2.2.3 Identification of priority intervention areas

Performance of all indicators

In order to identify the priority intervention areas and consider their levels of development, a profile of all indicators of the EPHF in the English-speaking Caribbean and Netherlands Antilles Region is presented below, classified in increasing order according to low, low-intermediate, high-intermediate, and high performance (Figure 87). In order to facilitate the analysis, the indicators for each function have been given a different color.

The principal critical areas of the subregion were observed in all of the indicators for the function of quality assurance in health services, in most of the aspects evaluated with regard to human resources development, and with regard to the capacities for orientation and regulation, except for the capacity for development of the regulatory framework. On the other hand, no country showed progress in preparing a national public health research agenda.

With regard to the most traditional areas in the performance of public health, significant weaknesses were observed in the capacity for timely response to threats to public health.

Evaluating the quality of information for monitoring health status was also a critical area in need of strengthening.

On the other hand, the principal strengths of the subregion were found in aspects related to emergency and disaster management, the existence of public health surveillance systems, and expertise in epidemiology at the NHA level.

Performance by intervention area

The primary *strengths* of the majority of the countries of the English-speaking Caribbean and Netherlands Antilles in performing the essential public health functions, and which should be maintained in the Regional plan, are as follows:

- Intervention in these important processes: developing standards and guidelines to reduce the impact of emergencies and disasters on health; surveillance systems to identify risks and threats to public health; coordination and partnerships with other agencies or institutions; promotion and action to improve access to necessary health services; and monitoring, evaluation, and modification of the regulatory framework.

- Intervention with regard to developing institutional capacities and infra-structure: expert support and the resources for monitoring and evaluating health status; and management of international cooperation in public health.

- The development of decentralized competencies: technical assistance and support for the subnational levels in reducing the impact of emergencies and disasters on health; and technical assistance and support for the subnational levels in public health surveillance.

On the other hand, the primary *weaknesses* of the English-speaking Caribbean and Netherlands Antilles Region which should be included in a public health strengthening program are as follows:

- Intervention in these important processes: developing a public health research agenda; upgrading human resources to ensure culturally appropriate delivery of services; improving user satisfaction with health services; evaluating the quality of information; responding to control public health problems in a timely and effective manner; enforcing health regulations; developing standards and evaluating the quality of personal and population-based health services; empowering citizens for decision-making in public health; defining national and subnational objectives; and promoting continuing education and graduate training in public health.

- Intervention to develop institutional capacities and infrastructure: technology management and health technology assessment to support decision-making in public health; and knowledge, skills, and mechanisms for reviewing, improving, and enforcing regulations.

- The development of decentralized competencies: technical assistance and support to the subnational levels to ensure the quality of services; and technical assistance and support to the subnational levels in developing and enforcing laws and regulations.

Performance according to the action priorities of the World Bank

The indicators have been regrouped in order to make the results of the measurement operational within the framework of international financing and co-operation strategies. The objective is to identify the action priorities based on: a) significant differences in the public health profile of the countries and b) investment needs. The categories that are considered and the results of the analysis are given below:

a) Development of health policies

In this area, the subregion made progress in defining public health objectives and promoting citizen participation in decision-making.

However, the health authorities of the countries of the English-speaking Caribbean and Netherlands Antilles need strengthening in aspects related to the quality of services, user satisfaction, and the ability to enforce regulations.

b) Collection and dissemination of information to guide health policy

The countries of the Region have made progress in regulating aspects related to monitoring and evaluating health status and institutional research capacity, but this has not been accompanied by adequate evaluation of the quality of information.

Technology management and, in particular, development of a public health research agenda, are areas that require strengthening on the part of the health authority.

c) Disease prevention and control

The subregion has developed a high capacity for monitoring threats to public health, based on strong laboratory support.

Nevertheless, in order to fulfill adequately the functions of disease prevention and control, the health authority must be able to respond in a timely and appropriate fashion to the threats detected.

d) Intersectoral intervention to improve health

In general, the English-speaking Caribbean and Netherlands Antilles Region has effectively developed intersectoral action, especially with respect to actions carried out by the health authority to promote adequate access to necessary services and to coordinate actions with other agencies and institutions.

However, significant weaknesses occur in the formation of partnerships for health promotion and in the efforts to promote citizen participation in health.

e) Human resources development and building institutional capacity in public health

The health authorities in the English-speaking Caribbean and Netherlands Antilles Region have made progress in providing support to the subnational levels for the execution of most of the essential public health functions. However, it is important to note the insufficiency of these actions in the areas of regulation and enforcement, especially with regard to the strengthening of skills and competencies.

The areas requiring significant efforts relate to continuing training and education in public health, development of the capacity to evaluate the quality of services and, especially, adaptation of human resources to the socioeconomic characteristics of the population.

2.2.3 Conclusions

This analysis of the performance of the EPHF in the English-speaking Caribbean and Netherlands Antilles Region demonstrates that while the countries of the Region display differences, they share certain areas of weakness, such as regulation and planning, management of resources, and support for the subnational levels in performing the essential public health functions.

The insufficient capacity to evaluate and prepare the information necessary for decision-making limits the process of developing policies and plans that are adapted to the changes proposed by the epidemiological pattern and emerging sanitary problems.

The lack of trained human resources hinders the performance of the functions, and this limitation is reflected particularly in the capacity to enforce the sanitary regulations and, thus, to ensure respect for the rights of the population with regard to health. In this area, efforts should be made to improve the quality of human resources and the management infrastructure, as well as

Figure 88 Performance of EPHF indicators in the English-speaking Caribbean and the Netherlands Antilles According to Intervention Priorities

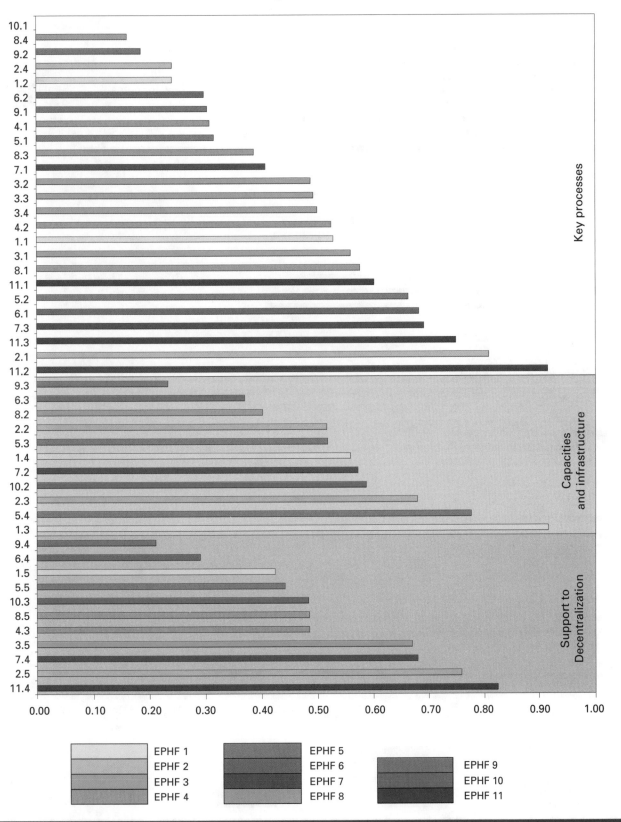

Figure 89 Performance of the EPHF indicators in the English-speaking Caribbean and the Netherlands Antilles Region According to the Intervention Areas Proposed by the World Bank

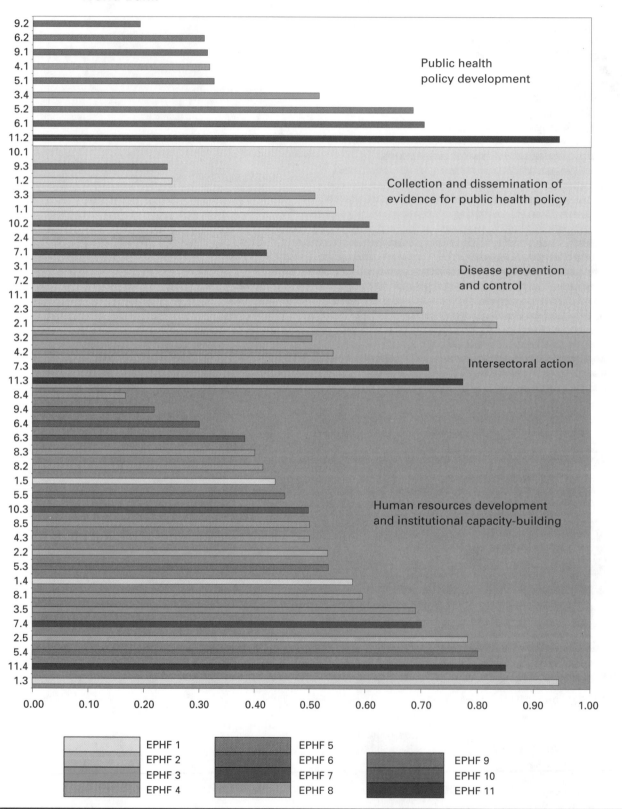

Figure 90   Performance of the EPHF in the Andean subregion

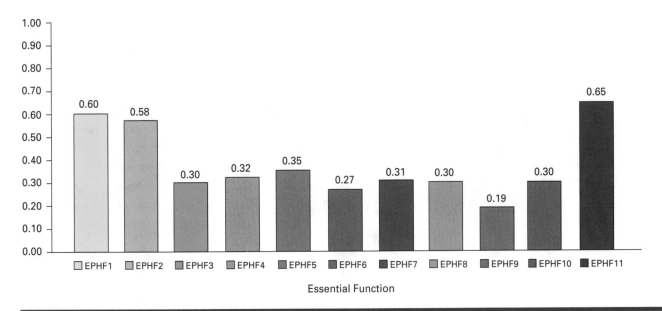

to strengthen the mechanisms for intra- and extrasectoral coordination.

Two elements, in particular, require an increased effort on the part of the health authorities of the English-speaking Caribbean and Netherlands Antilles countries: incorporating the measurement of user satisfaction as a variable to evaluate health system results, and adapting the health services to the sociocultural characteristics of the user population.

Finally, the lack of progress in defining a national public health research agenda makes this a priority area for strengthening, so that the available research capacities are oriented more effectively toward the sanitary objectives of primary concern to these countries.

2.3 Andean Countries

2.3.1 General results of the measurement

The results of the measurement in the countries of the Andean subregion,

composed of Venezuela, Colombia, Ecuador, Peru, and Bolivia, are presented below.

The overall performance of the countries of the subregion with respect to each of the EPHF evaluated is shown in Figure 90. Here the average is used as a summary measure in order to eliminate the influence of the extreme scores in a group of only five observations.

In general, the majority of the functions did not exceed a performance level of 40% of the defined standard for this measurement.

The EPHF that exhibited the best performance were: reducing the impact of emergencies and disasters on health (EPHF 11); monitoring, evaluation, and analysis of health status (EPHF 1); and public health surveillance, research, and control of risks and threats to public health (EPHF 2).

By contrast, the countries of the subregion exhibited the poorest performance

with respect to quality assurance in personal and population-based health services (EPHF 9).

The remaining EPHF exhibited a discreet level of performance with relatively similar results. These functions were: health promotion (EPHF 3), social participation in health (EPHF 4); development of policies and institutional capacity for planning and management in public health (EPHF 5); strengthening of institutional capacity for regulation and enforcement in public health (EPHF 6); evaluation and promotion of equitable access to necessary health services (EPHF 7); human resources development and training in public health (EPHF 8), and public health research (EPHF 10).

Generally speaking, this profile indicates that the countries of the Andean subregion exhibit the most satisfactory performance with respect to public health functions traditionally carried out by the public health authority. However, their relatively low level of performance with

Figure 91 Distribution of the Performance of EPHF in the Andean subregion

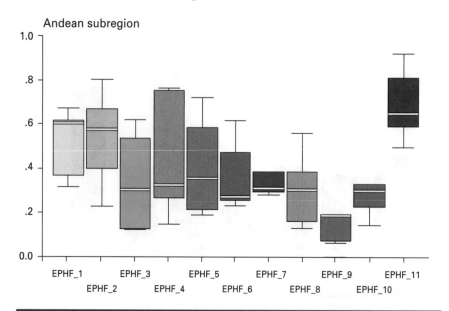

Andean subregion

respect to functions related to the steering role of the health authority, such as planning and regulation, among others, places these countries in a weak position to respond to the challenges presented by the sectoral reform process currently underway throughout the continent.

Within the same context, it is troubling to note the weakness of the countries in performing functions related to health promotion and social participation, which are major elements in achieving improvements in public health conditions. The same applies to the promotion of equitable access to necessary health services.

It is also troubling to note the subregion's poor performance with respect to human resources development, given that this function is vital to strengthening public health.

The overall performance of the group exhibits differences upon analysis of the dispersion in the performance of each

EPHF in the five countries of the subregion. The results show that two subgroups take shape for the first seven EPHF, one with performance generally above 50%, and another with performance near or below 40%. Nevertheless, this difference is smaller in EPHF 8 to 11. In addition, the performance of each country varies with respect to each of the EPHF, indicating that although some areas are critical in some countries, these same areas are more highly developed in others.

Figure 91 shows the average scores, the first standard deviation (representing 66% of the countries), and the maximum and minimum scores[13] for each function in the subregion.

As the Figure indicates, the most clearly well-performing function for the group is EPHF 11 (reducing the impact of emergencies and disasters). While EPHF

---

[13] Results identified as aberrant in the statistical analysis are excluded here.

1 (monitoring of health status) and EPHF 2 (public health surveillance) represent weaknesses for some countries.

The EPHF exhibiting discreet performance and high dispersion included EPHF 3 (health promotion), EPHF 4 (social participation), and EPHF 5 (development of policies and institutional capacity for planning and management). In some countries, particularly with respect to social participation, this level of performance may be considered a strength.

On the other hand, EPHF 9 (quality assurance in health services), EPHF 10 (public health research), and EPHF 7 (evaluation and promotion of equitable access to necessary health services), exhibited relatively similar performance, indicating them as weaknesses throughout the subregion.

2.3.2 Analysis of the results for each EPHF

The performance of each of the essential public health functions in the subregion is analyzed in detail below.

EPHF 1: *Monitoring, evaluation, and analysis of health status*
In the Andean subregion, average performance of the function for monitoring, analysis, and evaluation of public health status was approximately 60%.

The greatest strengths with regard to this function were technical support and assistance, assistance to the subnational levels of public health, and the institutional capacity for expert support and resources (Figure 92). All of the countries have access to computer equipment for managing current health status information in a timely fashion.

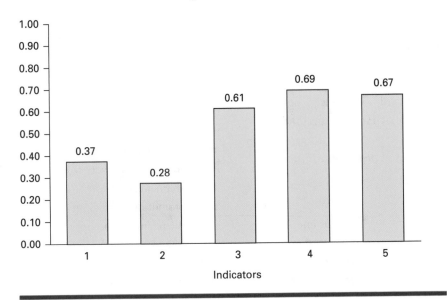

Indicators:

1. Guidelines and processes for monitoring health status

2. Evaluation of the quality of information

3. Expert support and resources for monitoring health status

4. Technical support for monitoring and evaluating health status

5. Technical assistance and support to the subnational levels of public health

Although progress has been made in the development of guidelines and processes for monitoring and evaluating health status, this function has not been fully developed in all of the countries of the subregion. The main deficiencies are the development of guidelines for the local level. There are no methodologies for processing and updating information, information is not periodically disseminated to the public, and genuine concern for protecting the confidentiality of personal information does not exist.

In addition, although all of the countries of the subregion have personnel with experience and training in epidemiology and statistics, the capacity to disseminate health status information is limited.

The area with the lowest overall development in the subregion is the evaluation of the quality of information, primarily because there are no entities devoted to this purpose and because audits to evaluate the quality of information are not performed periodically. One factor that heightens deficiencies in this area is that information on death certifications is untrustworthy in the majority of the countries.

EPHF 2: *Public health surveillance, research, and control of risks and threats to public health*

Performance of this function, although moderate, was among the best for the Andean subregion, with an average score of 58%.

The areas of greatest strength in the subregion were due to the existance of public health surveillance systems and technical support and assistance to the

Figure 93   Performance of the Indicators for EPHF 2 in the Andean subregion

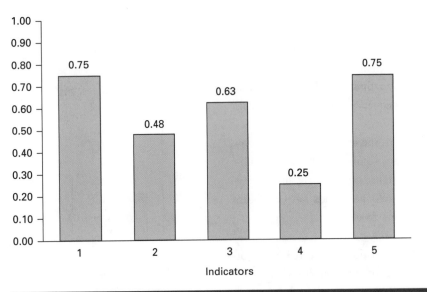

subnational levels (Figure 93). The surveillance systems are capable of identifying threats that require a response by the public health authority, are well-staffed at all levels, and have adequate procedures for disseminating information. The strength of technical support to the subnational levels is based on expert knowledge of the network, access to training, the existence of communication standards, and adequate dissemination of surveillance results.

Indicators:

1. Surveillance system to identify threats and harm to public health

2. Capacities and expertise in public health surveillance

3. Capacity of public health laboratories

4. Capacity for timely and effective response to control public health problems

5. Technical assistance and technical support for the subnational levels of public health.

By contrast, the area of greatest weakness in the Andean subregion was the capacity to respond in a timely and effective manner to control detected problems. Generally speaking, the capacity to analyze threats and harm has not been adequately developed, protocols have not been prepared, and the effectiveness of the emergency response system is not regularly evaluated. In addition, systems for regularly monitoring security response trends have not been adequately developed.

Lastly, regulation and certification of the quality of public health laboratories is limited throughout the subregion.

EPHF 3: *Health promotion*

The performance of the Andean subregion with respect to this function was generally low but its behavior very heterogeneous between countries.

In general, the subregion exhibited significant weaknesses in each of the evaluated areas. However, technical assistance to the subnational levels is more highly developed (Figure 94).

Indicators:

1. Support for health promotion activities, the development of norms, and interventions to promote healthy behaviors and environments

2. Building of sectoral and extrasectoral partnerships for health promotion

3. National planning and coordination of information, education, and social communication strategies for health promotion

4. Reorientation of the health services toward health promotion

5. Technical assistance and support to the subnational levels to strengthen health promotion activities.

In performing this function, the countries of the subregion have not made significant progress in acknowledging the importance of health promotion. This is evidenced by the fact that most of them exhibit weaknesses in formulating health promotion policies, in encouraging participation in health promotion activities, and in promoting healthy behavior and environments. Nevertheless, they have accepted the guidelines set forth at international conferences and have started to use tools that will foster the impact and accessibility of the public to health promotion.

Intersectoral coordination and coordination with the civil society is an area of weakness. The promotion of social and economic policies in support of health

Figure 94 Performance of the Indicators for EPHF 3 in the Andean subregion

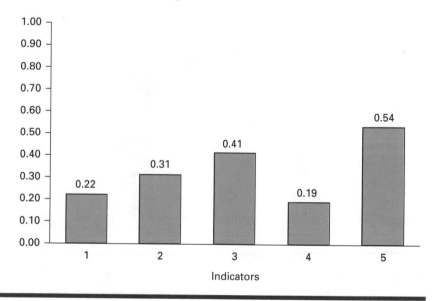

is an area of incipient development. Planning and coordination of communication strategies for health promotion is limited, as evidenced by the fact that there are no entities devoted to providing the general public with information and educational materials (which tend to be scarce).

In addition, strategies for the reorientation of the health services toward health promotion are slowly beginning to take shape. To this end, most of the countries are preparing clinical protocols with respect to health promotion activities at the individual level. Measures have still not been taken to strengthen primary care and human resources.

EPHF 4: *Social participation in health*

The countries of the Andean subregion exhibited low performance of this function, as reflected by the average score of 32%. However, this function was a strength for some countries.

The aspects that exhibited limited, but better development with respect to the performance of this function are related to strengthening social participation in health (Figure 95).

Indicators:

1. Empowering citizens for decision-making in public health

2. Strengthening of social participation in health

3. Technical assistance and support to the subnational levels to strengthen social participation in health.

Most of the countries of the subregion have formal entities for community consultation and participation, and some

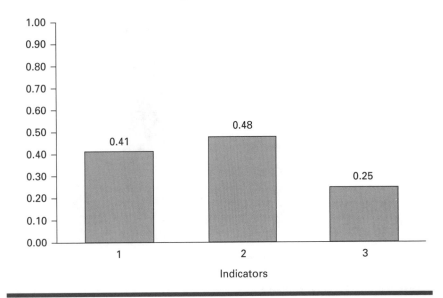

Figure 95 Performance of the Indicators for EPHF 4 in the Andean subregion

type of autonomous state institution that defends the rights of the public in the area of health. In addition, programs designed to inform and educate the public with regard to their health-related rights have been developed.

At all levels, the majority of the countries have community participation networks and staff trained in promoting community participation in individual and population-based health programs.

However, the development of policies aimed giving public participation a central role in the definition and pursuit of public health goals and objectives continues to be weak. Indeed, the ability of the countries to give account to the public regarding health status and the management of personal and population-based health services is limited, as are mechanisms for using public opinion with respect to these issues. Another area of limited development is the promotion of good practices with regard to

social participation in health. This problem is worsened by the difficulty of evaluating the health authority's capacity both to promote good practices and to provide the subnational levels with guidance and assistance in strengthening social participation activities that support decision-making in public health.

EPHF 5: *Development of policies and institutional capacity for planning and management in public health*

The countries of the Andean subregion exhibited low performance of this function, with an average score of 35%. The subregion exhibited a variable performance profile, with some countries indicating significant progress and others indicating significant weakness.

Of particular note is the subregion's high performance with respect to the management of international cooperation in public health, but limitations in the ability to define public health ob-

Figure 96 Performance of the Indicators for EPHF 5 in the Andean subregion

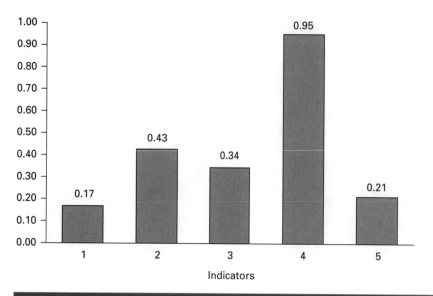

Indicators

Indicators:

1. Definition of national and subnational health objectives

2. Development, monitoring, and evaluation of public health policies

3. Development of institutional capacity for the management of public health systems

4. Negotiation of international cooperation in public health

5. Technical assistance and support to the subnational levels for policy development, planning, and management in public health.

Most of the subregion's national health authorities develop plans with goals and objectives for achieving health priorities, based on the health system profile, jectives, both at the national and subnational levels (Figure 96).

and have identified the parties responsible for implementing these plans at various levels. Nevertheless, there is a lack of leadership in the health improvement process, difficulty in developing financing mechanisms to implement these plans and programs, and limitations in the design and use of indicators to measure achievement of the proposed objectives.

All of the countries have implemented policies that have been translated into law, and all of them have trained personnel in these areas. In developing national plans of public health policy, although the health authorities seek and consider the opinions of other actors and recognize the national importance of agreements; they usually lack the ability to lead this process effectively limiting the participation of other sectors.

In most of the countries, although human resources trained in public health management are available, they have limited capacity to exercise leadership in this area. The institutional capacity for information-based decision-making is limited, primarily due to limited access to information systems. The majority of countries use strategic planning in management but acknowledge that this methodology is not used systematically. Human resources management is moderately well developed; however, most of the countries do not have the ability to reassign human resources based on priorities and necessary changes.

All of the countries of the subregion have resources, technology, and capacities with respect to the negotiation of international cooperation and are familiar with the mechanisms and requirements of the various international organizations for allocating resources. However, all of them exhibit deficiencies in the ability to systematically assess outcomes in collaboration with their counterparts.

The countries have personnel trained in providing technical assistance to the subnational levels, but serious limitations exist in providing assistance related to policy, planning, and management of public health activities, in addition to the inability to identify technical assistance needs at the subnational levels.

***EPHF 6:** Strengthening of institutional capacity for regulation and enforcement in public health*

The countries of the subregion exhibited low performance of this function, with the exception of one country for which it may be considered sufficiently developed.

The only area with respect to which the countries exhibited moderate development was the capacity of the NHA to

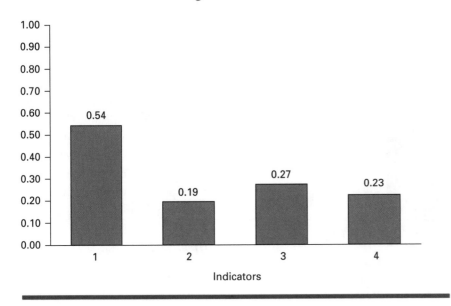

Figure 97 Performance of the Indicators for EPHF 6 in the Andean subregio

Indicators

prepare regulatory frameworks. The other areas exhibited limited development (Figure 97).

Indicators:

1. Periodic monitoring, evaluation, and modification of the regulatory framework

2. Enforcement of laws and regulations

3. Knowledge, skills, and mechanisms for reviewing, improving, and enforcing the regulations

4. Technical assistance and support to the subnational levels of public health in developing and enforcing laws and regulations

In the effort to perform this function, most of the countries of the Region have adequate resources and technical assistance to formulate regulations, but timely and periodic studies of the impact or adverse effects of current regu-

lations are not always performed. All of the countries acknowledge as a weakness the fact that the regulatory framework is usually not reviewed or modified in a timely fashion, but rather in response to external pressure.

Although the countries of the Andean subregion have personnel in charge of enforcement tasks, the health authorities do not have systematic processes for enforcing regulations. This is evidenced by the absence of guidelines for the enforcement process, the irregular development of bodies devoted to providing training and education with regard to regulatory compliance, and the lack of incentives for compliance. In general, policies and plans aimed at preventing corruption in the public health system and abuse of authority by inspectors have not been developed.

Although most of the countries have sufficient institutional capacity to perform regulatory and inspection func-

tions, competent and skilled enforcement teams, and institutional resources, significant obstacles exist to obtaining sufficient financial resources to enforce the regulatory framework. Inspectors are provided with orientations, but ongoing inspector training programs do not exist.

The health authorities of most of the countries have developed mechanisms for providing support to the subnational levels in the event of complex enforcement situations. However, technical assistance is usually not provided for drafting and enforcing laws and regulations, protocols for providing managerial support have not been developed, and technical assistance that has been provided is not periodically evaluated.

EPHF 7: Evaluation and promotion of equitable access to necessary health services

The countries of the Andean subregion exhibited limited performance of this function, with an average of score of 37% of the optimal score for this measurement.

In performing this function, the countries have achieved moderate progress in promoting access to necessary health services and in taking actions to improve it, but they do not exhibit acceptable levels of development in other areas (Figure 98).

Indicators:

1. Monitoring and evaluation of access to necessary health services

2. Knowledge, skills, and mechanisms for improving access by the population to necessary health services

Figure 98 Performance of the Indicators for EPHF 7 in the Andean subregion

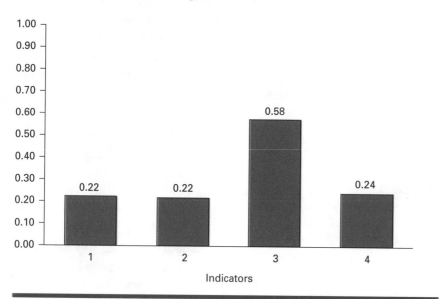

3. Advocacy and action to improve access to necessary health services

4. Technical assistance and support to the subnational levels to promote equitable access to health services.

Although information is available in the majority of the countries of the Region, the national authorities exhibit weaknesses in evaluating access to personal and population-based health services at the national level. Many of them do not have indicators and have a limited capacity to identify obstacles to accessing health care.

Only some countries have personnel with training in reaching the community and providing guidance in the use of health services.

The countries of the subregion carry out activities to promote policies or regulations designed to increase access for the neediest segment of the population. To this end, strategic partnerships have been formed with other sectors and institutions, particularly in the area of human resources, with respect to which weaknesses are generally understood. Some countries have established incentives for service providers designed to increase equitable access to services. In addition, the majority of the countries have national programs aimed at eliminating barriers to access.

The countries of the Andean subregion have partially defined a basic package of personal and population-based services that should be available to the entire population, and they have developed complementary programs for promoting equitable access by the population to services; however, the subnational levels are provided with little assistance in promoting these initiatives.

EPHF 8: *Human resources development and training in public health*

All of the countries of the Andean subregion exhibited relatively low performance of this function.

Performance of each aspect of the function was limited, particularly with regard to improving the quality of the workforce, which was the greatest weakness of this function (Figure 99).

Figure 99 Performance of the Indicators for EPHF 8 in the Andean subregion

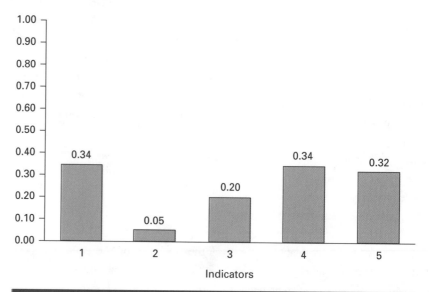

Indicators:

1. Description of the public health workforce

2. Improving the quality of the workforce

3. Continuing education and graduate training in public health

4. Upgrading human resources to ensure culturally appropriate delivery of services

5. Technical assistance and support to the subnational levels in human resources development.

Some of the countries of the subregion have undertaken actions aimed at determining the characteristics of the workforce and defining the required skills for performing the essential functions and collective public health services. They have also begun to identify differences in the composition and availability of the workforce that must be overcome.

All of the countries, with greater or lesser limitations, tend to periodically evaluate the characteristics of the existing public health workforce. However, only one has carried out a qualitative analysis of these characteristics, and none have prepared job profiles.

Nearly all of the countries have developed strategies for improving the quality of the public health workforce, although these strategies are limited by the lack of accreditation standards and guaranteed levels of training. Incentives for professional service careers, programs that include ethical issues, and performance evaluation systems have not been established in the subregion.

Continuing education programs are not frequently promoted, and their impact is not frequently evaluated.

Most of the countries have undertaken the process of upgrading human resources to take into account the characteristics of users, particularly the sociocultural characteristics of users.

The countries of the Andean subregion provide the subnational levels with partial support in developing human resources, particularly through decentralized management mechanisms.

EPHF 9: Quality assurance in personal and population-based health services

The countries of the Andean subregion exhibited their lowest performance with respect to this function, with an average score of 19% of the optimal standard for this measurement.

They exhibited low performance in all areas of this function, particularly with

respect to technological management and health technology assessment to support decision-making in public health and with respect to improving user satisfaction (Figure 100).

Indicators:

1. Definition of standards and evaluation to improve the quality of population-based and personal health services

2. Improving user satisfaction with the health services

3. Systems for technological management and health technology assessment to support decision-making in public health

4. Technical assistance and support to the subnational levels to ensure quality improvement in the services.

Some of the countries have partially developed policies with respect to continu-

Figure 100 Performance of the Indicators for EPHF 9 in the Andean subregion

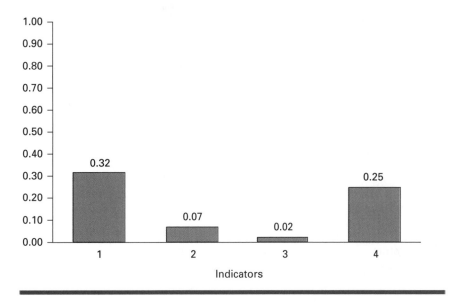

ously improving the quality of health services. Standards have not been sufficiently developed, and national performance goals for population-based services have not been established. The quality of personal health services is certified and inspected with some regularity. However, the use of instruments to measure results is limited, and results are usually not divulged. None of the countries have an independent agency devoted to evaluating and certifying quality.

With regard to the evaluation of user satisfaction, some countries have developed mechanisms for gauging the general response of the public through surveys. These evaluations do not refer to specific personal or population-based services. Unfortunately, the results of these limited efforts have not been used to make decisions with respect to improving health services or upgrading health personnel.

Efforts to develop technological management systems or health technology assessment mechanisms are at a very early stage throughout the subregion.

The subnational levels are provided with some technical assistance in collecting and analyzing information on the quality of population-based health services. Little technical assistance is provided for technology assessment.

EPHF 10: *Public health research*

The Andean subregion exhibited low performance of this function, with an average score of 30%, a score shared by four of the five countries of the Region.

The countries demonstrated the least progress with regard to developing a research agenda. They exhibited moderate

Figure 101 Performance of the Indicators for EPHF 10 in the Andean subregion

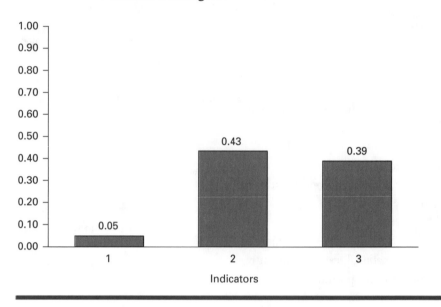

performance with regard to the development of institutional research capacity and providing technical assistance to the subnational levels (Figure 101).

Indicators:

1. Development of a public health research agenda

2. Development of institutional research capacity

3. Technical assistance and support for research in public health at the subnational levels

With regard to the development of a public health research agenda, some countries were only able to identify a particular department of the public health authority with the capacity to oversee this program. With few exceptions, national research agendas have not been formulated with the full participation of the affected parties, and they have not been evaluated.

To some extent, all of the countries of the Region have implemented strategies for the development of institutional research capacity, but only three are ready to engage in dialogue with other research organizations. The majority of the countries stated that they have autonomous capacity to do research in public health, a process for which protocols have been partially established in two countries and for which they have equipment and computer programs. The main limitation is the number of personnel trained to analyze and update the available information.

To a greater or lesser extent, the health authorities of the Andean subregion have the capacity to provide the subnational levels with technical assistance concerning research methodology, particularly in areas related to epidemic outbreaks. Only one or two countries provide technical assistance in order to study the effectiveness population-based interventions, health services, or community health.

The same observations apply to the interpretation of results. Limited support is provided for research at the subnational levels and for using results to improve public health practices.

EPHF 11: *Reducing the impact of emergencies and disasters on health*

The countries of the Andean subregion exhibited their best performance with regard to this function, with some achieving very satisfactory scores.

The lowest level of development in this function is in the area of management. The remaining areas showed moderately high levels of development. (Figure 102).

Indicators:

1. Reducing the impact of emergencies and disasters

2. Development of standards and guidelines that support emergency preparedness and disaster management in health

3. Coordination and partnerships with other agencies and/or institutions

4. Technical assistance and support to the subnational levels to reduce the impact of emergencies and disasters on health.

Although all of the countries of the subregion have institutionalized national plans to support emergency preparedness and disaster management in health, as well as units within the health authority in charge of this area, the quality and coverage of the plans vary. This is primarily due to deficiencies in sectoral coordination and in mechanisms for periodically evaluating the plan.

Health personnel receive training in this area, but it is still not part of professional development programs.

All the countries of the subregion have designed strategies and developed health standards for the national plan of emergencies that encompass most of the pertinent aspects, generally excluding those related to the construction and maintenance of physical infrastructure.

The countries of the Region have generally not established standards for dealing with the aftermath of disasters, except for standards designed to facilitate the delivery of services during emergencies, which is the most important function of the health sector in these situations.

Coordination between the health authority and other sectors or agencies does take place throughout the subregion, although the level of coverage and commitment varies. Coordination is usually handled by the national civil defense organization or by other bodies with multisectoral responsibility. All of the countries have established international partnerships in order to address emergencies.

The majority of the countries provide adequate assistance to the subnational levels in reducing the impact of emergencies and disasters. To varying degrees, the countries collaborate with the subnational levels with regard to building response capacity, preparing regulations, and identifying the parties responsible for managing emergency plans. General weakness was observed in the ability to evaluate needs at the subnational levels.

2.3.3 Identification of priority intervention areas

Performance of all indicators

In order to identify the priority intervention areas and consider their levels

Figure 102   Performance of the Indicators for EPHF 11 in the Andean subregion

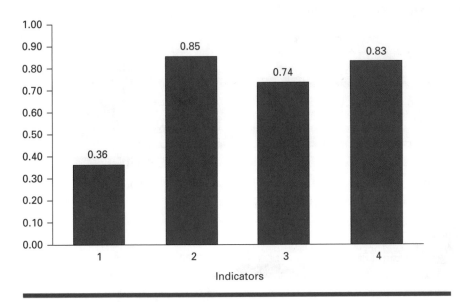

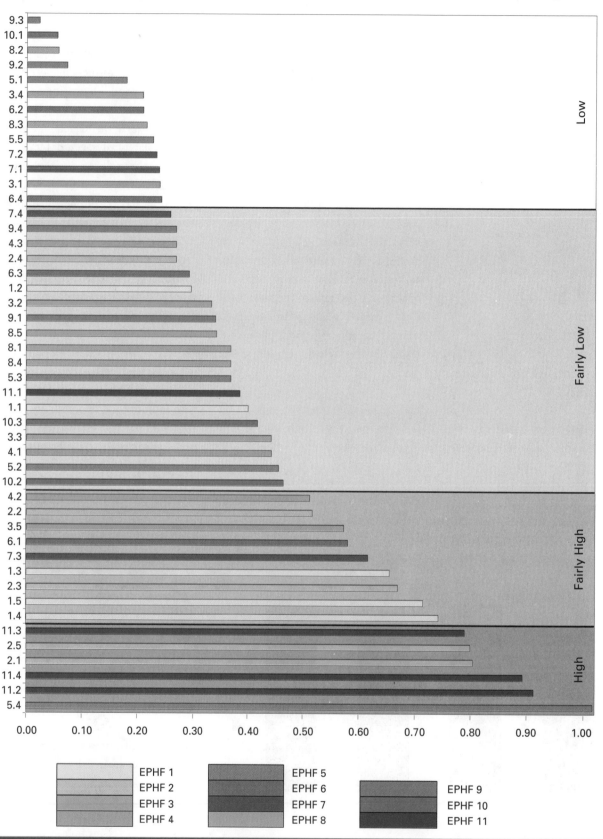

of development, a profile of all indicators of the EPHF in the Andean subregion is presented below, classified in increasing order according to low, low-intermediate, high-intermediate, and high performance (Figure 103). In order to facilitate the analysis, the indicators for each function have been given a different color.

The general profile indicates significant weaknesses in the Region with respect to virtually all of the indicators for EPHF 9 (quality assurance), particularly concerning the improvement of user satisfaction. With regard to human resources development, it is especially critical to improve the quality of human resources and to improve continuing education and training activities. In particular, weaknesses were noted in levels of knowledge and expertise for the development of strategies to improve public access to health services and activities aimed at enforcing the health regulatory framework.

The institutional capacity for public health management and sectoral management in the event of emergencies and disasters are also regarded as critical areas.

In general, efforts to define national and subnational health objectives to guide public and sectoral policy are in a very early stage of development. Weaknesses were also noted with respect to developing and enhancing health policies that are in accord with new health challenges.

As in other subregions of the Americas, limited progress has been made with respect to developing national health research agendas, evaluating the quality of information used to monitor health status, and developing the capacity to respond to public health threats in a timely and effective manner.

The subregion's primary strengths were noted in the management of international cooperation, in the other indicators related to disaster management, and in the availability of public health surveillance systems.

Performance by area of intervention

The primary **strengths** of the majority of the countries of the Andean subregion in performing the essential public health functions, which should be maintained in the subregional plan, are as follows:

- Intervention in these important processes: developing standards and guidelines to reduce the impact of emergencies and disasters on health; surveillance systems to identify risks and threats to public health; and coordination and partnerships with other agencies or institutions to reduce the impact of emergencies and disasters on health.

- Intervention with regard to developing institutional capacities and infrastructure: management of international cooperation in public health.

- The development of decentralized competencies: technical assistance and support for the subnational levels in reducing the impact of emergencies and disasters on health; and technical assistance and support for the subnational levels in public health surveillance, research, and the control of risks and threats to public health.

On the other hand, the primary **weaknesses** of the Andean subregion, which should be included in a public health strengthening program, are as follows:

- Intervention in these important processes: developing public health research agendas; improving user satisfaction with health services; defining national and subnational public health objectives; reorienting health services toward health promotion; enforcing health regulations; continuing education and graduate training in public health; monitoring and evaluating access to necessary health services; supporting health promotion activities and developing standards and interventions to encourage healthy behavior and environments; responding to control public health problems in a timely and effective manner; evaluating the quality of information; establishing sectoral and extrasectoral partnerships for health promotion; defining standards for and evaluating the quality of personal and population-based health services; describing the public health workforce; upgrading human resources to ensure culturally appropriate delivery of services; managing activities aimed at reducing the impact of emergencies and disasters; and maintaining guidelines and processes for monitoring and evaluating health status.

- Intervention to develop institutional capacities and infrastructure: technology management and health technology assessment systems to support decision-making in public health; improving the quality of the workforce; knowledge, skills, and mechanisms improving access by the population to programs and services; knowledge, skills, and mechanisms for reviewing, improving, and enforcing regulations; and developing institutional capacity

Figure 104 Performance of EPHF indicators according to the priority areas of intervention

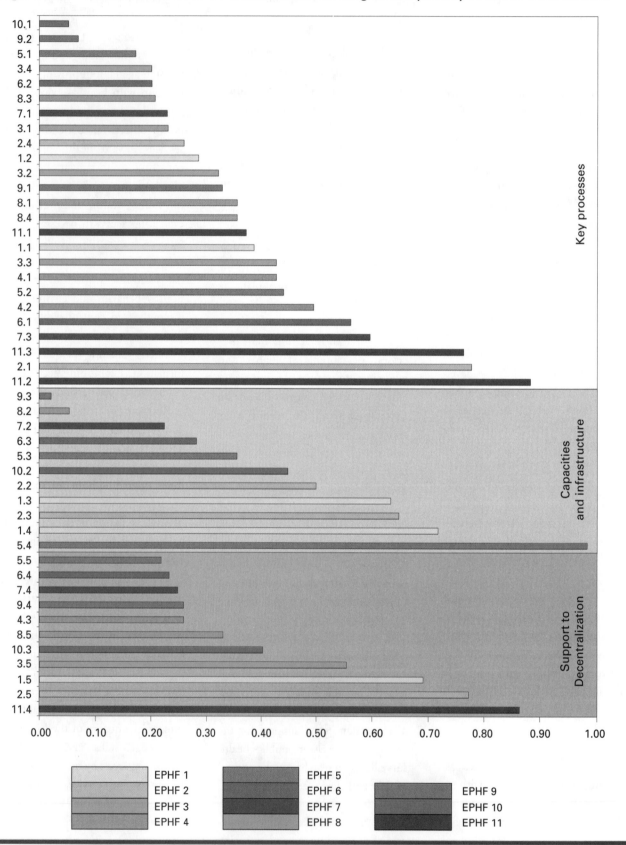

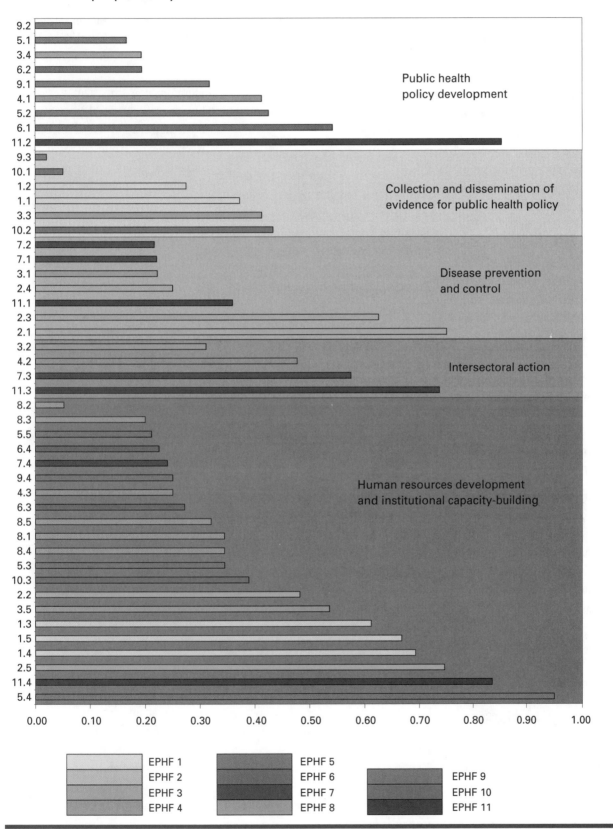

for the management of public health systems (Indicator 5.3).

- The development of decentralized competencies: technical assistance and support to the subnational levels in policy development, planning, and management in public health; technical assistance and support to the subnational levels in developing and enforcing laws and regulations; technical assistance and support to the subnational levels to promote equitable access to health services; technical assistance and support to the subnational levels to strengthen social participation in health; technical assistance and support to the subnational levels to ensure quality improvement in the services; technical assistance and support to the subnational levels in human resources development; and technical assistance and support for research in public health at the subnational levels.

Profile according to the action priorities of the World Bank

The indicators have been regrouped in order to make the results of the measurement operational within the framework of international financing and cooperation strategies. The objective is to identify action priorities based on: *a*) significant differences in the public health profile of the countries, and *b*) investment needs. The categories that were considered and the results of the analysis are given below.

a) Development of health policies

In this area, the subregion exhibited weakness in defining public health objectives, and exhibited little progress in designing policies to improve user satis-

faction and reorienting public health services toward health promotion.

In addition, policies related to the enforcement of regulations must be strengthened.

b) Collection and dissemination of information to guide public health policy

The countries of the subregion have made progress in providing technical assistance for monitoring and evaluating health status, but this has not been accompanied by evaluations of the quality of information.

An area of limited development is the national public health research agendas. There is also little concern in the area of technology management and assessment.

c) Disease prevention and control

The subregion has a good surveillance system, but there are deficiencies in the speed and appropriateness of responses to public health threats.

In addition, the NHA have not demonstrated the ability to improve access to services or to sponsor promotional activities aimed at improving the population's quality of life.

d) Intersectoral intervention to improve health

The Andean subregion has good mechanisms for intersectoral coordination, but it must strengthen efforts to form partnerships designed to improve the implementation of health promotion activities.

e) Human resources development and building institutional capacity in public health

In this area, the subregion demonstrated good management of international cooperation, as well as good capacity for providing technical assistance to subnational levels with regard to the essential public health functions.

However, it is important to note that human resources development needs to be strengthened in several respects. This is because the countries have not yet succeeded in adequately defining and describing the public health workforce, which weakens the already limited access of the workforce to continuing education and guidance with regard to managing the more complex public health functions, such as developing regulatory policies and mechanisms, guaranteeing equitable access to services, and carrying out health promotion and social participation activities.

It should be noted that the NHA have taken little action to adapt human resources to the socioeconomic characteristics of the population, or to study the quality of care and service providers.

2.3.4 Conclusions

This analysis of the performance of the EPHF in the Andean subregion demonstrates that while the countries of the subregion display differences, they share certain areas of weakness, such as regulation and planning, social participation, and health promotion.

One critical area common to all the functions that should be underlined is the insufficient ability to manage information, which hinders the policy development and planning process and makes it difficult to monitor and evaluate strategies aimed at making these policies and plans more operational. Consequently, this area should be strengthened. In addition,

Figure 106 Performance of the EPHF in the Southern Cone and Mexico subregion

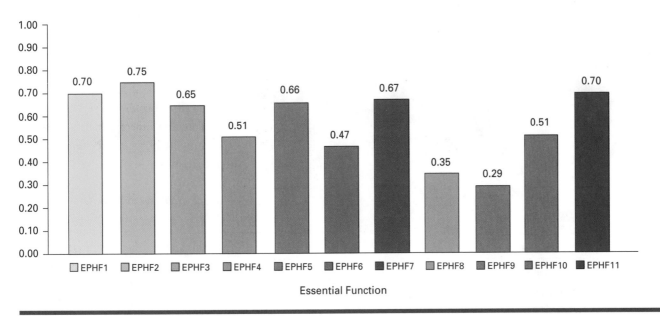

efforts must be made to achieve qualitative improvements in the human resources and management infrastructure, and to strengthen intra- and extrasectoral communication mechanisms.

2.4 Southern Cone and Mexico

2.4.1 Overview of EPHF Performance

In this chapter, we look at the measurement results for the six countries of the Southern Cone (Argentina, Brazil, Chile, Paraguay and Uruguay) and Mexico[14] subregion.

Figure 106, above, shows the overall performance achieved by countries in the subregion for each evaluated EPHF. As this subregion comprises only six countries, the average value has been

---

[14] Mexico is included in this group of countries because of its geopolitical similarity with the countries of the Southern Cone.

used as a global measurement, in order to avoid the influence of extreme values.

This subregion scores over 50% of the pre-established measurement standard in 8 of the 11 essential functions.

As Figure 106 illustrates, the better-performing EPHF are those related to: public health surveillance, research, and control of risks and threats to public health (EPHF 2); monitoring, evaluation and analysis of health status (EPHF 1); and reducing the impact of emergencies and disasters on health (EPHF 11).

The worst performance by countries in the subregion is found for EPHF 9 (ensuring the quality of personal and population-based health services) and for EPHF 8 (human resource development and training in public health).

For the remaining EPHF, the performance level is average. In decreasing order, they are: evaluation and promotion of equitable access to necessary

health services (EPHF 7); development of policies and institutional capacity for planning and management in public health (EPHF 5); health promotion (EPHF 3); social participation in health (EPHF 4); and strengthening of institutional capacity for regulation and enforcement in public health (EPHF 6).

In general, the success achieved in public health research (EPHF 10) is higher than for other subregions and higher than for the entire Region.

This shows that the countries of the Southern Cone and Mexico have achieved levels of performance in essential public health functions not only in traditional areas, such as epidemiological surveillance and the monitoring of health status, but also in other, newer areas, which have been promoted as part of sectoral reform processes. These areas include health promotion and evaluation of equitable access of the population to health services. Significant progress has also been made in the plan-

Figure 107 Distribution of the Performance of each EPHF in the Southern Cone and Mexico subregion

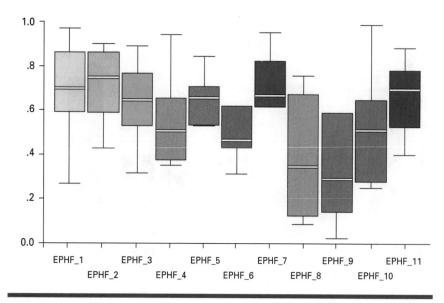

source development), where overall development levels are regarded as average, and EPHF 9 (ensuring quality of services), which scores the worst overall performance in the subregion. In this case, the performance of these functions may be regarded as a strong point in some of the countries analyzed, but a weakness in others. This suggests that there is room for cooperation between the countries.

2.4.2 Analysis of Results for Each EPHF

In this section, the performance of each essential public health function is analyzed in the context of the subregion, and its constituent elements identified and described.

EPHF 1: Monitoring, Evaluation and Analysis of Health Status

In the Southern Cone and Mexico, the function "monitoring, evaluation and analysis of the people's health status" achieves 70% of the expected standard, according to the average value. Variation between the countries in the subregion is limited.

Indicators:

1. Guidelines and processes for monitoring and evaluating health status;

2. Evaluation of information quality;

3. Expert support and resources for monitoring and evaluating health status;

4. Technical support for monitoring and evaluating health status;

5. Technical assistance and support to the subnational levels of public health.

ning and management functions, as well as in the promotion of equitable access to health services.

The functions that probably require greater impetus are those related to more qualitative aspects of the steering factors of the of the health sector such as the regulation and enforcement of compliance with health regulations, human resource development and, in particular, ensuring the quality of services offered to the population.

With regard to the 11 essential public health functions, all countries of the Southern Cone and Mexico show certain weaknesses and strengths in public health. This suggests the possibility of promoting cooperation between countries in the subregion in order to improve public health practice.

Figure 107 shows the results in terms of average value, the first standard deviation (equivalent to 66% of the coun-

tries), and maximum and minimum values [15] for each function.

The Figure 107 shows also, EPHF 5 (planning and management in public health), and EPHF 7 (evaluation and promotion of equitable access to necessary health services) show the least dispersion. We may therefore conclude that these two functions generally represent strengths for all countries analyzed.

EPHF 6 (strengthening of institutional capacity for regulation and enforcement in public health) generally demonstrates an average to low performance level with less variability. We may therefore conclude that this is a critical area, which should be strengthened in most countries in the subregion.

The biggest variations in performance levels are found for EPHF 8 (human re-

[15] For the purposes of this analysis, certain results identified in the statistical analysis as aberrant values have been excluded.

Figure 108 Performance of Indicators for EPHF 1 in the Southern Cone and Mexico subregion

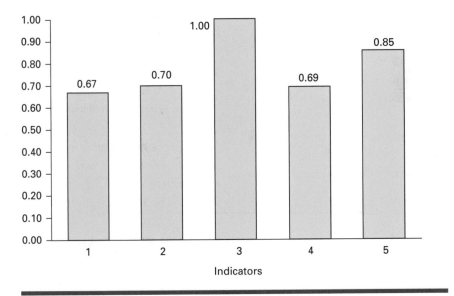

All areas of this function demonstrate a satisfactory performance level (Figure 108), especially those related to the availability of experts and resources for monitoring and evaluation. In contrast to the rest of the Region, this subregion is especially noteworthy for the good result achieved in the evaluation of the quality of information.

In the aspects related to guidelines and processes for monitoring and evaluation, the periodic revision and updating of its contents is not optimum and there are difficulties in adequately disseminating the information that is produced.

With regard to the evaluation of the quality of information, the countries do recognize that the institutions appointed to carry out this function are not sufficiently independent of the health authority.

The subregion has an adequate supply of expert support and resources to monitor the health status of the population.

The strong performance achieved with respect to the technological support provided to carry out this function is limited by the fact that such support is not widely used locally and by the difficulties involved in having adequate access to maintenance.

Technical assistance provided to the subnational levels for the performance of this function is problematical only in terms of the timeliness of such actions.

EPHF 2: *Public Health Surveillance, Research, and Control of Risks and Threats to Public Health*

This function demonstrates the best performance level in the subregion, achieving an average value of 75%. This Figure is relatively constant across all countries analyzed.

All areas demonstrate a level of high performance, except for the one related to capacity and expertise in epidemiology, which achieves only average levels (Figure 109).

Indicators:

1. Surveillance system to identify risks and threats to public health;

2. Capacities and expertise in public health surveillance;

Figure 109 Performance of Indicators for EPHF 2 in the Southern Cone and Mexico subregion

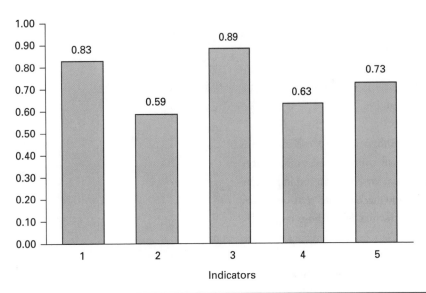

3. Capacity of public health laboratories;

4. Capacity for timely and effective response to control public health problems;

5. Technical assistance and support for subnational levels of public health.

The surveillance system used by health authorities demonstrates a good performance level in countries of the subregion, but tends not to include quality of life indicators. The system has some difficulties in obtaining information feedback and tends not to use the information produced by other national agencies or institutions that also deal with surveillance.

The poorer performance level exhibited with respect to expertise in epidemiology is linked to the limited use of geoFigureic information systems by health officials of countries in the subregion, and this is compounded by the lack of training in mental and occupational health. Another limitation is the frequency with which data analysis is carried out.

With regard to public health laboratories, most countries have a consolidated network, but present certain shortcomings with respect to certification of laboratory quality.

Health authorities' response capacity is high for all countries in the subregion. Difficulties arise only in the implementation of mechanisms that recognize good performance by those responsible for surveillance and emergency response.

Technical assistance at subnational levels is adequate, but health authorities tend not to receive reports on these lev-

els regarding the surveillance situation in their areas.

EPHF 3: *Health Promotion*

The performance of the subregion for this function is average. The average value of 65% is relatively constant for all countries.

The subregion scores an average performance in all areas. Worthy of note is the good result achieved in the formulation of standards and interventions to encourage healthy behaviors and environments (Figure 110).

Indicators:

1. Support for health promotion activities, development of norms, and interventions to promote healthy behaviors and environments;

2. Building of sectoral and extrasectoral partnerships for health promotion;

3. National planning and coordination of information, education and com-

munication strategies for health promotion;

4. Reorientation of health services toward promotion;

5. Technical assistance and support to the subnational levels to strengthen health promotion activities.

All countries have formulated promotion policies that include international recommendations and incorporate information technologies in an effort to encourage promotion. Those policies define both short-term and long term goals. Health authorities are not always successful in eliciting the commitment of all levels and all actors, and application of these policies is not regularly evaluated. All countries promote development of standards and interventions aimed at fostering healthy behaviors and environments.

All countries in the subregion have set up a coordinating entity that brings together other sectors in order to meet targets, but not all have prepared a plan

Figure 110 Performance of Indicators for EPHF 3 in the Southern Cone and Mexico subregion

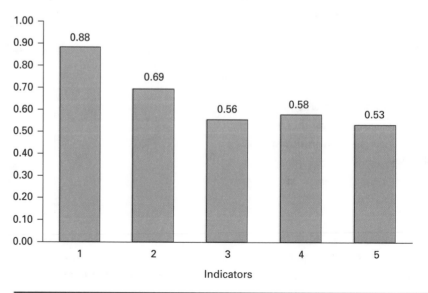

212

of action. Most countries have difficulties in monitoring joint activities and in analyzing the impact of social and economic policies. Nevertheless, one of the subregion's strengths lies in its efforts to promote the incorporation of these areas in health policies and in policies on health promotion, in particular.

There are community-education programs that are implemented jointly with other sectors and institutions in an effort to improve the people's health status. Unfortunately, promotion campaigns are not often evaluated. The subregion does not have specific entities responsible for informing the people and providing educational materials.

One topic of discussion within health sector decision-making institutions is the refocusing of health services toward promotion. This is reflected in the presence of project-financing mechanisms created for that purpose. Application of other strategies in the subregion is limited. Such strategies might include payment mechanisms encouraging promotion of insurance systems, whether public or private; design of clinical protocols; or strengthening of primary care through the creation of health teams that are trained in promotion, are responsible for specific population groups and carry out specific promotion programs.

Health authorities do have expert personnel to provide technical assistance at the subnational levels. There is only a limited amount of material incorporating cultural diversity and limited evaluation of the needs of specialists in health education at the subnational level. There is coordination with other social actors at this level. Moreover, good use is made of national tools for strengthening the impact of, and access to health promotion.

EPHF 4: *Social Participation in Health*

For this function, the countries of the Southern Cone and Mexico exhibit an average performance, as reflected in the average value (51%). There is little variation between countries.

The area that exhibits a better (though average) performance level for this function is the strengthening of social participation in health (Figure 111).

Indicators:

1. Empowering citizens for decision-making in public health;

2. Strengthening of social participation in health;

3. Technical assistance and support to the subnational levels to strengthen social participation in health.

With a view to strengthening social decision-making power in public health, average progress has been made toward implementation of mechanisms for consulting with citizens and taking their opinions into account, both within formal entities and at all levels. Procedures for responding to the opinions of civil society have not yet been set up.

Most countries have introduced the institution of the independent public defense counsel with the legal status to protect the health rights of the citizen.

All countries, to varying degrees, give public account of the population's health status and the management of health services. Citizens are not, however, encouraged to offer feedback.

With respect to the strengthening of social participation in health, most countries express the importance of this as a key element in defining and implementing the objectives and goals of public health. Accordingly, they have created formal entities, usually at the intermediate and local levels. Unfortunately, very few countries offer programs for informing citizens about their rights in health-related matters, which

Figure 111   Performance of Indicators for EPHF 4 in the Southern Cone and Mexico subregion

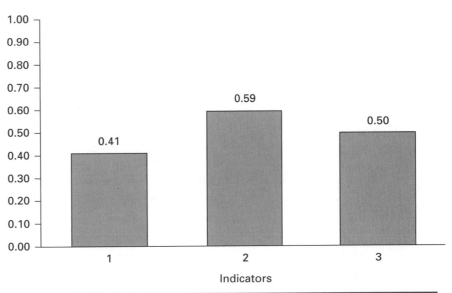

is among the fundamental areas of enabling people to assume responsibility for their own health.

All countries in the subregion employ staff who are trained to promote citizen participation and good practices for social participation in health. Most allocate resources to organizations involved in developing public health programs.

There is broad calling about the need to promote participation in health, but this capacity is seldom evaluated.

With regard to technical assistance at the subnational levels, all countries have the capacity to promote the development of mechanisms for participation in decision-making on public health, but show evidence of difficulties in evaluating the impact of these actions and ensuring a response that is adequate for the needs expressed by the population at those levels.

EPHF 5: *Development of Policies and Institutional Capacity for Planning and Management in Public Health*

Performance for this function in the subregion is average. The average value of 66% is fairly uniform across the five countries concerned.

With regard to this function, particularly noteworthy is the high level achieved in the monitoring and evaluation of public health policies and in the management of international cooperation in public health. However, the capacity of the NHA to assist in these matters at the subnational levels is somewhat more limited (Figure 112).

Indicators:

1. Definition of national and subnational health objectives;

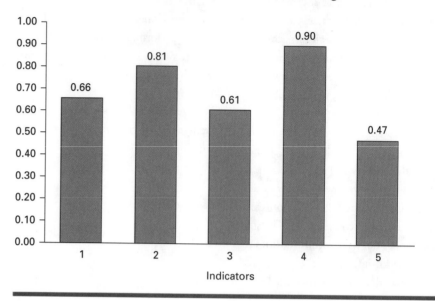

Figure 112 Performance of Indicators for EPHF 5 in the Southern Cone and Mexico subregion

2. Development, monitoring and evaluation of public health policies;

3. Development of institutional capacity for the management of public health systems;

4. Negotiation of international cooperation in public health;

5. Technical assistance and support to the subnational levels for policy development, planning, and management in public health.

Most countries in the subregion develop plans with goals and objectives related to health priorities, based on the health system profile. This process is led by the health authority and complemented by officials appointed to implement those goals and objectives at the different levels. The design and use of indicators for measuring compliance with the proposed objectives is generally good. Nevertheless, problems do arise with funding mechanisms that tie management to certain health objectives.

All countries in the subregion have applied policies that are reflected in bodies of law, for which they have trained staff. Development of the national plan for public health policies is a process spearheaded by the health authority, with the participation of other sectors. Moreover, the capacity for monitoring and evaluating those policies is generally high.

There is evidence of strong leadership in health management. Consequently, most countries do have technical expertise, while planning, decision-making and evaluation of activities are usually based on data. Furthermore, there is generally adequate coverage in terms of information-systems (which are deficient only in terms of quality), personnel trained to use such systems, and mechanisms for supervision and evaluation. However, this subregion still does not make use of performance indicators that make it possible to continue improving management in public health.

Organizational development, which exhibits shortcomings in all areas, is one of the areas of least progress in the countries under consideration.

With respect to resource management, most countries in the subregion have adequate capacity as well as experience in reallocating resources according to health priorities and observed needs.

Management of international cooperation is adequate in all countries in the subregion, thanks to the fact that they have the necessary resources, technology, and capacities, and are familiar with the various international organizations' mechanisms and requirements for the allocation of resources. Only one of the countries analyzed exhibits certain shortcomings in this area.

With regard to technical assistance at the subnational level, the countries under consideration do have trained staff, but demonstrate certain shortcomings in the areas of policy definition, strategic planning and ongoing improvement of management. The greatest difficulties demonstrated by the subregion are linked to the inability to detect technical assistance needs at those levels.

EPHF 6: *Strengthening of Institutional Capacity for Regulation and Enforcement in Public Health*

In this subregion, performance for this function is among the poorest of the 11 EPHF under consideration. The average value is 47%, and there is limited variation among the countries concerned, which confirms its position of weakness across the subregion.

Of particular note for the group of countries in the subregion are the high level of development of processes for monitoring regulations and the strong capacity for enforcement. However, as

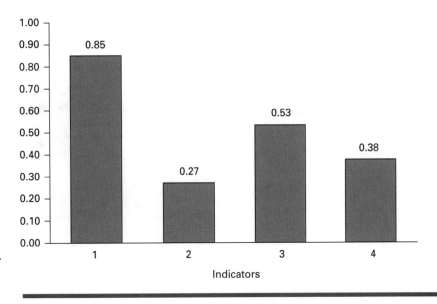

Figure 113   Performance of Indicators for EPHF 6 in the Southern Cone and Mexico subregion

Figure 113 illustrates, this is not reflected in the results, which show a low performance for institutional ability to enforce norms.

Indicators:

1. Periodic monitoring, evaluation and modification of regulations;

2. Enforcement of laws and regulations;

3. Knowledge, skills, and mechanisms for reviewing, improving and enforcing regulations;

4. Technical assistance and support to the subnational levels of public health in developing and enforcing laws and regulations.

In order to perform the function of regulation and enforcement in public health, most countries of the Southern Cone and Mexico have adequate resources and technical assistance for the formulation of regulations, although

those regulations are not always reviewed on a sufficiently timely and regular basis to study the impact or adverse effects of the regulations established.

Although in the subregion those responsible for overseeing compliance of regulations have been identified and guidelines to support them have been made available, health authorities do not establish systematic procedures to enforce regulations. This is reflected in the lack of supervision for the enforcement process, the absence of regular activities by training and education bodies regarding compliance with regulations and the provision of incentives for compliance. In general, policies and plans to prevent corruption in the public health system have not been developed.

Most countries exhibit sufficient institutional capacity to perform regulatory and enforcement functions, and have competent and skilled teams and institutional resources. However, they exhibit marked limitations in terms of ac-

215

cess to the financial resources needed to enforce regulations and in terms of the volume of human resources needed to perform this function. Orientation activities are provided for enforcement officials, but long-term training plans are not provided.

In their dealings with the subnational levels, health authorities in most countries of the subregion have developed support mechanisms for complex enforcement situations, but there is generally no technical assistance for the formulation and enforcement of laws and regulations. Protocols that support the management at subnational level have not been developed, and there is no regular evaluation of the technical assistance provided.

EPHF 7: *Evaluation and Promotion of Equitable Access to Necessary Health Services*
Performance for this function is average. The average value is 67% and there is little dispersion among countries in the subregion.

In the performance of this function, the best-performing areas are the provision of technical assistance at the subnational levels (which achieves very high levels), followed by promotional efforts and actions to improve access to necessary health services. However, there is less compliance in the monitoring and evaluation of access to necessary services (Figure 114).

Indicators:

1. Monitoring and evaluation of access to necessary health services;

2. Knowledge, skills, and mechanisms for improving access by the population to necessary health services;

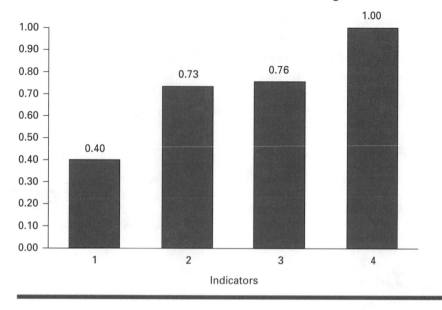

Figure 114 Performance of Indicators for EPHF 7 in the Southern Cone and Mexico subregion

3. Advocacy and action to improve access to necessary health services;

4. Technical assistance and support to the subnational levels to promote equitable access to health services.

Health authorities in the subregion manage the evaluation of access to essential services on an irregular basis, with respect both to personal and population-based services. This is mainly because the process does not generally involve collaboration with other agencies or institutions, and obstacles to access are not fully identified (in general, variables related to ethnicity, culture, religion, language, or physical or mental disability are not included). Also, not all countries analyzed use methodologies for the detection of inequalities. Consequently, there is less promotion of equity in access to essential health services.

There are enough staff who are trained to work with the community and advise the population on how to use health services, although there are flaws in the methods used to inform society. Moreover, health authorities do not evaluate this capacity often enough.

Countries in the subregion carry out actions to promote policies or regulations to increase the access of the neediest population. Strategic partnerships have been set up for this purpose with other sectors and institutions, especially in the area of human resources. There is generally an awareness of inequalities. In this context, three countries have introduced incentives for service providers in an effort to reduce inequalities in access to services. Most countries do have national programs to resolve access problems.

Health authorities in the Southern Cone and Mexico have enough capacity to provide assistance at the subnational levels in all areas, such as in the definition of the basic package of personal and population-based services that should be available to the whole population, identification of unmet needs and obstacles to access, and development of complementary programs for working with the community to promote equitable access to services.

EPHF 8: Human Resources Development and Training in Public Health

This is one of the poorer-performing functions in the subregion, with an average value of 35%. Nevertheless, there are major differences between the different countries, which means that it is a satisfactory performance function in some of them.

The Southern Cone and Mexico subregion exhibits a good overall performance both in the definition of the characteristics of the public health workforce and the provision of technical assistance at the subnational levels. This is contrasted by countries' low scores for improving the quality of, and providing continuing education to human resources, as well as training aimed at responding to users' changing needs (Figure 115).

Indicators:

1. Description of public health workforce;

2. Improving the quality of the workforce;

3. Further education and graduate training in public health;

4. Upgrading human resources to ensure culturally appropriate delivery of services;

5. Technical assistance and support to the subnational levels in human resources development.

Health authorities in the subregion have sufficient capacity to define the needs of staff in the public health sector, by describing its profile and identifying the skills required. They are successful in identifying differences at the national level. However, there are problems with the evaluation of the existing workforce, notably the limited access to informa-

tion systems that can show the distribution of the workforce and produce an up-to-date and complete inventory. There is little coordination with other institutions to evaluate the quantity and quality of public health workers.

In the countries of the Southern Cone and Mexico, health authorities formulate accreditation and certification regulations to facilitate the hiring of public health workers. Compliance with these regulations is evaluated regularly. There are also well-defined training policies, which are supported by teaching institutions, and with which the basic public health education plans have been developed.

Unfortunately, the impact of these policies is not evaluated often enough. This is also the case with plans to improve the quality of the public health workforce.

Although health authorities provide opportunities to develop leadership in public health and have the ability to identify potential leaders, no effort is made to encourage leaders to remain over the long-term, and there are no incentives to improve the capacities of their public health workers.

The area that exhibits the least development on the part of health authorities in the countries under consideration is the availability of systems to evaluate the performance of public health workers. This evaluation is carried out only on a partial basis in two of the five countries in the subregion.

In order to promote continuing education and graduate training in public health, a certain degree of coordination has been developed with educational

Figure 115 Performance of Indicators for EPHF 8 in the Southern Cone and Mexico subregion

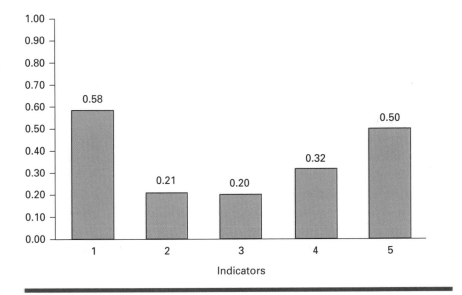

entities, but trained staff are not monitored, and no strategies have been implemented to ensure that they remain in their jobs over the long term.

In this subregion, adaptation of human resources to provide services that correspond to users' characteristics is poor. This is mainly due to ignorance of the existing obstacles and the lack of policies for hiring a culturally appropriate workforce.

Nevertheless, technical assistance provided for human resources development at the subnational level is generally good. Strategies are applied to ensure access to continuous training programs that take into account local sociocultural characteristics and to ensure development of the capacity for decentralized planning and management of these resources, as well as the implementation of measures to support them.

EPHF 9: *Ensuring the Quality of Personal and Population-based Health Services*

This is the function with the lowest performance level in the countries of the Southern Cone and Mexico, with an average value of 29%. However, there is a significant amount of performance dispersion, and two countries achieve average performance levels.

The performance of countries in this subregion is low in all the relevant areas, except in the definition of standards and in the evaluation to improve the quality of personal and population-based health services (Figure 116).

Indicators:

1. Definition of standards and evaluation to improve the quality of per-

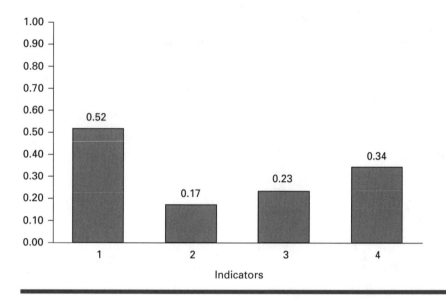

Figure 116 Performance of Indicators for EPHF 9 in the Southern Cone and Mexico subregion

sonal and population-based health services;

2. Improving user satisfaction with health services;

3. Systems for technological management and health technology assessment to support decision-making in public health;

4. Technical assistance and support for the subnational levels to ensure quality of services.

All countries, to varying degrees, implement policies for the continuous improvement of health services, which take into account standards and performance goals at the national level, and whose implementation is evaluated on a more or less regular basis. This process incorporates the use of new methodologies for quality assessment and includes evaluation of user satisfaction. National authorities have achieved good progress with such strategies, both for personal and population-based services. Unfortu-

nately, there are problems with disseminating evaluation results to providers and users. Four of the five countries have an autonomous and independent agency for the accreditation and evaluation of individual service quality.

Only in two countries in the subregion have health authorities succeeded in encouraging the community to evaluate user satisfaction with the health services provided. This evaluation, both of personal and population-based services, is carried out with limited frequency and does not involve all pertinent actors. The results, which generally make it possible to orient strategies toward improving access, are not disseminated to the community or to providers.

Technical management and assessment of technologies is an area of limited development in the Region. Although health authorities have tried to promote them and have identified the responsible entities, their opinions are not generally taken into account in decision-making or in the formulation of health policies.

Furthermore, strategies are not implemented to ensure that the existing system of technology management operates adequately. Only in three countries is there a certain degree of assessment of available technologies and advocacy of their use by decision-making bodies.

Support to the subnational levels to ensure quality of services is limited. Although technical assistance in methodologies of data collection and analysis is good, only one of the countries analyzed promote the use of tools for the management and evaluation of technologies.

EPHF 10: *Research in Public Health*

The public health research function exhibits an average performance in the subregion, with an average value of 51% and limited variation among the different countries.

Of the three areas, the one that exhibits the least progress relates to the development of a public health research agenda.

Institutional capacity and technical assistance at the subnational levels, on the other hand, demonstrate an adequate performance level (Figure 117).

Indicators:

1. Development of a public health research agenda;

2. Development of institutional research capacity;

3. Technical assistance and support for research in public health at the subnational levels.

All countries in the subregion have developed a public health research agenda, but its content is generally limited to an awareness of the existing potential funding sources and cooperation agencies. Implementation is evaluated in only one of the five countries analyzed.

In the Southern Cone and Mexico exists there is good development of the institutional capacity for public health

research, thanks to the availability of technical teams capable of conducting autonomous research, as well as instruments for qualitative and quantitative analysis for research into public health problems and for support of appropriate information systems.

The health authorities of the countries in the subregion do provide adequate technical assistance to the subnational levels regarding methodologies for operational research in public health and the interpretation of results. Furthermore, efforts are made to promote participation of professionals at those levels in national research. What has still not been achieved, however, is the creation of a network of institutions that might benefit from the results of pertinent research.

EPHF 11: *Reducing the Impact of Emergencies and Disasters on Health*

This is one of the functions with a good performance in the countries in the subregion, with an average value of 70% and limited dispersion.

In the performance of this function, countries have achieved high performance levels in technical assistance at the subnational levels and the development of standards and guidelines. It is noteworthy is the low level achieved in reducing the impact of emergencies and disasters (Figure 118).

Indicators:

1. Reducing the impact of emergencies and disasters;

2. Development of standards and guidelines that support emergency preparedness and disaster management in health;

Figure 117   Performance of Indicators for EPHF 10 in the Southern Cone and Mexico subregion

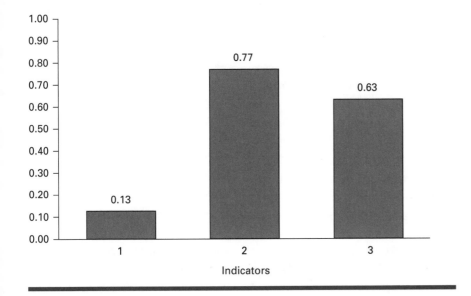

Figure 118 Performance of Indicators for EPHF 11 in the Southern Cone and Mexico subregion

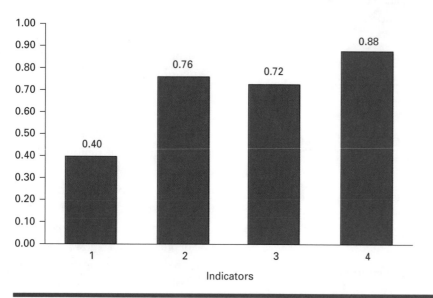

3. Coordination and partnerships with other agencies and/or institutions;

4. Technical assistance and support to the subnational levels to reduce the impact of emergencies and disasters on health.

All countries in the subregion have an institutional national plan for reducing the impact of emergencies and disasters on health, a unit responsible for this area at the health authority level, and an allocated budget. Nevertheless, health authorities lack the capacity to coordinate the whole sector, even though they have communication and transportation networks, whose operation tends not to be evaluated. The responsible staff is trained appropriately, but these contents are still not integrated into vocational training.

Health authorities in the Southern Cone and Mexico have achieved an adequate development level of strategies for reducing the impact of emergencies and disasters, which includes the preparation

of health standards for a national emergency preparedness plan. The areas that exhibit less progress in this area are those related to mental health, standards for donation of drugs and medical supplies, and the construction and maintenance of the health infrastructure.

Especially noteworthy is the good level achieved by three of the five countries in the development of standards for the delivery of health services during emergencies.

Coordination between the health authority and other sectors or agencies is present in all countries in the subregion, with a good level of coverage and commitment, primarily at the national level. There is generally coordination with the respective national civil defense organization or other multisectoral agencies and the creation of international partnerships for dealing with emergencies.

Assistance at the subnational levels for reducing the impact of emergencies and

disasters is carried out adequately, both with respect to collaboration with those levels in order to establish a response capacity, and with respect to support for the drafting of regulations and the identification of staff to manage emergency plans. Unfortunately, even though health authorities do have the ability to detect needs at the subnational levels, the resources needed to respond to those needs are not forthcoming.

2.4.3 Identifying Priority Intervention Areas

2.4.3.1 Performance of All EPHF Indicators

In order to identify the priority intervention areas and consider their development level, a profile of all EPHF indicators for the subregion is presented below, classified in ascending order according to whether their performance level is low, low-intermediate, high-intermediate or high (Figure 119). In order to facilitate the analysis, the indicators for each function have been given a different color.

As this overview shows, the main critical areas are human resource development (especially quality improvement and efforts to improve continuing education and graduate training); the absence of a national public health research agenda to help direct research toward health priorities; the low level of concern about user satisfaction; the incipient progress in assessment of health technologies; shortcomings in the enforcement of existing health regulations, and the capacity for management to deal with emergencies and disasters.

On the other hand, there is a very good subregional performance in the provision of support to decentralized entities

Figure 119 Performance of all EPHF Indicators in the Southern Cone and Mexico subregion

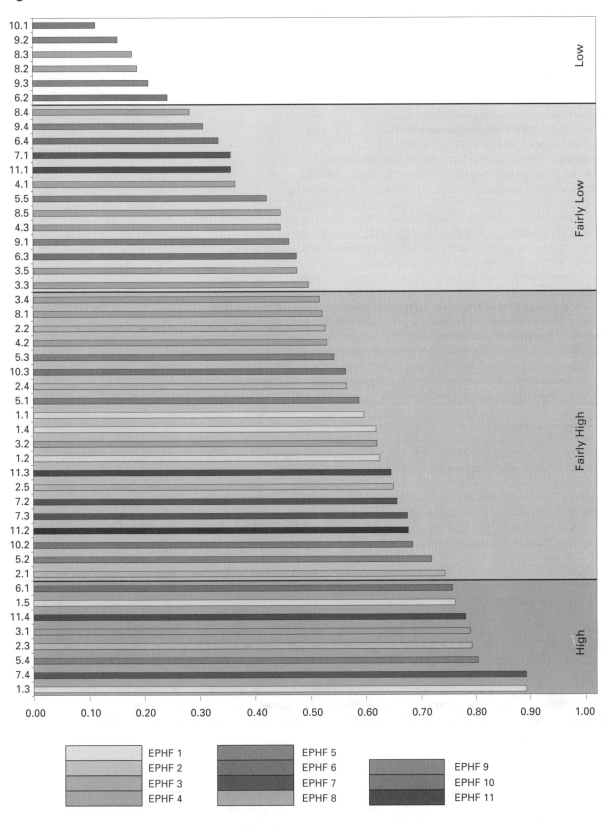

221

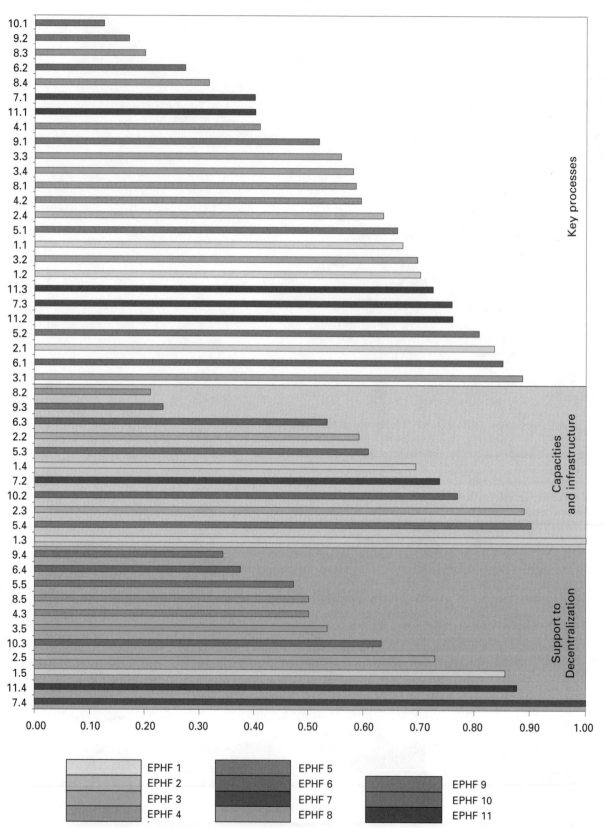

in order to ensure access to health services, the capacity and expertise to monitor health status and public health surveillance, the capacity to manage international cooperation, and the development of national and subnational health promotion plans.

2.4.3.2 Performance by Intervention Area

The primary **strengths** of most countries of the Southern Cone and Mexico in performing the essential public health functions, which should be maintained in the subregional plan, are the following:

- Intervention in the following important processes: support for health promotion activities; preparation of standards and interventions designed to encourage healthy behaviors and environments; development of standards and guidelines to help reduce the impact of emergencies and disasters on health; coordination and partnership with other sectors and actors to reduce disasters; evaluation of quality of information; follow-up, evaluation, and modification of regulations; promotion and action to improve access to necessary health services; surveillance system to identify risks and threats to public health; and development, monitoring, and evaluation of public health policies.

- Intervention to develop institutional capacities and infrastructure: expert support and resources for the monitoring and evaluation of health status; development of the institutional capacity for research; capacity of the public health laboratories; knowledge, aptitudes, and mechanisms to bring programs and services closer to the population; and management of

international cooperation with regard to public health.

- Development of decentralized competencies: technical assistance and support at the subnational levels of public health with regard to the promotion of equitable access to health services; technical assistance and support at the subnational levels for reducing the impact of emergencies and disasters on health; technical assistance and support at the subnational levels with regard to public health surveillance; and technical assistance and support at the subnational levels of public health.

On the other hand, the primary **weaknesses** exhibited by the subregion, which should be part of a program for improving public health in the Southern Cone and Mexico, are the following:

- Intervention in the following important processes: development of a public health research agenda; continuing education and graduate training in public health; improving user satisfaction with health services; enforcing health regulations; monitoring and evaluating access to necessary health services, and sectoral management to reduce disasters.

- Intervention to develop institutional capacities and infrastructure: improving the quality of the work force; improving human resources for the delivery of culturally appropriate health services; technology management and health technology assessment systems to support decision-making in public health.

- Development of decentralized competencies: technical assistance and support to the subnational levels of public health for the drafting of laws

and enforcement of regulations; and technical assistance and support to the subnational levels to ensure quality improvement in health services.

2.4.3.3 EPHF Performance by World Bank Action Priorities

These indicators have been regrouped in order to make the results of the measurement operational within the framework of international financing and cooperation strategies. The objective is to identify action priorities based on: *a*) significant differences in countries' public health profile, and *b*) investment needs. The categories considered and the results of the analysis are given below:

a) Development of Health Policies

In this area, the subregion exhibits a good general performance level, but there is a need to apply strategies to strengthen the power of the health authority to enforce health regulations. Furthermore, one area that needs to be strengthened is the implementation of policies to improve user satisfaction with the services provided.

b) Collection and Dissemination of Information to Guide Public Health Policy

In order to develop this area adequately, health authorities of countries in the subregion should advance in the formulation of a comprehensive research agenda and promote technological management and technology assessment, in order to take advantage of their existing technical capacity and infrastructure.

c) Disease Prevention and Control

Overall, this area represents a strength in the subregion. However, there are some areas that can be improved, espe-

Figure 121 Performance of EPHF Indicators according to priority Areas of Intervention proposed by the World Bank in the Southern Cone and Mexico subregion

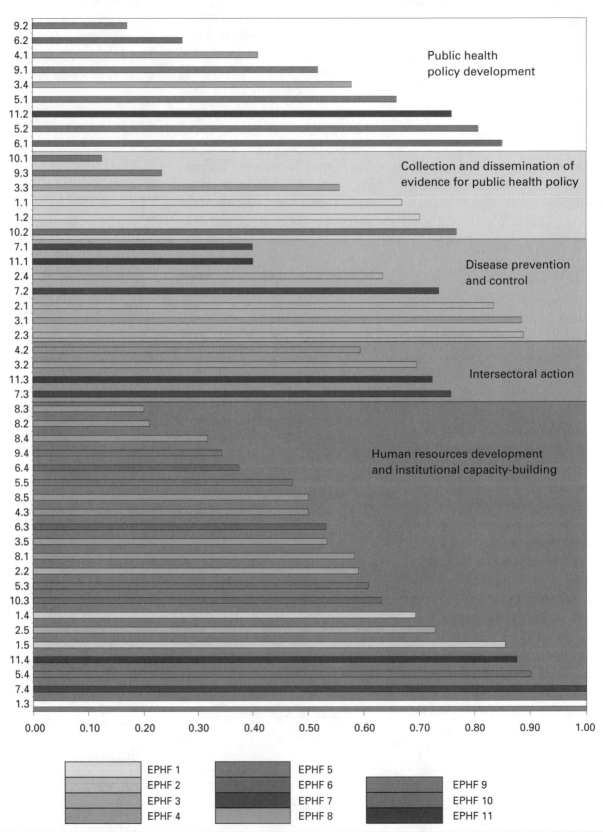

cially in monitoring access to necessary services and managing the impact of emergencies and disasters.

d) Intersectoral Action to Improve Health

This is a good area of development overall, but more progress still needs to be made in creating partnerships and strengthening social participation in health.

e) Human Resources Development and Building Institutional Capacity in Public Health

Although the development of human resources exhibits a level of high-intermediate progress in most countries in the subregion, health authorities must strengthen decentralized institutional competencies regarding regulation and enforcement, and policy planning and design, which are the two weakest areas. With regard to the public health workforce, quality-improvement policies must be strengthened, notably through adequate monitoring, the promotion of continuing education institutions, and further efforts to adapt to the sociocultural characteristics of the population.

2.4.4 Conclusions

Analysis of EPHF performance in the subregion indicates a good performance level in most functions, with certain variations that are not very pronounced.

However, there are common areas of weakness, such as the ability to enforce regulations, the strengthening of human resources (especially with regard to quality), assessment of the population's satisfaction with the services offered, and the decision-making power of citizens with regard to health. The latter area, which is linked to the limited progress achieved

in technological management, limits decision-making in the delivery of services that are able to meet people's needs and that are based on data that can improve the population's level of health.

The opportunity to advance in the preparation of national research programs in public health will direct institutions' efforts according to countries' health needs and priorities and to improve public health practice.

Cooperation can be initiated between countries in the subregion, in most EPHF. In that way, those that exhibit greater strengths in certain areas can help address the weaknesses of the others.

3. Major conclusions from the first performance measurement of the EPHF in the Region

The purpose of the first evaluation of the "Public Health in the Americas" (PHA) Initiative was to provide Member States with a profile of the current state of public health practice. Using a common instrument, a self-evaluation was carried out in each country of the Americas on performance of the essential public health functions, based on pre-established optimum standards. The objective of this measurement exercise was to identify the fundamental areas that require priority actions and the elements that hinder or facilitate the development of public health in the Americas.

This comprehensive review, based on the consensus of a group of expert representatives in each country, is intended to provide an overview of the current state of public health in the Americas in order to spur advances toward improving public health in the future, thus

strengthening the leadership of the health authorities in relation to the entire health system.

Sectoral reforms face the challenge of strengthening the steering role of the health authority, and an important part of that role consists of exercising the EPHF that are the responsibility of the State at its central, intermediate, and local levels.

The objective of identifying the strengths and weaknesses of public health practice in the Americas is to offer the countries an operational diagnosis of areas that require greater support in order to strengthen public health infrastructure, understood in its broadest sense to include human competencies and the facilities and equipment necessary for good performance.

The measurement exercise does not attempt to establish a classification of countries but rather offer both a Regional and subregional overview, of the principal areas of greatest weakness, in order to provide data to support policies and plans for the development of public health in national, subregional, and Regional contexts.

The decision was made to not prepare a composite indicator comprising all the EPHF, given that each function has its own value and includes pertinent competencies for the development of public health in the countries. It would therefore not be appropriate to construct an average using the scores on all the EPHF to reflect the broad reality of public health in each country or in the entire Region.

Notwithstanding these considerations, the presentation of an overall picture allows decision makers to compare their reality with that of other countries and to define areas of collaboration toward common objectives of improving public health in their respective areas of responsibility.

The instrument is not intended to have validity in the strict scientific sense of the term, given the possibility of error in the positive or negative response to each specific question, if that response is contrasted with the reality as depicted by another observer or by independent arbitration. The responses reflect the opinions of the participants in the measurement exercise, which means that readers of the results who believe they know the national situation could disagree with these judgments. But despite these limitations with regard to validity, the instrument presents a reasonably accurate overview of the fundamental areas for the development of public health in the Region.

Special attention was given to constructing a common picture based on the consensus of a broad and representative group of national experts regarding the status of the EPHF in each country, and preparing a profile of the status of public health in the Region, through an analysis of those practices that are most clearly defined and representative for the entire group of countries. This also allows each country to review internally other characteristics that show greater variability in results.

The reports of each country reflect this important emphasis and allow national authorities to make decisions based on more precise data concerning their respective situations.

3.1 Profile of the Region

The principal conclusions, derived from all 41 countries taking part in the self-evaluation exercise, were as follows:

- An analysis of the performance profile of the essential public health functions shows that all the countries have areas of better performance and other areas that are more critical; these areas differ from one country to another. With a few exceptions, one cannot point to countries with consistently better or worse performance on all the functions evaluated.

- In general, the profile shows intermediate to low performance on the overall set of EPHF. Two functions had relatively better performance: reducing the impact of emergencies and disasters on health (EPHF 11) and public health surveillance (EPHF 2). Nevertheless, no function exceeded 70% fulfillment in relation to the standard used for the evaluation.

- The following functions showed lower performance levels: ensuring the quality of personal and population-based health services (EPHF 9) and human resource development and training in public health (EPHF 8). These two functions also showed less variability of results among countries, which underscores the need to strengthen these areas in the great majority of countries of the Region.

- Although EPHF 5 (health policies and management) shows an intermediate level of performance, it is important to note that there is a high correlation between this and the performance level of almost all the other functions, especially health promotion (EPHF 3) and strengthening of capacity for regulation and enforcement (EPHF 6). This highlights the importance of making focused efforts

to improve the fundamental areas of this function throughout the Region.

- An aspect of public health that constitutes a fundamental function of the health authority is that of ensuring access to necessary health services (EPHF 7), especially for the neediest groups. The high correlation of performance levels of this function with performance levels of other functions considered to be "emerging" (health promotion, social participation in health, ensuring the quality of services) suggests that, in the current context, strengthening these new public health functions has a key role in guaranteeing access to health.

- The evaluation points to priority areas that should be promoted within the framework of health policy development. These include the definition of national health objectives, together with relevant actors including the private sector and social security, as well as ensuring compatibility of these objectives with decisions on how to structure the health system. It should be noted that one of the greatest weaknesses is the failure to define indicators that can be used to evaluate achievement of the national objectives over time.

- Efforts to collect and disseminate data for decision-making need to advance. There should be a shift from an approach centered on delivery and use of health services—usually only those of the public sector—to a comprehensive view of health systems, con-

---

[16] Health technologies are understood here in the broadest sense, as including not only equipment and medicines but also health care processes, clinical practice, etc., as defined by PAHO/WHO.

centrating on the areas of technological management and evaluation of health technologies[16] to provide data on safety, risk, effectiveness, efficiency, and the economic and quality impact of using such data to guide decisions (by health personnel, patients, funding entities, insurers, planners, service administrators, and political decision-makers, among others).

- With respect to disease control and prevention, the principal shortcomings are found in the adaptation of surveillance systems to new epidemiological challenges: mental health, risk factors for chronic diseases, occupational health, and the environment. Although there is concern about access to health services, mechanisms are not available to identify obstacles to access or, in particular, problems of inequitable access. The absence of intersectoral coordination among public and private subsectors, as well as limited progress in the overall development of the primary health care strategy, are areas that need to be strengthened in the Region.

- When levels of performance across all functions are compared, several common fundamental areas are seen that affect a set of essential public health functions and that should be established as priorities for strengthening performance of the NHA in the majority of the countries. These common fundamental areas that need strengthening are as follows:

  - Evaluation and monitoring: In general, the countries do not periodically and systematically carry out actions to evaluate and monitor initiatives they have planned and implemented, a weakness that hinders improvement of strategies designed on the basis of accomplishments.

  - Performance incentives: Where the existence of incentives is measured as part of the performance of the EPHF, this appears as a critical area in all the countries of the Region. This weakness is important because lack of incentives undermines efforts to promote and reward good performance and thereby reinforce improvements in public health work.

  - Information management: In order to raise performance on several of the essential public health functions, it is necessary to improve the conditions of collection, analysis, and dissemination of information, especially quality control of data used to prepare public health indicators that, ultimately, guide the authorities in making decisions on health priorities.

1. There are certain general characteristics of countries, such as a small rural population, higher levels of school enrollment, and higher total health expenditure, that are broadly associated with better performance of the EPHF.

2. Although indicators of harm to health depend on a broad set of health and quality of life factors, those countries that show better performance of the functions linked to ensuring access to and quality of health services also have better indicators of infant and maternal mortality and mortality from infectious diseases.

3. Although financial restrictions, stemming from the economic crises suffered by countries of the Region in recent decades, have revealed the serious limitations of health institutions in managing their resources, it is interesting to note that the countries with greater inequity in income distribution (and thus more poverty) show a relatively better performance of the EPHF. This conclusion suggests that it is possible (or at least cannot be ruled out) that in those countries with a larger at-risk population, governments have made stronger efforts in the field of public health.

4. In general, performance of the EPHF in the countries with integrated public health systems is better than in countries with other health systems (or very similar, in the case of EPHF 2). The regulated mixed system shows the lowest level of performance of public health functions (except for EPHF 11).

5. In this regard, it is necessary to review more thoroughly how health system reforms implemented in the Region, oriented to regulated mixed (public-private) systems, have affected public health performance. It is known that the separation of functions in health, strengthening the health authority and giving it a role in regulating and supervising the performance of other actors in the health system (insurance companies and providers), has been a difficult process. It is still very far from achieving optimal performance, which, in this case, also affects performance in public health.

6. There is a set of factors, consistent with those identified in the evaluation of the countries of the Region carried out under the Health for All strategy, that stand in the way of bet-

227

ter public health performance. They include the following:

– Limited institutional capacity for ensuring adequate interaction on health matters among the State, civil society, and the general population, to support the development of public health.

– Excessive centralization of decision-making and available resources that has considerably limited development of the decentralized subnational levels, impeding creation of innovative strategies that are close to the population.

– Weakness of mechanisms for intersectoral coordination, undermining the integration needed to define and set priorities and carry out action strategies focused on the neediest groups, thereby hindering the synergy of efforts that public health requires.

– Insufficient development of mechanisms for monitoring and evaluating the impact of public and structural policies that affect health, resulting in reactive responses by the health authorities rather than proactive public health measures to improve the well-being of the population.

3.2 Specificities of each subregion

Since the Regional profile is also valid for the subregions, the section below summarizes only those elements most characteristic of each subregion.

The Southern Cone and Mexico subregion, in general, shows good performance on the majority of the EPHF, with relatively minor variations. The principal areas of weakness that should be addressed are: increasing the decision-making power of citizens with respect to health, increasing user satisfaction, monitoring access of the population to services, and advancing the preparation of a national program of public health research, provided the institutional capacity is available to do so.

In the Caribbean, identified areas of weakness include the capacity for timely and effective response to public health problems and support to the subnational levels in the performance of the EPHF. No country in the subregion shows progress in development of a national research program. On the other hand, the countries of the Caribbean show notably good performance on the function of guaranteeing access to necessary health services, especially in terms of encouraging provider institutions to ensure access to health care.

The Central America subregion has a profile that is very similar to that for the entire Region of the Americas, with efforts to promote social participation in health and empower citizens in public health standing out as areas of achievement. None of the countries show progress in assessment of health technologies to guide decision-making.

Finally, the countries of the Andean Area show low levels of performance in all the functions, except for EPHF 1, 2, and 11. The principal areas that should be strengthened are probably those related to the development of

health policy and institutional capacity for regulation.

3.3 Bases for the preparation of a public health strengthening plan

This diagnosis suggests several priority areas for strengthening public health:

1) For the definition of new functions of the national health authority and strengthening the State's steering role in health, the following, at minimum, should be considered:

• Definition of national health objectives

• Sectoral management in accordance with equitable access to health

• Strengthening the capacity for regulation of the health system

• Financing of priority health interventions to achieve national health objectives

• Harmonization of service delivery, with particular attention to strategies having greatest impact on personal and population health

• The modulation of insurance regimes, with emphasis on the universal guarantee of necessary individual and collective health services.

In short, all this involves challenges focused on the inclusion of public health areas in health sector reform plans.

2) Development of information systems, including efforts in:

- Improvement of data quality and standardization of information on public health, essential for decision-making

- Orientation of information systems to reduce equity gaps and promote equal opportunities for the entire population with respect to health

- Development of capacity for information analysis, with special attention to public health monitoring that integrates epidemiological surveillance and performance evaluation of the health services

- Strengthening of essential areas of information for higher-level management of the health system, such as systems of national health accounts that provide information on how the economic resources of the health system are used.

3) Development of institutional competencies for management of public health policies, with a view to:

- Strengthening data-based decisions and improving management control systems

- Strengthening public accountability mechanisms in health

- Promoting institutional development of the health ministries, especially the definition of roles, structure, functions, and human and material capacities needed for the exercise of authority in health

- Increasing competencies for the design and evaluation of public policies that promise greater impact on population health

- Strengthening the leadership capacity of the health ministries through strategies such as definition of national health plans and promotion of a reorientation of health sector reforms based on the principles of equity, quality, effectiveness, and sustainability.

4) Human resources development and training in public health that includes:

- Formation of partnerships with human resources training centers to strengthen continuing education and advanced and graduate studies in public health

- Improvement of human resources management by promoting the decentralization of competencies, the capacity for promotion and articulation of policies, research and production of technologies, technical cooperation, leadership, and conflict resolution

- Definition of professional profiles necessary for performance of the EPHF and development of strategies to retain trained staff

- Development of incentive systems for improving the performance of public health personnel.

5) Reorientation of health services toward health care and maintenance, including:

- Development of individual and collective health services consistent with defined health objectives

- Creation of real incentives for promotion and protection of the health of population groups, families, and individuals

- Priority assignment of resources to primary care

- Incentives to strengthen the commitment of citizens to their health and promote their involvement in decision-making on local and general health policies.

6) Quality assurance for personal and population-based health services that strengthens development of:

- Assessment of health technologies and technological management in health

- Methodologies for development of data-based actions in public health

- Accreditation of providers and institutions

- Strategies to guide health services toward greater user satisfaction.

7) Innovation in public health should include:

- Creation of national research programs that respond to the country's health priorities

- Strengthening of essential research

- Promotion and development of public policies favoring health and based on the health objectives

With respect to international cooperation, steps can be taken to:

- Promote technical cooperation through an exchange of successful experiences from other countries, the Region, and the world, making it possible to establish networks for strengthening public health.

- Support the process of health sector reform, thereby strengthening public health programs.

- Reinforce the leadership of the health authorities in all spheres of development related to health, especially the essential common areas of performance of the EPHF in the countries of the Region, as outlined previously.

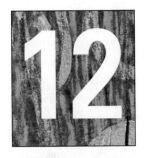

A Case Study in Performance Measurement at the Subnational Level: United States of America

1. Public Health in the United States of America

1.1 Essential Public Health Functions

In 1988, the Institute of Medicine identified the functions of public health in its landmark report, *The Future of Public Health*, (1988). The Institute identified assessment, policy development, and assurance as the "core functions of public health." These core functions, although meaningful to public health leaders in the United States, did not resonate with legislators and the general public. The inability to universally interpret the core functions and health care reform in the 1990's prompted public health leaders to describe the core functions with more precision.

In 1994, the United States Surgeon General (Dr. Jocelyn Elders) and the Associate Secretary for Health (Dr. Phillip Lee) co-chaired a Core Functions Steering Committee. This Committee was assembled to characterize the role of public health in the United States. The Steering Committee and a complementary workgroup were assembled: 1) to develop a taxonomy of the essential services of public health; and 2) to develop methods to address the deficiencies identified in the 1988 Institute of Medicine report. A consensus statement describing the mission, vision, activities, and services of public health in the United States resulted from the collaboration of the Core Functions Steering Committee, its workgroup, representatives of public health service agencies and major public health organizations. The consensus document is commonly known as the "Public Health in America Statement". The public health functions outlined in this statement are transformed into health outcomes through implementation of the ten essential public health services.

In 2001, 70% of local public health agencies reported the provision of adult and childhood immunizations, communicable disease control, community outreach and education, epidemiology and surveillance, food safety, restaurant inspections, and tuberculosis testing. Generally, public health agencies at the state and local level prevent epidemics and the spread of disease; protect against environmental hazards; prevent injuries; promote and encourage healthy behaviors; respond to disasters and assist communities in recovery; and assure the quality and accessibility of health services.

1.2 Public Health Administration

The Department of Health and Human Services is the principal government agency responsible for protecting the health of all Americans. The Department, state, local, and tribal governments and various agencies administer health services. There are eleven operating divisions in the Department, including the National Institutes of Health, Food and Drug Administration, the Centers for Disease Control and Prevention (CDC), the Indian Health Service, the Health Resources and Services Administration, the Substance Abuse and Mental Health Services Administration, the Agency for Healthcare Research and Quality, the Centers for Medicare & Medicaid Services (formerly the Health Care Financing Administration), the Administration for Children and Families, and the Administration on Aging.

The Centers for Disease Control and Prevention (CDC), in collaboration with states, provides a system of health surveillance to monitor and prevent disease outbreaks, implements strategies to prevent disease, and maintains national statistics. In addition, CDC provides for the prevention of international disease transmission, national immunization services, workplace safety, and environmental disease prevention.

The United States health care system has unique characteristics that distinguish it from all others in the world. "U.S. healthcare is not delivered through a network of interrelated components designed to work together coherently, which one would expect to find in a veritable system. To the contrary, it is a kaleidoscope of financing, insurance, delivery, and payment mechanisms that remain un-standardized and loosely coordinated." Because public and private health systems are not logically integrated, a national framework for evaluation is essential to ensure equitable service provision. National Public Health Performance Standards provide a logical evaluation framework to improve collaboration and service integration among health care organizations.

1.3 Public Health Systems

In 2001, a National Association of City and County Health Officials (NAC-

CHO) database contained 2,912 entries for local public health agencies. According to NACCHO, a local public health agency is "an administrative or service unit of local or state government concerned with health and carrying some responsibility for the health of a jurisdiction smaller than a state." The relationship of a local public agency to the state-level public health agency varies from state to state. Generally, state public health systems are organized in either a centralized, decentralized, shared or mixed framework as shown below:

- Centralized (15 states)—Local public health agencies are operated by the state or the state provides local health services directly without local health agencies.

- Decentralized (2 states)—Local health agencies are managed by local governments.

- Shared (2 states)—The state exercises some control over the local health agencies. This could include the appointment of a health officer or requiring the submission of an annual budget or health improvement plan.

- Mixed (9 states)—Both centralized and decentralized frameworks. The state serves as the local health agency if none exist. A mixed framework is commonly found where a local government chooses not to form a local health agency and the state must provide services.

At the local level, public health jurisdictions are established in accordance with governmental units. Local jurisdictions may correspond with counties, cities, towns, townships, special districts or any combination of these categorizations.

The existence of multiple state and local operational frameworks adds complexity to the task of evaluating public health systems.

The National Public Health Performance Standards Program (NPHPSP) was created in 1997 to establish excellence in public health practice. State and local public health agencies are not independently evaluated in the National Public Health Performance Standards Program. Rather, public health system effectiveness is evaluated to determine if essential public health services are adequately provided. A "public health system is a complex network of people, systems, and organizations working at the national, state and local levels. The public health system is distinct from other parts of the health care system in two key respects: its primary emphasis on preventing disease and disability, and its focus on the health of entire populations." Local public health systems are subunits of state health systems. State public health systems are subunits of the national health system. Collectively, national, state, and local health systems ensure the provision of the essential public health services and living conditions that are conducive to health.

Partners in the National Public Health Performance Standards Program include: the American Public Health Association, the Association of State and Territorial Health Officials, the National Association of County and City Health Officials, the National Association of Local Boards of Health, the Public Health Foundation, and the Centers for Disease Control and Prevention. Academic partners representing the Association of Schools of Public Health also made considerable contributions. CDC and national public health organizations presented the first set of drafts for the performance standards to the public in June 1999.

The overall goal of the NPHPSP is to improve the practice of public health by providing leadership in research, development, and implementation of optimal, science-based performance standards. The specific goals of the NPHPSP are: 1) to improve quality and performance of public health systems, 2) to increase accountability, and 3) to further develop the scientific foundation for public health practice. These goals are achieved, in part, through the systematic implementation of nationwide surveys of public health systems and intervention to address service delivery gaps. The Public Health Practice Program Office of the CDC administers the NPHPSP in collaboration with national public health organizations.

2. Public Health Assessment

2.1 Theoretical Framework

A public health system includes public, private, and voluntary entities, as well as individuals and informal associations that contribute to the delivery of essential services of public health. Performance measurement for public health systems is guided by principles established for the National Public Health Performance Standards Program to facilitate comparable data collection from discrete state and local public health systems. The guiding principles of the National Public Health Performance Standards Program are:

- Performance standards include process and outcome measures.

- Public health system improvement is the primary goal and as such, a minimum standards approach is not ac-

ceptable. Minimum standards potentially create a ceiling for performance with few incentives to advance beyond this threshold.

- Public health standards apply to all communities.

- Performance standards should be used not only to measure public health capacity but also as a tool for achieving consensus on the role and function of public health.

- Performance standards reflect the roles of public health agencies as essential, but inadequate to address comprehensive public health needs. The local public health system is a term that describes the constellation of organizations and individuals that help achieve public health goals within communities. A similar concept is used to describe the state public health system where the primary distinction is the locus of action. The goal is not to minimize the role of official government public health organizations but rather to promote the inclusion of other organizations that contribute to public health practice.

2.2 Assessment Methodology

National Public Health Performance Standards surveys are voluntary self-assessments for state and local public health systems and local boards of health. Data collection during the early phase of the NPHPSP was accomplished using hardcopy surveys. After the content and format were refined, a web-based local public health system survey was developed in April 1999. When respondents contact the CDC to complete a NPHPSP survey, a user identification number is assigned to allow access to web-based instruments.

The National Public Health Performance Standards Program is a forum for public health agencies to serve as catalysts and facilitators for public health improvement. State and local agencies take a lead role in organizing data collection. A liaison is designated within the state health department to facilitate the data collection process. CDC and national public health organizations coordinate with state liaisons to arrange regional orientation conferences and develop a time line for data collection, analysis, and reporting.

Survey data is collected at the state and local levels. Local level public health agencies are categorized as county, city, city-county, township or multi-county/district/r. The most common type of local public agency is county-level. Separate surveys are administered to state public health systems, local public health systems and local boards of health. Ideally, representatives of the state or local public health system convene to complete the NPHPSP surveys.

During the data collection process, the CDC, Public Health Practice Program Office, provides technical assistance to answer questions about the surveys and to resolve issues that emerge with data entry and submission. NPHPSP web-based surveys cannot be submitted for analysis unless every question is answered. Data is not registered in the CDC database until data is fully submitted for each of the ten essential services. Web-based data entry is the method of choice; however, hardcopy surveys are available if technology prohibits electronic data submission.

Data analysis generates quantitative scores for each essential public health service, relevant indicators and measures. Data extraction, analysis and re-

233

port generation is accomplished using Statistical Analysis Software. Summary reports include quantitative scores and a descriptive analysis that describes strengths, weakness, opportunities and threats. Numerical scores are calculated to provide a mechanism to compare similar public health systems across the nation. Scores less than 0.80 indicate opportunities for improvement or gaps in service delivery. Hardcopy reports depicting data in histograms, tables, and narrative summaries are sent to respondents.

The National Public Health Performance Standards Program is a developmental activity that will continue to evolve over time. Ultimately data analysis and reporting will be fully automated. CDC personnel and staff from national public health organizations conduct site visits at the conclusion of each data collection to review results and answer questions. With full implementation of the NPHPSP in 2002, site visits will be conducted as federal resources permit. Results from National Public Health Performance Standards surveys characterize the status of public health in the United States.

2.3 Survey Instruments

The CDC and national public health organizations developed three complementary assessment instruments for the NPHPSP:

1. The local public health system performance assessment instrument (local instrument)

2. The state public health system performance assessment instrument (state instrument)

3. The local public health governance performance assessment instrument (governance instrument)

The survey instruments are designed for public health systems to conduct voluntary self-analysis. State public health systems administer the state instrument to obtain an analysis of strengths, weaknesses, opportunities, and threats. The local instrument is similarly designed for local public health system assessment. In both instances, the state or local public health agency convenes other members of the public health system to conduct a comprehensive, collaborative assessment. Public health governing bodies, such as local boards of health, are components of local public health systems. A separate survey, the governance instrument, is specifically designed to assess organizational effectiveness of public health governing bodies.

Each assessment instrument is divided into ten sections each corresponding with an essential public health service. Table 1 provides an outline of the survey format. Essential public health service titles are followed by a brief description

---

Table 1 Design Inquiry of National Public Health Performance Standards Program

Level I:	Essential Public Health Service
Level II:	Indicator
Level III:	Model Performance Standard
Level IV:	Stem Question (Measure)
Level V:	First tier sub-measure
Level VI:	Second tier sub-measure
Level VII:	Third tier sub-measure

---

of the scope of the service. At the next level, a maximum of four indicators describe the attributes of each essential service. Each indicator has a corresponding model performance standard.

Performance standards represent expert opinion concerning actions and capacities that are necessary to optimize public health system effectiveness. Each model standard is followed by a series of questions that serve as measures of performance. An example of an essential service with a corresponding indicator, model standard, and measures is shown in Table 2.

2.4 Data Collection

Three strategies exist for data collection in the National Public Health Performance Program:

- *National Data Collection:* CDC may systematically collect data to assess and monitor the development of public health infrastructure throughout the nation. In this instance, participation is prescribed by research protocols.

- *Mobilizing for Action Through Planning and Partnership (MAPP):* MAPP is a strategic planning tool principally developed through a cooperative agreement between the National Association of City and County Health Officials and the CDC. The local instrument is one of four assessments in the MAPP strategic planning process for communities.

- *Public Health System Self-Assessment:* Public health systems and local boards of health may voluntarily collect data using surveys developed for

Table 2 Sample Essential Public Health Service with an Indicator, Model Standard, and Measures

EPHF 10: Research for New Insights and Innovative Solutions to Health Problems

For the Local Public Health System (LPHS), this service includes:

- A continuum of innovative solutions to health problems ranging from practical field-based efforts to foster change in public health practice, to more academic efforts to encourage new directions in scientific research.
- Linkages with institutions of higher learning and research.
- Capacity to mount timely epidemiological and health policy analyses and conduct health systems research.

Indicator 10.1: Fostering Innovation

Local Public health System Model Standard:

Organizations within the local public health system foster innovation to strengthen public health practice. Innovation includes practical field-based efforts to foster change in public health practice as well as academic efforts to encourage new directions in scientific research.

- Enable staff to identify new solutions to health problems in the community by providing the time and resources for staff to pilot test or conduct experiments to determine the feasibility of implementing new ideas.
- Propose to research organizations one or more public health issues for inclusion in their research agenda.
- Research and monitor best practice information from other agencies and organizations at the local, state, and national level.
- Encourage community participation in research development and implementation (e.g., identifying research priorities, designing studies, preparing related communications for the general public).

Please answer the following questions related to Indicator 10.1:

Sample Measures

10.1.1 Do LPHS organizations encourage staff to develop new solutions to health problems in the community?
If so,

    10.1.1.1 Do LPHS organizations provide time and/or resources for staff to pilot test or conduct experiments to determine new solutions?

    10.1.1.2 Have LPHS organizations identified barriers to implementing innovative solutions to health problems within the community?

    10.1.1.3 Do LPHS organizations implement innovations determined to be most likely to lead to improved public health practice?

---

the National Public health Performance Standards Program.

To initiate the data collection process, a state liaison is designated by the state health officer. The state liaison and CDC organize a 1-day regional conference for members of state and local public health systems. Regional conferences are planned to include participation according to the Department of Health and Human Services Regions, (see figure 1). Conference attendees are oriented to the NPHPSP, key concepts, such as the public health system framework, and the data collection process.

After the regional conference, the state liaison and CDC establish a time line for data collection and analysis. CDC provides technical assistance to facilitate survey completion during the empirical phase of the process.

To generate reliable data that represent the status of public health systems, state and local agencies convene staff and representatives of other public health organizations. In this forum, public health system representatives develop consensus responses to survey questions. Survey completion at the state or local level may encompass several meetings. The time allowed for data collection varies since public health systems across the nation are diverse. Generally, the local instrument requires 24 hours for orientation, consensus meetings, data collection and submission. State instrument completion requires 15 hours and the governance instrument requires 6 hours. Web-based data entry and scoring facilitate data analysis and dissemination of results. A quantitative performance score is assigned for overall performance and scores are also calculated for each subdivision of the instrument. Qualitative comments are provided in summary reports to highlight opportunities for public health system improvement.

2.5 Field Testing

The first draft of the local instrument was introduced to the public health community in June 1999. Since that time, primarily as a result of validity studies and field tests, the state, local and governance instruments have been substantially revised. The local instrument has undergone the most rigorous testing. Figure 2 depicts state and local public health systems that have participated in

Figure 1 Department of Health and Human Services Regional Map

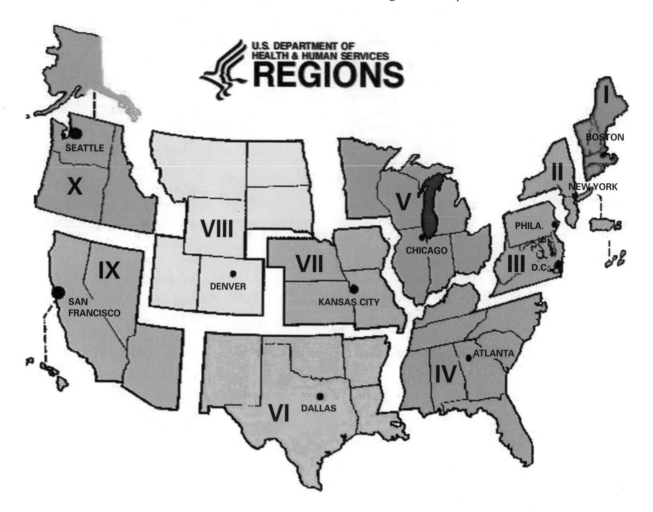

the National Public Health Performance Standards Program. Data from these state and local public health systems are not readily comparable since multiple versions of the instruments were used over time and public health systems differ by jurisdiction types, governing bodies, population served, workforce composition and funding sources and levels.

As a part of the National Public Health Performance Standards Program field test in 2000, Hawaii, Minnesota and Mississippi completed the state instrument. Subsequently, the Indian Health Service in New Mexico also completed the state instrument to assess public health service provision. Local agencies

in New York, Minnesota, Mississippi, Hawaii and San Diego, California participated in the local instrument field test using version 5b of the local instrument. The governance instrument was piloted in Massachusetts.

Field tests were designed to evaluate the adequacy of preparation for data collection, the efficiency of the data collection process, survey format, and content validity. Of special interest to CDC and national public health partners, was the feasibility of convening representatives of state and local public health systems to collaborate and complete survey instruments. The goal of data analysis was to develop methodology to

monitor and promote public health system improvement over time. Evaluation questions were developed to assess the utility of results generated by the NPH-PSP survey instruments. A series of recommendations emerged from the field test experience.

Several state and local public health agencies self-nominated to evaluate the usefulness of draft performance standards. In the pre-testing phase of survey development, health officials representing state and local agencies completed the surveys and provided recommendations to improve the surveys and the data collection process. To assess the validity of responses, the University of Kentucky

Figure 2 National Public Health Performance Standards Program State and Local Public Health System Participation

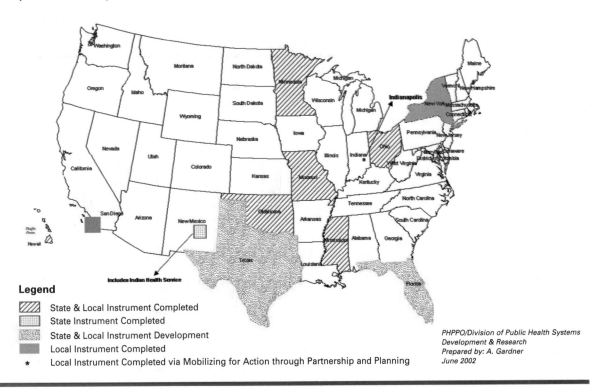

Legend

▨	State & Local Instrument Completed
▦	State Instrument Completed
▩	State & Local Instrument Development
■	Local Instrument Completed
★	Local Instrument Completed via Mobilizing for Action through Partnership and Planning

PHPPO/Division of Public Health Systems Development & Research
Prepared by: A. Gardner
June 2002

deployed a team of researchers to conduct a retrospective study of selected performance indicators. The researchers concluded that evidence was available to support data generated by self-assessment using the local instrument.

2.6 Data Limitations

The most frequently used methodology for data collection in research is self-administered questionnaires. Data collection is accomplished in the National Public Health Performance Standards Program through self-administered surveys.

Although widely employed, advantages and disadvantages are inherent in this approach to data gathering. Cost effectiveness and simplified administration are obvious benefits. Using web-based

surveys in the National Public Health Performance Standards Program extends the capacity of CDC and its partner organizations to generate a national dataset to describe the capacity and limitations of existing public health systems.

The disadvantage of voluntary assessment is that, collectively, self-nominated respondents may form a non-representative convenience samples for the nation. The field test survey frame was limited to a convenience sample of field test states. This sample may not be representative of the nation; therefore results cannot be generalized.

Response rates are also less predictable with self-administered surveys. Field test experience with survey instruments in the National Public Health Performance Standards Program demon-

strated that literacy, language barriers, and clarity of questions influenced results. Response options are limited to "Yes", "high partially", "low partially" or "No". A high degree of subjectivity is introduced with responses limited to these four options without explanatory remarks or quantitative data to support answers.

All survey results are subject to non-sampling errors, random and non-random. Random non-sampling errors result from various interpretations of the survey questions. Some randomness is also introduced when respondents estimate capacity based on program experience, current documentation and the collective expertise of public health system representatives. Non-random sampling errors can also arise from difficulty interpreting questions, non-response, partial responses, or incorrect information. Survey instruments in the National Public Health Performance Standards Program are completed on-site and submitted electronically. Survey data is not processed unless every question is answered. This quality measure limits non-random sampling errors. The allowance of partial answers conversely contributes to non-sampling error.

Nominal survey data was analyzed using descriptive statistics. Mean scores were calculated for each essential service. The data presented in figures 3, 4, and 5 was obtained by tabulating an average score for indicators that support each essential service.

Measurement error may be generated by the survey format (self assessment) and the inconsistent administration of the survey at the local level. Some field test respondents reported completion of the instruments without involvement by other public health system representatives. Additional reliability and validity testing is warranted to ensure that performance scores represent the true capacity of public health systems to deliver the essential public health services.

2.7 Format and Process Revisions

Self-assessment of the "public health system" has proved to be a new concept for many local agencies. Consistently, respondents commented that additional information on the components of the system would facilitate the data collection process. Respondents also expressed an interest in a separate section within the tools that would generate and assessment of the agency in addition to the system analysis. Current instruments retain the system focus, however, two Likert questions now follow

each indicator to assess the respondents' perception of the contributions of the public health system and the direct contribution of public health agencies.

Public health agencies convened public health system representatives to complete state and local instruments. In many instances, participants reported

Figure 3　Distribution of EPHS Scores for Local Level Agencies

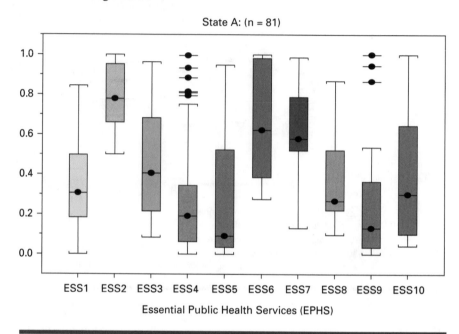

Figure 4　Distribution of EPHS Scores for Local Level Agencies

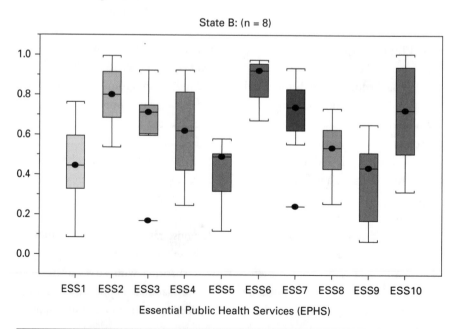

Figure 5 Distribution of EPHS Scores for Local Level Agencies

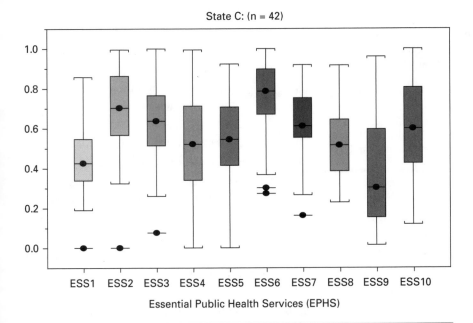

State C: (n = 42)

Essential Public Health Services (EPHS)

that they did not have an adequate amount of time to engage system partners. Feedback on evaluation forms clearly indicated that respondents also needed more time for orientation activities. As a result of these findings, the time required to review, complete, and submit the local instrument was adjusted from 8 to 24 hours. Time allowances for the completion of the state and governance instruments were also increased as a result of consistent feedback from field test state and local participants. Many of these comments are similar to those received during the evaluation of the Latin America and Caribbean exercise.

The feasibility of convening representatives of state and local public health systems to collaborate and complete survey instruments proved to be a challenge in almost every instance. Various methods were employed to generate responses. Some local agencies completed the entire instrument, others divided the in-strument for various divisions within the agency to complete, and others engaged a few key organizations. More work is needed to assist state and local agencies with stakeholder analysis and the use of effective techniques to engage public health system partners. Although participants believed the assessment instruments were time and labor intensive, the consensus among respondents was that the results of the process would be beneficial for overall evaluation and strategic planning activities. Most respondents agreed that the instruments should be completed in collaboration with other public health system representatives, not independently by public health agencies.

While field test respondents agreed that the survey instruments have value, participants recommended reducing the subjective nature of questions. Field test participants also consistently identified a need to explain terminology used in the assessment instruments. A comprehen-sive glossary and reference section was developed for the instruments to improve face validity. The state, local and governance instruments were re-tooled after field-testing to reduce subjectivity and improve face validity. Additionally, model standards were simplified and summarized in bulleted statements that correspond with stem questions.

Reports were retooled to "retain the information in the data" by providing guideposts to improve performance.

Initially there were three response options for NPHPSP survey questions: "Yes", "Partial" or "No". Evaluation feedback indicated that the partial category was too broad. Respondents were confused by an intermediate "partial" category offered as one response option. To clarify the response options, the assessment instruments were revised to include 4 response options with numerical quartiles assigned to each category as shown in table 3.

Regarding the efficiency of the data collection process, field test participants who completed the web-based survey encouraged its continued use. Participants were satisfied with the availability of technical assistance on a customer care hotline established for field test support.

3. Data Utilization

3.1 State Experiences

The State of Texas has been actively involved with the development of the National Public Health Performance Standards Program. Texas used the National Public Health Performance Standards as a template to dissect assessment questions that were most relevant to its state and local public health systems. Texas

Table 3 Possible answers on the evaluation tool

Response	Description
"Yes"	Greater than 75 percent of the activity described within the question is met within the local public health system.
"High Partially"	Greater than 50 percent, but no more than 75 percent of the activity described within the question is met within the local public health system.
"Low Partially"	Greater than 25 percent, but no more than 50 percent of the activity described within the question is met within the local public health system.
"Low"	No more than 25 percent of the activity or resource described within the question is met within the local public health system.

has created a state-specific version of the local instrument to enhance the preparedness of local public health agencies to respond to public health threats and emergencies. In addition, the 76th Texas Legislature passed House Bill 1444. The essential public health services are now incorporated into the Texas Health and Safety Code with House Bill 1444.

State and local agencies that participated in the field test planned to use the results for strategic planning, in grant applications to illustrate needs, to justify increased funding to expand the workforce, and to justify funds to develop community health improvement plans. Respondents completing the local tool strongly recommended sharing results with elected officials, local boards of health and other organizations within the public health system.

In Minnesota, considering data limitations, National Public Health Performance Standards results were shared with the State Department of Health and local public health partners to initiate discussion on potential opportunities to develop the workforce, improve technology and evaluation methods. Minnesota used the model standards to support and improve the State system for community health services. The model

standards provided a framework for statewide discussion of public health improvement and for strengthening the partnership between state and local agencies. Minnesota participants believed that patterns in the data could also potentially be used to identify state and regional strengths and needs for capacity building. Minnesota noted that performance scores were consistently low throughout the state for essential service 1, 8 and 9. The Minnesota State Community Health Services Advisory Committee planned to use performance standards information to further analyze policy strategies to address gaps, focus on staff development and direct strategic planning.

The State of Mississippi used performance standards to educate their Legislative Sunset Review Body on public health and its role. Mississippi also used assessment data to support development of a bond bill for capital facilities improvement. The bill was presented to the State legislature to improve information systems and public health laboratory systems. Performance standards data was also used to develop grant applications for bio-terrorism and environmental health. Mississippi found the performance standards data useful in strategic planning at the State level. Performance standards

data is used to familiarize new health officers with opportunities for public health infrastructure improvement.[1]

3.2 Local Level Gap Analysis

Assessment results and respondent evaluation forms from several states were reviewed and summarized at the CDC in the summer of 2000. Figures 3, 4, and 5 illustrate the distribution of performance scores for three field test states, 131 local public health systems. Overall scores ranged from 0.40 to 0.62 with 1.00 representing optimal performance. Figures 3, 4 and 5 are box plots with the range of possible scores on the vertical axis and the factors of interest, the essential public health services, on the horizontal axis. Each figure contains ten box plots, each representing an essential service. The box plot identifies the median, a lower quartile (the 25th percentile) and an upper quartile, (the 75th percentile). Additionally an interquartile range, (the difference between the upper and lower quartile-IQ) was calculated as shown below:

(L1) Lower quartile 1 = lower quartile – $1.5 \times IQ$

(L2) Lower quartile 2 = lower quartile – $3.0 \times IQ$

(U1) Upper quartile 1 = upper quartile + $1.5 \times IQ$

(U2) Upper quartile 2 = upper quartile + $3.0 \times IQ$

In figures 3, 4 and 5, a line is drawn from the lower quartile to the smallest point that is greater than L1. Likewise, the line from the upper quartile to the maximum

---

[1] Personal Communication. Kage W. Bender, RN, PhD, FAAN, Deputy State Health Officer.

was drawn to the largest point smaller than U1. Points between L1 and L2 or U1 and U2 are drawn as small circles. Points less than L2 or greater than U2 are drawn as large circles.

Field test results demonstrated wide variation among states and within essential service categories. State A represents a centralized state-local public health system framework and State C is organized in a shared framework. In State B, the state health department serves at the local level in a manner similar to but not synonymous with a centralized system. Average scores by essential service at the local level for 131 local public health systems are provided in figures 6, 7, and 8.

With the exception of essential service 6 (State B), essential service scores for these field test states consistently fell below the standard of 0.80. A range of 65 exists between the highest and lowest essential service score, (0.22-State A, essential service 9; 0.87-State B, essential service 6). Opportunities for improvement are more readily apparent in some areas; however, this wide variation in scores indicates potential risks to public health in every category of service delivery.

Abbreviated state profiles are provided in table 4. Factors that impact public health, such as population density, metropolitan/non-metropolitan population distribution, gross state product, health care expenditures and the percent of persons below the poverty level are provided to characterize each state.

Without calculating correlation coefficients, one can observe an apparent relationship between performance scores, predominantly metropolitan population, gross state product and health

Figure 6 State A Profile of Essential Public Health Service Scores for Local Level Agencies

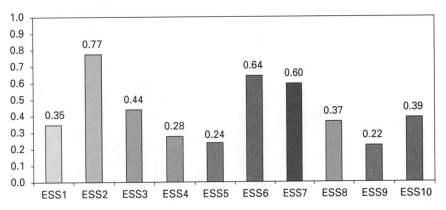

ESS1   **Monitor** health status to identify community health problems.
ESS2   **Diagnose and investigate** health problems and health hazards in the community.
ESS3   **Inform, educate, and empower** people about health issues.
ESS4   **Mobilize** community partnerships to identify and solve health problems.
ESS5   **Develop policies and plans** that support individual and community health efforts.
ESS6   **Enforce** laws and regulations that protect health and ensure safety.
ESS7   **Link** people to needed personal health services and assure the provision of health care when otherwise unavailable.
ESS8   **Assure** a competent public and personal health care workforce.
ESS9   **Evaluate** effectiveness, accessibility and quality of personal and population-based health services.
ESS10 **Research** for new insights and innovative solutions to health problems.

Figure 7 State B Profile of Essential Public Health Service Scores for Local Level Agencies

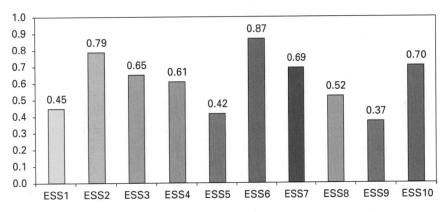

ESS1   **Monitor** health status to identify community health problems.
ESS2   **Diagnose and investigate** health problems and health hazards in the community.
ESS3   **Inform, educate, and empower** people about health issues.
ESS4   **Mobilize** community partnerships to identify and solve health problems.
ESS5   **Develop policies and plans** that support individual and community health efforts.
ESS6   **Enforce** laws and regulations that protect health and ensure safety.
ESS7   **Link** people to needed personal health services and assure the provision of health care when otherwise unavailable.
ESS8   **Assure** a competent public and personal health care workforce.
ESS9   **Evaluate** effectiveness, accessibility and quality of personal and population-based health services.
ESS10 **Research** for new insights and innovative solutions to health problems.

Figure 8 State C Profile of Essential Public Health Service Scores for Local Level Agencies

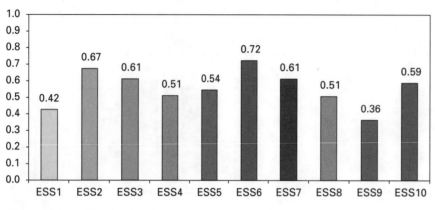

ESS1 **Monitor** health status to identify community health problems.
ESS2 **Diagnose and investigate** health problems and health hazards in the community.
ESS3 **Inform, educate, and empower** people about health issues.
ESS4 **Mobilize** community partnerships to identify and solve health problems.
ESS5 **Develop policies and plans** that support individual and community health efforts.
ESS6 **Enforce** laws and regulations that protect health and ensure safety.
ESS7 **Link** people to needed personal health services and assure the provision of health care when otherwise unavailable.
ESS8 **Assure** a competent public and personal health care workforce.
ESS9 **Evaluate** effectiveness, accessibility and quality of personal and population-based health services.
ESS10 **Research** for new insights and innovative solutions to health problems.

care expenditures. Population density is nearly constant at 60.3 for State A and 61.8 persons per square mile for State C. The overall performance score for State A (0.44) is barely more than half the standard 0.80. State A is predominately non-metropolitan with a lower gross state product and lower personal health care expenditures, but higher poverty rates than State C, (see table 5). State C has a substantially higher overall performance score (0.60). State C

expenditures for personal health care are twice as much as State A. State C also has a gross state product that is more than double that of State A and poverty rates are twice as low in State C. State A scores consistently fell below 0.50 for seven out of ten essential public health services. State C scores were consistently higher than 0.50 for 8 out of ten services. This data suggests that health care expenditures and gross state product may influence public health

performance capacity and ultimately health outcomes such as infant mortality. Infant mortality in State A in 1998 was 10.1 and in State C 5.9 deaths per 1,000 live births.

Scores were in close approximation on essential service 1 (Figures 6, 7, and 8), with a range of 10. For essential service 1, the three states received similar scores: 0.35, 0.45, and 0.42. The first filter in the NPHSPS, the essential service, points these states in the direction of improved methodology for community assessment and health monitoring. The three indicators for essential service 1, (population-based community health profile, access and use of current technology, maintenance of population health registries), provide additional details for gap analysis related to health status monitoring.

Since surveillance is an old tenet of public health practice, one expects to see high scores for essential service 2. Each of the three states scored better than .60 on essential service 2 with a range of 12. Mean scores were 0.77, 0.79, 0.67 respectively for State A, B and C. State A performed best overall on essential service 2.

Survey questions for essential service 3 are designed to assess public health system capacity to inform, educate and

Table 4 Abbreviated State Profiles

	NPHPSP Overall Average	Population Density	Metropolitan %	Non-metropolitan %	Gross State Product*	Personal Health Care Expenditure**	Population Below Poverty Level %
State A	.44	60.3	34.0	64.0	62.2	8,882	16.1
State B	.56	188.6	72.3	27.7	39.7	4,658	10.9
State C	.60	61.8	70.4	29.6	161.4	20,313	7.2

Source: U.S. Census Bureau, 2001 Statistical Abstract of the United States. * In billions **In millions

Table 5 Comparison of state profiles

	NPHPSP Overall Average	Population Density	Metropolitan %	Non-metropolitan %	Gross State Product*	Personal Health Care Expenditure**	Population Below Poverty Level %
State A	.44	60.3	34.0	64.0	62.2	8,882	16.1
State C	.60	61.8	70.4	29.6	161.4	20,313	7.2

Source: U.S. Census Bureau, 2001 Statistical Abstract of the United States.   * In billions   **In millions

empower communities. Wider variation among the states on this essential service may correlate with the percent of persons below the poverty level or inadequate resource availability for health education. State A had the largest percent of persons below the poverty level 16.1% and the highest infant mortality. State A also had the lowest score (0.44)

on essential service 3, while states B & C scored 0.61 and 0.65 respectively. Poverty levels for State B & C levels were substantially lower, 10.9 and 7.2, respectively. Infant mortality was also lower in States B (5.9) and C (6.9).

The widest variation among the three states was observed for essential service

4, mobilizing community partnerships. With a range of 33, scores fell between 0.28 and 0.61. Developing partnerships is a recent addition to the gestalt of public health concerns that can be traced back to ancient Greece. Public health has the most experience linking environmental conditions to diseases, and inconsistent experience developing partnerships to accomplish essential services.

Table 6 Essential Public Health Services

Essential Service # 1:   Monitor Health Status to Identify Community Health Problems

Essential Service # 2:   Diagnose and Investigate Health Problems and Health Hazards in the Community

Essential Service # 3:   Inform, Educate, and Empower People about Health Issues

Essential Service # 4:   Mobilize Community Partnerships to Identify and Solve Health Problems

Essential Service # 5:   Develop Policies and Plans that Support Individual and Community Health Efforts

Essential Service # 6:   Enforce Laws and Regulations that Protect Health and Ensure Safety

Essential Service # 7:   Link People to Needed Personal Health Services and Assurethe Provision of Health Care when Otherwise Unavailable

Essential Service # 8:   Assure a Competent Public and Personal Health Care Workforce

Essential Service # 9:   Evaluate Effectiveness, Accessibility, and Quality of Personal and Population-Based Health Services

Essential Service # 10:   Research for New Insights and Innovative Solutions to Health Problems

Essential Service 5 is focused on the development of policies and plans that support individual and community health efforts. Scores on essential service 5 also varied widely from 0.24 for State A to 0.54 for State C. Extremely low scores for this essential service signal opportunities to improve strategic planning for community health improvement. The gap analysis provided by the NPHPSP is intended to complement, not replace local efforts to conduct community health assessments and develop community health improvement plans. Both are critical to establish effective system-wide partnerships to address issues that result in poor health outcomes. Gross state product and personal health care expenditures may limit resource availability for individual and community health efforts. Data provided in table 4 illustrates the budget climate for these states in terms of gross state product and personal health care expenditures. Further investigation in this area with a larger data set may confirm the hypothesis that a direct correlation exists between these expenditures and organizational capacity to deliver the essential public health services.

Most public health systems have honed their skills in compliance enforcement and the delivery of direct services, essential service 6. State B (0.87) and State C (0.72) scored highest on essential service 6. The performance score for State A was slightly lower at 0.64. Since areas of peak performance are not mirrored state-to-state at the local level, public health may not be sustaining the benefits of past success. Continuous quality improvement focused on delivering the essential public health services at the local level remains a national priority to ensure effective public health action.

Essential service 7 scores varied within a range of 0.08. Scores for State A, B, and C were 0.60, 0.69 and 0.61 respectively. Serving as a "safety net" provider of direct health care, for individuals without access to care, is an established function of public health systems. Essential service 7, scores are demonstrative of consistent capacity in these three states.

Workforce development is an emerging competency for public health systems. State scores varied from 0.37 to 0.53 with a range of 15 on essential service 8. Workforce assessment is a process that many local public health systems need to add to the credentialing and licensure process to ensure workforce competency.

Evaluation was a weaker component of service provision for this sample of states. Each state scored below 0.40 on

essential service 9. Strategies that are agency specific may not succeed in isolation to combat public health threats, emerging infections or bio-terrorism. Public health systems must collaborate to evaluate the combined influence on community health. Effective program evaluation is a systematic way to improve public health actions by involving procedures that are useful, feasible, ethical and accurate.

Research is not a traditional function for local public health systems. In addition to environmental health, preventive medicine, epidemiology, and disease control, local public health systems have primary responsibility for direct medical care, advocacy, school health, crisis response, family planning, care of the poor, dental care, licensure and certification, mental and home health care. Often the workforce is stretched to provide these services on a limited budget. Local public health systems in close proximity to academic institutions are more likely to engage in research activities.

State A, with 64% of the population living in non-metropolitan areas, scored lowest on essential service 10 (0.36). The majority of residents in State B (72.3%) and State C (70.4%) live in metropolitan areas. State B and C scored .70 and 0.59 on essential service 10 respectively. The correlation between rurality and the capacity to participate in research warrants future analysis.

The NPHPSP is a nation-wide program to identify elements of public health infrastructure that lack adequate capacity and resources. The information generated by the assessment process is intended for use by decision makers to create robust information technology

systems to share data, develop the public health workforce and enhance organizational capacity. These are the essential elements of public health infrastructure.

4. Lessons Learned

The NPHPSP field test experience taught many lessons. Priorities that emerged from the experience included the need for:

1. Case examples of successful state and local public health systems

2. Detailed gap analyses

3. Improved evaluation mechanisms

Participants encountered difficulty with the notion of meeting with health partners from the community to assess their combined capacity to deliver the Essential Services. As a result, the NPHPSP will incorporate case examples from around the nation in the orientation package for program implementation. Gap analysis for field test sites needed fortification with specific recommendations to improve performance in each Essential Service. Hardcopy and electronic resources have been identified to provide specific recommendations to address gaps that may emerge in Essential Service delivery. A stronger evaluation component for all phases of implementation (orientation, survey administration and data analysis) also emerged as a priority. A formal evaluation process with regular intervals of data analysis has been implemented to identify barriers to excellence in public health system assessment.

5. Conclusion

The intent of the National Public Health Performance Standards Program is to provide focus and direction for proactive, rather than reactive, public health system development. Performance assessment is one step in a comprehensive strategic planning process for public health systems. "Without standard performance indicators and systematic comparisons, public health lacks useful benchmarks for improvements." The National Public Health Performance Standards Program outlines benchmarks for public health improvement in accordance with the essential services of public health. The performance standards program provides a consistent framework to assess the performance of public health systems and governing bodies such as local boards of health. Although state and local public health agencies take the lead in the data collection process, they serve only as catalysts to initiate involvement by system partners. The full responsibility for data interpretation and application of results lies with state and local public health systems throughout the nation. Full implementation of the National Public Health Performance Standards Program will facilitate the development of a skilled public health workforce, development of robust information and data systems, and effective health departments and laboratories. The CDC and its national public health partner organizations plan to implement the National Public Health Performance Standards Program in 2002. This system of national data collection will allow public health leaders to monitor trends over time as the United States strives to achieve national health objectives outlined in Healthy People 2010.

Bibliography

Institute of Medicine. The future of public health. Washington, D.C: National Academy Press; 1988.

Harrell JA, Baker EL. The essential services of public health. Leadership in Public Health 1994; 3(3):27–31.

Hajat A, Brown C, Fraser M. Local public health infrastructure: a chartbook. Washington, DC: National Association of City and County Health Officials; 2001.

Department of Health and Human Services. HHS: what we do. 2002; [5 screens]. Available at: http://www.hhs.gov/news/press/2002pres/profile.html. Accessed May 7, 2002.

Leiyu S, Singh DA. Delivering health care in America, a systems approach. 2nd ed. Gaithersburg, MD: 2001. p. 5–6.

Pickett G, Hanlon JJ. Public health administration and practice. 9th ed. St. Louis, MO: Times Mirror/Mosby College Publishing; 1990. p. 104–105.

Department of Health and Human Services. Public health's infrastructure: a status report. Atlanta, GA: Centers for Disease Control and Prevention. 2000, p. 4.

Turnock B. Public health, what it is and how it works. 2nd ed. Gaithersburg, MD: Aspen Publications; 2001. p. 338.

Halverson P. Performance measurement and performance standards: old wine in new bottles. J Public Health Management Practice 2000 Sep; 6(5): vi–ix.

Bouroque LB, Fielder EP. How to conduct self-administered and mail surveys. Thousand Oaks, CA: SAGE Publications; 1995.

Local Public Health System Performance Assessment Instrument. 2001; [78 screens]. Available at: http://www.astho.org/phiip/pdf/pmlocal.pdf. Accessed June 7, 2002.

State Public Health System Performance Assessment Instrument. 2001; [110 screens].

Available at: http://www.astho.org/phiip/pdf/pmstate.pdf. Accessed June 7, 2002.

Local Public Health Governance Performance Assessment Instrument. 2001; [82 screens]. Available at: http://www. nalboh.org/perfstds/govfinal.pdf. Accessed June 7, 2002.

A strategic approach to community health improvement: mobilizing for action through planning and partnership. Washington, DC: National Association of City and County Health Officials; 2001.

Cleveland, William S. Visualizing Data. Summit, NJ: Hobart Press; 1993. p. 5.

State Community Health Services Advisory Committee, Assessing Organizational Capacity Workgroup. The public health performance assessment field test: Minnesota's experience and recommendations. St. Paul, MN: Minnesota Department of Health; 2001. p.15.

U.S. Census Bureau 2001 Statistical Abstract of the United States-Vital Statistics, 2001; [110 screens]. Available at: http://www.census.gov/prod/2002pubs/01statab/vitstat.pdf. Accessed June 7, 2002.

U.S. Census Bureau 2001 Statistical Abstract of the United States-Population, 2001; [56 screens]. Available at: http://www.census.gov/prod/2002pubs/01statab/vitstat.pdf. Accessed June 7, 2002.

Milstein RL, Wetterhall SF. Framework for program evaluation in public health. Atlanta, GA: Centers for Disease Control and Prevention; 1999.

Healthy People 2010. 2000; [25 screens]. Available at: http://www.health.gov/healthypeople/Document/word/volume 2123phi.doc. Accessed June 12, 2002.

PART IV

From Measurement to Action

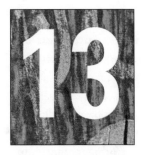

13 Institutional Strengthening for the Performance of the EPHF

1. Introduction

Based on the results obtained in the EPHF measurement exercise in the Region of the Americas, the challenge of encouraging member countries to develop national plans for the institutional strengthening of their national health authorities is addressed in an effort to improve public health practice in each country.

In preparing those national plans, it is essential that the actors involved understand the relationship between EPHF performance measurement and the institutional work of the NHA, so that progress may be made toward achieving the strategic objectives proposed by the Initiative:

1. to improve public health practice

2. to develop the infrastructure to improve the performance of EPHF, and

3. to strengthen the steering role of the national health authority.

The design and implementation of strategies and actions aimed at achieving these objectives and, consequently, bridging the existing gaps between the optimal standard and the degree of performance obtained in the measurements of EPHF are fundamental for this purpose.

Measuring the degree to which the EPHF are carried out in each country utilizing a common instrument has made it possible to identify critical areas shared by two or more EPHF and others that are specific to each function. Accordingly, it should be recognized that these weaknesses may require both immediate action for improvement and the identification of the principal elements that favor or hinder the development of public health in the countries of the Region.

This diagnosis is a starting point—that is, the baseline or point of departure representing the current level of public health performance in the countries—and its realization is what will make it possible to make solid progress with a clear vision toward the preparation of plans for strengthening public health institutions.

2. Guidance in Moving From Diagnosis to Action

A preliminary finding of the diagnosis is that some countries are stronger in some areas, while others are weaker. Thus, there are situations that call for complementary synergistic exercises between neighboring countries, or even countries with similar political, demographic, and socioeconomic features.

This reveals the great potential for establishing partnerships in the Region and underscores the potential for stimulating cooperation among countries to improve performance in public health. The opportunity to establish or consolidate opportunities for sharing experiences, as well as to intensify efforts for the socialization of satisfactory practices in the field of public health, emerges immediately as a primary recommendation for initiating the move from diagnosis to action.

Notwithstanding the initiatives programmed or undertaken by each country according to its capacities, problems, and priorities, the fact is that an analysis of the average obtained for the Region following application of the measurement instrument indicates three essential functions that require a redoubling of efforts for improvement at the national, subregional, and regional levels, since they are highly relevant to the preparation of plans for strengthening the EPHF. They are, in order of importance: Quality Assurance Personal and Population-based Health Services (EPHF 9); Human Resources Development and Training in Public Health (EPHF 8); and Development for Policies and Institutional Capacity for Planning and Management in Public Health (EPHF 5).

In addition, an aspect of public health that is a primary function of the health authority is ensuring access to necessary health services (EPHF 7), especially for the most disadvantaged populations. Its high correlation with the performance of other functions considered to be "incipient", including health promotion (EPHF 3) and social participation (EPHF 4), leads to the conclusion that strengthening these public health functions is fundamental to guarantee access to health services and expand social protection in health to the population ex-

cluded for economic, social, geographical, or cultural reasons.

Notwithstanding the different profiles deriving from the regional and subregional analyses discussed in detail in the previous chapter, it must be ensured that critical aspects of the performance of EPHF revealed by the diagnosis will be given national priority in each country, so that programs appropriate to each national reality can be formulated to orient public health action in a particular manner specific to the country. In this regard, a number of questions that can guide this discussion should be considered, namely:

• What are the main findings of the diagnosis and what is their relevance to the country?

• How do the results of the performance evaluation affect the national health authority?

• What decisions should be made to correct the deficiencies encountered and to reinforce favorable processes?

Decisionmakers should establish parameters and have criteria at their disposal that enable them to use the results to identify the critical problems and determine their priority. This presupposes that each country define the **threshold of differentiation** between strengths and weaknesses; this will permit an objective distinction between the scores considered problematic—that is, those corresponding to weaknesses—and those that are relatively satisfactory—that is, the strengths of the public health system.

In selecting the method to define the threshold and determine the corresponding reference values, it is preferable

to use consensus or collective decision-making among the key national actors who have assumed responsibility for evaluating the performance of the EPHF, since this will encourage representativeness and objectivity in prioritizing problems and thus increase the viability of the approach and the feasibility of executing the strategies and lines of action selected.

Once the principal **critical areas** have been identified, prior to determining the strategies for the national plans, the future vision and desirable scenarios should be defined in order to direct efforts toward the expected results. To this end, the **performance optimums** of the different measurement indicators of EPHF should be analyzed and adapted to the national reality, under the definition of a **possible optimum** that leads, within well-defined and reasonable terms, to the institutional vision crafted by each country.

After specifying the most positive and least satisfactory aspects in the performance of EPHF based on the national analysis, it is also advisable to identify **opportunities and threats**—that is, the external factors that can positively or negatively affect the viability of the interventions to overcome weaknesses or reinforce strengths in the performance of EPHF. A criteria to define a factor as external is the impossibility to affect it directly in order to modify it, making it a condition, rather than an object of management.

3. Design of Systemic Actions

For each country that initiates the planning process to develop institutional capacities for the performance of EPHF,

Figure 1 Relationship between diagnosis of the EPHF, planning, and intervention for the development of institutional capacity

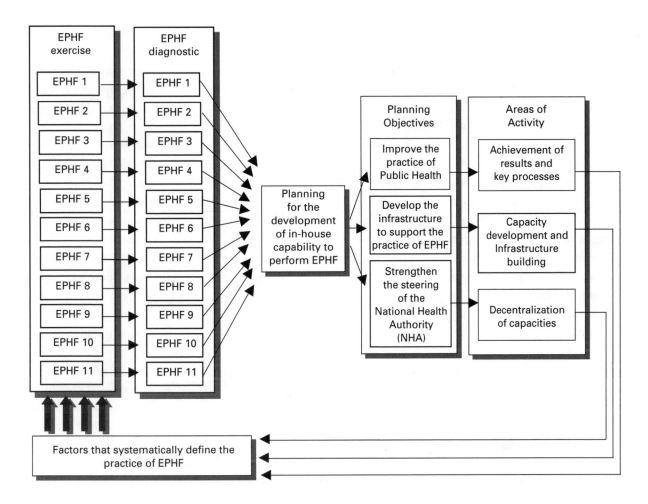

the results of their diagnosis will be the starting point or primary input. Subsequently, a logic with a synthetic approach should be utilized to incorporate these results into the planning process aimed at generating interventions, recognizing that the level of performance of the various EPHF responds to some elements that are common to other functions or even to the EPHF as a whole and may be affected by them.

The methodology followed in measuring the performance of the EPHF and the diagnostic instrument facilitate the progression from the analytical-diagnostic approach to the synthetic ap-

proach of the intervention, making it possible to group the results into three strategic intervention areas:

1. adequate performance of key processes and the securing of results;

2. development of institutional capacities and strengthening of infrastructure, and

3. support for the development of decentralized competencies.

This logic was used in the design of the measurement indicators and, accordingly, the indicators have been organ-

ized in a manner consistent with those categories. Thus, the principal strengths and weaknesses that should become the basic input in preparing the plans to improve public health are inferred from the diagnosis, based on the strategic objectives defined by each country, each subregion, or the Region of the Americas as a whole (see Figure 1).

As observed in this figure, **systemic factors** affect the area of several EPHF or all of them; that is, represented graphically, they affect the EPHF horizontally or cross through them because they have a significant influence in promoting or impeding the EPHF. This graphic representation makes it possible to observe how the planning of interventions or actions for improvement uses planning objectives as referents and establishes a link with the areas of intervention that may be considered.

4. Specific Areas of Intervention to Improve the Performance of EPHF

In addition to identifying the systemic interventions that affect the performance of various EPHF and that impact on institutional capacities in general, such as the training of human resources or the upgrading of infrastructure, it is also essential to identify **the weaknesses and strengths specific** to each function that are relevant to addressing the particular elements necessary for each case.

Some examples of this type of intervention may include the strengthening of the public health laboratory network, the design of timely mechanisms for responding to public health hazards, and the improvement of health sector management in emergencies and disasters. The special features of these areas are both the resources and specific interventions in public health stemming from the diagnosis, as well as the specialization of the actors involved and the sphere of action that will be affected.

These areas are highly significant and thus should not be overlooked when designing the plans, although they could produce strategies that are more isolated and, in some cases, very restricted in their sphere of action or more limited in terms of their capacity to bring together the actors involved.

Human resource development and training in public health (EPHF 8) re-

quires special mention as a specific area of action whose improvement simultaneously results in the overall strengthening of action in public health, as stated in Chapter 15.

The results of the diagnosis indicate that within the context of each nation and the regional scenario, it is urgent that countries implement strategies to correct the weaknesses encountered.

5. Setting Priorities

In setting priorities, it is useful to ensure that the formulation of strategic objectives for the national plan corresponds to the interests, objectives, and expertise of the key actors in the national, subnational, and local contexts who will be in charge of this effort or affected by it. Accordingly, it is particularly important to convene a full meeting with the representation of these actors.

In order to achieve practical validation of the priorities set in the strategies and lines of action, an analysis of causal relationships among the problems identified or critical areas requiring intervention should be performed. To establish an objective order of priority, the following taxonomy, which allows problems to be classified for subsequent analysis and prioritization, can be used:

- *Urgent.* These are cases that, due to their exigency, magnitude, and importance, cannot be postponed.

- *Systemic and serious.* These respond to systemic factors involving several EPHF and demand significant actions over time.

- *Of high vulnerability.* These are problems of a specific or systemic nature

whose improvement is technically and financially feasible; they can be addressed effectively within the limits of the resources available immediately or in the short term;

- *Multidimensional and highly complex.* These are problems in which the specific area to be addressed is difficult to pinpoint; they require the efforts of numerous actors and entail financial and technical difficulties.

Once the priorities of the national plan have been set, an analysis of the institutions, agencies, and actors involved should be performed, through the preparation of a **political map of participants** that enables the strategies and mechanisms that guarantee its viability to be incorporated into the plan.

To perform that analysis, a list of stakeholders, or people affected by the implementation of the plan, should be prepared. As part of this process, the position and specific weight of each stakeholder in the public health system should first be identified. Finally, the political map resulting from the stakeholder analysis should reflect the significance and function of each actor and entity in fulfilling the contents of the plan and contain information that permits an analysis of the situation and outlook.

Finally, since setting priorities for the national plan to improve public health goes beyond the health sector's sphere of action to include the entire set of stakeholders that comprise the different levels of government and social actors involved, it must employ an intersectoral approach with broad social participation to allow the plan to be incorporated into national development strategies.

It is therefore essential to forge concrete ties between these priorities and the political, social, and economic development strategies of each country, maintaining the plan within the national public policy framework to promote joint responsibility with the entire realm of actors and entities, governmental and nongovernmental alike, that participate in the national effort and are relevant to the success of this initiative.

6. From Diagnosis of the Performance of EPHF to the Development of the Institutional Capacity of the Health Authority

The starting point for articulating the diagnosis and plan for improving public health in the countries is the recognition that exercising the EPHF is one of the basic missions of the national health authority.

The nature of the EPHF has been widely discussed in earlier chapters and the level of importance and significance of this effort has been confirmed. In order to move toward action based on the measurement of EPHF performance, the health sector and relevant institutions in the country should raise at least the following questions:

What is the operative definition of each EPHF in the country?

What value does each EPHF have or what does each represent for the practice of the sector?

What does each EPHF represent for the practice of each participating institution?

Who are the primary and most significant actors in each EPHF?

How will the people and institutions make a commitment to carrying out each EPHF?

Based on this analysis, a practical, objective relationship can be established with the principal elements and dimensions of the development of the NHA's institutional capacity.

7. Institutional Development for the Exercise of EPHF

The meaning and scope of the concept of **institutional development** imply a focus on the continuous improvement of the capacities, competences, and aptitudes of the work force and of the means and instruments that support public health systems in their task of exercising the essential functions properly, effectively, efficiently, and in a sustained manner.

Institutional capacity cannot be developed without appropriation of the concept of EPHF by national and subnational institutions, recognizing also that the performance of an individual, team, or organization is a systemic function that includes both internal and external factors and, naturally, affects the actors directly involved.

It is important to establish a link between the **institutional capacity** and **infrastructure** of the public health system and ensure their adaptation to one another. Although on certain occasions these two basic components are managed separately, we know that they represent complementary notions that overlap.

The area of institutional capacity or development encompasses three broad components:

1. worker competence;

2. information and data systems, and

3. organizational capacity.

These components are closely linked; deficiencies in each have an impact on the others and, thus on the entire system. Therefore, the strategic interventions aimed at strengthening institutional capacity should be directed at the components as a whole. Institutional capacity should respond in a timely and adequate manner and operate systemically, articulating information, material, human, and financial resources.

Information resources include data collection systems and communication technologies utilized as a result of this institutional capacity. Human resources contribute the talent and skills needed to carry out the work of public health.

There are two distinctive features that should be considered in analyzing and dealing with organizational capacity for institutional development of the public health system. On the one hand, we have the fact that in many countries, the national ministry of health is responsible for the delivery of health services to both individuals and the population at large.

On the other hand, a precedent has been set in linking public health almost exclusively to certain specific or programmatic activities—for example, the *eradication* of malaria, the prevention and control of cholera, and the prevention and control of HIV/AIDS.

Thus, it is important to carefully examine the relationship between these programmatic activities and the system's institutional capacity and infrastructure, in order to determine the connections between institutional development, the adequacy of infrastructure, and effectiveness in the execution of EPHF.

Institutional capacity based on a strong and functional public health infrastructure is considered an essential element in the effectiveness of programs and services. The goal of that infrastructure is to deliver complete and quality services. That goal can be attained more easily if the construction and development of the system's infrastructure follows an explicit conceptual definition of the essential public health functions and services.

Unfortunately, this network of people, organizations, resources, and systems suffers from different weaknesses in different countries and has been under stress for many decades. Thus, a frame of reference that is sufficiently documented in terms of the evolution of public health in each context becomes a particularly valuable input for an adequate and objective evaluation of the existing infrastructure: this can yield greater dividends or clarifications regarding the strategic planning exercise to be carried out.

This analysis becomes even more important if we consider that these actions to strengthen the national health authority represent varying degrees of evolution, budgetary sufficiency, and cumulative experience among the different countries of the Hemisphere.

Programmatic activities cannot be carried out in a vacuum, but must have a system to support them in their different processes if they are to function properly. An appropriate infrastructure that supports the institutional ability to provide services can act like a "circuit board," which handles differentiated, constant, and specific demands to which it responds in a timely and effective manner, appropriate to the moment and type of need presented.

For example, in the case of chronic disease surveillance, a developed institutional capacity based on a solid infrastructure will allow the public health system to acquire more reliable data with a superior power of analytical inference. Using the essential public health functions as a frame of reference also facilitates and gives greater emphasis to the development of strategic interventions to solve problems completely, and not just with isolated responses that meet the needs of only certain specific programs: this promotes the implementation of more integrated methods with a greater response capacity to address public health issues and needs.

8. Worker Capacity and Competence

The linchpin of institutional capacity development is a trained public health workforce—that is, as proposed in Chapter 15, health workers whose competencies and aptitudes are those required by the tasks they will perform. Lack of a formally trained work force poses obstacles to the development of the system and public health in general.

A 1997 study in the United States indicated that 78% of the local Department of Health directors did not hold graduate degrees in public health. That same study revealed that these professionals also lacked opportunities for continuous education in their fields. This reveals the existence of a gap, which demands more from the workforce in coping with change and increasingly complex needs and requires that workers be provided with the technology, instruments, and training necessary to meet these growing needs.

In this regard, it is necessary to creatively articulate: 1) the use of public health competencies to develop educational and in-service training programs based on practice; 2) a framework for certification and accreditation; and 3) the use of telematic media and appropriate technology to provide public health education and foster health promotion.

9. Information and Data Systems

Strengthening institutional capacity implies systematically formalizing and reinforcing the ties among the different areas and institutional responsibilities of public health practice. It is therefore essential that all components of the system be able to share information among themselves and have access to multiple data sources. A number of studies have reported serious deficiencies in the facility with which public health information can circulate rapidly through the system. Other studies have revealed the existence of gaps in the utilization of the technology infrastructure.

Deficiencies in the basic information infrastructure are an obstacle, not only because they prevent public health agencies from communicating among themselves in a timely manner, but also because they hinder communication among public health workers, private physicians, and other sources of information about emerging health problems. These basic gaps in communication also fragment surveillance systems because of the great differences in the countries' communications infrastructure.

Health institutions need to address aspects related to strengthening the capacity of the information and data infrastructure in their public health systems. Much more is required for this purpose than the acquisition of equipment. One of the major decisions to be made involves obtaining the human resources necessary to operate the equipment and properly maintain it.

10. Organizational Capacity

Capacity may be defined in many ways, but as it pertains to the field of health, it could be defined as follows:

The capacity of a health professional, team, organization, or system is its ability to effectively, efficiently, and sustainably exercise the functions established for it to contribute to the institutional mission and vision and to the policies and strategic objectives of the health team, organization, and system. The public health system has numerous components that should work in unison to achieve the common goal of implementing quality public health functions and activities. Strengthening capacity and organization in these circumstances can pose a challenge, because in the process, the system must not become the result of piecemeal solutions with many variants in its ability to function.

The first step in strengthening organizational capacity consists of evaluating the strengths and weaknesses of the organizations or systems, in addition to analyzing the threats and opportunities that they face. Many instruments are cur-

rently available for performing this type of public health system evaluation. For example, the National Public Health Performance Standards Program (NPH-PSP) of the United Kingdom has designed three tools for measuring the results of state and local systems, including measurement of the effectiveness of local health institution Governing Councils. These tools and the methods for utilizing them will be discussed in greater detail in the following chapters.

International and local organizations have become aware that, while technical and financial inputs are fundamental to help improve the operation of systems, they do not by themselves ensure that the system is sufficiently flexible to adapt to a changing and significantly dynamic environment. This strengthening of capacities implies that the organization or system is capable of performing the basic functions and of including and meeting its own development needs in a broad context and a sustainable manner in four dimensions. This concept is based on identifying the capacities that are indispensable to strengthening the capacity of any organization. The four dimensions referred to above are described as follows:

Human and institutional capacities are indispensable for competent staff performance. If the organization where people work has serious deficiencies—such as the lack of a precise mission and vision, inadequate structures, anomalous practices, management, and systems, a lack of incentives, and an environment that does not facilitate high levels of performance—the performance of its staff is probably inadequate, at the margin of its knowledge and aptitudes. The methods and steps required for

building human and institutional capacities should be different.

Capacities for planning and execution differ in nature, but are interdependent. The close link between policies, plans, and their execution is fundamental. Both capacities must be cultivated without sacrificing one for the other.

Micro and macro dimensions reveal the need for diagnosing capacity in terms of the appropriate level. Different capacities are required at the micro level (for example, within a program) than at the highest level, where policy and planning capacities should be emphasized.

In the cognitive and practical dimensions, the need to increase capacities beyond the level that can be achieved through formal or informal training must be underscored. Learning by trial-and-error or on-the-job, conceiving new practices and systems, and assimilating work modes are some of the methods for applying and adapting knowledge and are part of the strengthening of capacities. This learning takes a long time, which explains the need for a long-term perspective.

As the above classification makes clear, the capacities related to some of these dimensions can be strengthened more rapidly than others. Thus, while the order of priority for these dimensions may vary, it should not be overlooked that strengthening capacity requires a solution for each of these dimensions at some point in the process. This is particularly important for smaller countries that lack enough technical specialists to strengthen their capacities.

In cases where external technical assistance is required, it would be advisable to include these dimensions in a plan of action to define the critical needs for which this level of expertise is required. A useful resource for obtaining external help is the network of WHO Collaborating Centers, which offer a wide variety of technical assistance. These Centers are the national institutions designated by the Director-General of WHO to be part of an international collaboration network charged with carrying out activities that support the WHO mandate to work in international health, as well as its programmatic priorities. The directory of these centers can be found on at following website: http//whqlily.who.int-search.asp.

The strengthening of true capacities throughout the system can be a challenge, given the structural inequalities that tend to exist among its components. Hence, there is a need to establish a process to measure system performance and evaluate its total capacities. Deficiencies at any point in the system thus become evident and can be systematically detected and corrected.

Any plan for strengthening organizational capacity should include improvements in the entire organization. This implies developing the leadership skills of managers, strengthening effective systems for financial and human resources planning, and developing processes that promote institutional, programming, and financial sustainability. Depending on these improvements, NGOs, community organizations, and public sector health programs make good management decisions and provide high-quality, sustainable health services. This approach fosters the strengthening of capacities in the community and promotes the most satisfactory expansion and integration of

general capacity. This expansion in the community can be achieved through the formation of long-term associations and plays an inestimable role in the sustainability of the capacity-strengthening process.

The organizations have described strategies to strengthen organizational capacity. Outside of those strategies, it is always important to have a mechanism in place for supervising and evaluating the system, with the purpose of obtaining feedback to improve system performance and make adequate use of operations. This surveillance and evaluation function is particularly important in health sector reform, since changes in institutional responsibilities and the duties of personnel may be introduced as a consequence of health system restructuring (figure 2). It would be very easy for essential processes to disappear during restructuring and, instead of strengthening system capacities, for the opposite to occur.

It is therefore recommended that the planning process for the institutional strengthening required for the exercise of the EPHF include the active participation of sectoral actors as the agents responsible for the financial support of the process, with a vision that goes beyond the traditional organizational boundaries of the NHA.

Although the objectives, strategies, and actions are aimed at developing the capacity for performance of EPHF, the interventions required for their achievement ultimately depend on developing concrete areas for the institutional work of the NHA. Some practical examples of potential areas of intervention for the performance of EPHF, based on the diagnosis performed, are the following:

- development and technological expansion of information, management, and operating systems, and development of the regulatory and political framework;

- strengthening of the institutional organization of the NHA;

- strengthening of management capacity;

- development of human resources in public health;

- organization of the budget relative to the performance of EPHF;

- strengthening of institutional infrastructure capacity;

- development and technological expansion of information, management, and operating systems, and

- expansion of social participation in sectoral decision-making and oversight.

In the process of identifying the most relevant intervention options to be included in the national plans for improving public health, it should be determined whether the proposal envisions some of the elements that, based on institutional development experiences around the world, have been the most effective in achieving satisfactory development of institutional capacity, including:

- Development of skills to manage the process of institutional change, based on the organizational culture.

- Recognition and consideration of incentives and limitations external to the change.

- Definition of the phases of the process of change, taking into account contextual limitations, existing strengths, and cultural or functional rigidities.

- A guarantee that the national interest translates into sustained investment, meaning that international cooperation will have to be complementary, while promoting the creation of broad participatory networks and partnerships.

- Confirmation that all participants understand the purposes of the initiatives, thus ensuring their commitment.

- Promotion of an environment open to experimentation in the development of processes at different levels, with clear objectives and priorities that can be translated into concrete plans.

At the conclusion of this process, it should be clear which interventions could be undertaken to secure the expected results, **defining the horizon** that will characterize the country once the limitations detected and prioritized have been overcome.

Subsequently, progress should be made toward definition of the work aimed at developing the EPHF, justifying the reason for the institutional strengthening, specifying the necessary strategies and courses of action, and indicating who benefits, what services and actions will be carried out, and who will be responsible for them. This type of design should be consistent with the framework of the three basic goals of the Initiative: 1) to improve public health practice; 2) to develop the infrastructure for performance of EPHF; and 3) to strengthen the steering role of the national health authority.

In order to facilitate the entire process of planning and preparing the national plans, PAHO/WHO has put together a practical guide containing a set of tools available to the countries.

11. Development of Lines of Action

The framework for preparing the national plan to strengthen the essential public health functions should include two simultaneous and synergistic lines of action: a) the development of national health objectives, and b) the development of the institutional objectives of the NHA to improve public health practice in the countries.

There are interesting examples of the definition of national health objectives in the Region (the United States, Canada, the United Kingdom, Chile, Uruguay), all of which concur in the formulation of two major general objectives: to prolong healthy life and reduce inequities in health. The major problematic areas tend to be related to chronic diseases, injuries, environmental and mental health, and other illnesses related to lifestyle. Furthermore, the need to coordinate activities with other social sectors is emphasized, since many of the determinants of health are not the responsibility of the health sector.

This framework of health challenges, which by and large are common to the countries of the Region, should be the basis for reorienting the sectoral reform processes currently under way, making the population's health problems the central element in the orientation of health policies. Without neglecting the timely care of disease, the emphasis on health protection underscores the im-

portance of making public health a priority area of action.

From these national health objectives, strategies are derived to achieve the expected results, which are directly related to ensuring the fulfillment of EPHF, the execution of population-based interventions to prevent and reduce specific risks in priority areas (tuberculosis, etc.), and the maintenance of satisfactory strategies to control disease in each country and address new threats to public health.

Considering all of the above, the *institutional objectives to improve the practice of the NHA* should be geared toward, and incorporated in, health objectives. This implies the challenge of designing new institutional arrangements for the NHA consistent with these national health challenges.

Without detriment to the priorities established by each country for strengthening the institutional capacity of the NHA, based on the identification of critical areas in the performance of EPHF, the regional diagnosis and the subregional analyses suggest certain courses of action that can contribute to the repositioning of the NHA.

Strengthening the steering role of the NHA requires, in large measure, resolution and improvement of the performance of EPHF at both the central and subnational (intermediate and local) levels. Reorienting health care to reduce inequities and barriers to access, designing strategies that provide social protection in health for ever-growing groups of people who remain unprotected today, ensuring greater effectiveness and quality in health interventions to promote the efficient use of always-limited available resources, reorienting health care models toward health promotion to prevent growing harm, and promoting public policies that protect and improve the health of the population are some of the areas that need improvement and whose fulfillment is not only fundamental to improve the levels of health and quality of life of the population, but is also part of the State's regulatory responsibility in health.

In addition, ensuring the supply of public goods with positive externalities for health—including semiprivate or private goods whose impact on public health is a significant factor—and ensuring that they are consistent with national epidemiological priorities should also be part of any plan to strengthen the NHA to improve national public health practice.

Developing greater competencies and skills to improve public health practice also requires the development of strategies to upgrade the workforce in public health, adopting new educational approaches, new practices and forms of training, and upgrading public health personnel, as well as other human resources who may contribute to public health practice in general (see Chapter 15).

Pointing the compass that separates sector functions toward the strengthening of regulatory and supervisory functions, while improving management in health services delivery, emerges as a priority for better performance of the EPHF. All this, together with public accountability, helps to strengthen the image of the health authority in the eyes of the citizenry.

Another action that helps to promote the role of the NHA is to move forward with the harmonious development of the regulatory capacity, in the area of care (public and private health care providers) as well as the environment and occupational health, to increase the health impact and attempt to place the well-being of the population ahead of the pressures that may be exerted by the various interest groups.

Improving the evaluation of access to health services; promoting knowledge, skills, and the development of mechanisms to bring health programs and services closer to the population; and increasing access to services, within a framework characterized by multiple public and private actors responsible for access to health, become fundamental to reduce the vulnerability of the most susceptible populations at the greatest risk of disease. In this regard, efforts to establish explicit rights in health through mechanisms that guarantee benefits; the creation of regulatory systems to ensure their faithful fulfillment; and the facilitation of necessary information for users are other areas for strengthening the institutional capacity of the NHA that should be among the priorities in the national plan.

The challenge of adequately integrating public health actions to ensure the anticipated health impact of these health promotion and disease prevention measures, in an environment marked by the growing differentiation of functions and actors within the health systems, also implies the need for the organizational and functional redesign of public health programs to achieve the successes envisioned.

The management of sectoral action to strengthen the NHA's capacity to formulate, organize, and direct the execution of the national health policy through processes that include the definition of objectives, the preparation and imple-

mentation of strategic plans that articulate the efforts of the sector's public and private institutions, as well as other social actors, the establishment of participatory mechanisms, and the building of partnerships and consensus to make the proposals viable and facilitate the mobilization of the necessary resources to carrying out the proposed actions require stronger NHA leadership in health.

Finally, the importance of including a framework for monitoring and evaluation in the national plan should be emphasized. To this end, indicators must be established to describe institutional performance, define responsibilities for monitoring and evaluation, and allocate specific resources that make it possible to verify fulfillment of the programmed actions, establish accountability, introduce the necessary corrections, and take away lessons in this regard.

Bibliography

Bryson JM. Strategic Planning for Public and Nonprofit Organizations. San Francisco: Jossey-Bass; 1995.

Centre for Development and Population Activities. Planificación estratégica, un enfoque de indagación. Serie de Manuales de Capacitación de CEDPA; 2000.

Fundación Acceso. Metodología de ACCESO de Planificación Institucional. San José.

Ganeva I, Marín JM, Segovia M. Capacidad de negociación en el sector salud. Guatemala: Proyecto Subregional de Consolidación e Incremento de la Capacidad Gerencial de los Servicios de Salud, Organización Panamericana de la Salud; 1993

Milén A. What do we know about capacity building? An overview of existing knowledge and good practice. Geneva: World Health Organization, Department of Health Service Provision; 2001.

Organización Panamericana de la Salud/ Organización Mundial de la Salud, Centers for Disease Control, Centro Latinoamericano de Investigaciones en Sistemas de Salud. Guía para la aplicación del instrumento de medición del desempeño de las Funciones Esenciales de Salud Pública. Iniciativa "La salud pública en las Américas", Medición del Desempeño de las Funciones Esenciales de Salud Pública. Washington, D.C.: OPS; 2001.

Organización Panamericana de la Salud/Organización Mundial de la Salud. Desarrollo institucional de la capacidad de rectoría en salud. Washington, D.C.: OPS, División de Desarrollo de Sistemas y Servicios de Salud. (In press.)

Organización Panamericana de la Salud/Organización Mundial de la Salud, Centers for Disease Control, Centro Latinoame-

ricano de Investigaciones en Sistemas de Salud. Instrumento para la medición del desempeño de las Funciones Esenciales de Salud Pública. Iniciativa "La salud pública en las Américas". Washington, D.C: OPS; 2001.

Organización Panamericana de la Salud/Organización Mundial de la Salud. Fortalecimiento del desempeño institucional de las FESP. Guía metodológica para el diseño de planes nacionales. Washington, D.C.: OPS. (In press.)

Reich MR. Applied Political Analysis for Health Policy Reform. Current Issues in Public Health 2:186–191;1996.

Reich MR and Cooper DM. PolicyMaker: Computer-Aided Political Analysis. (Version 2.3.1). Brookline Massachussetts; 2000.

USAID Center for Development Information and Evaluation. Selecting Performance Indicators. Performance Monitoring and Evaluation TIPS, #6. Washington, D.C.: PN-ABY-214; 1996.

Valladares R and Forrtín A. Sistema de Monitoreo del Proyecto de Acceso a la Educación Bilingüe Intercultural (PAEBI): Descripción del Modelo Global. Guatemala World Learning/USAID, GSD Consultores Asociados. (In preparation.)

Estimate of Expenditures and Financing for EPHF and Mechanisms for Determining Cost and Budgeting

1. Estimate of expenditures and financing

1.1 Introduction

Among other factors, the performance of the essential public health functions (EPHF) in each country is determined by the management of the institutions and organizations that implement them, the capacity of the human resources involved in the process, and the availability and distribution of economic resources allocated to their financing.

In the process of State and, particularly, health sector reform in the Americas, the level of resources allocated to EPHF has been affected by the introduction of modalities—both organizational and financial—that result in differentiated care. The introduction of those modalities was attributable to an economic model that initially advocated "reducing State intervention." The effort made to diminish the role of the State neglected

the importance of reviewing and strengthening its obligation to guarantee citizens' rights to have access to a series of benefits and services, for which the market has proven to be a poor administrator of resources in terms of equity and social well-being.

One explanation may lie in the fact that until now, no instrument was available to measure the "output" of health systems with respect to EPHF. That deficiency hinders the ability to allocate resources based on the criteria of rationality or, ideally, profitability.

In terms of the analysis of expenditure and financing, EPHF have not received adequate attention. With regards to health care, for many years the sector studies in the different countries maintained a tradition of concentrating on problems related to expenditure. As a result, the information was usually guided by how much was spent on the different levels of care, and the conclusions took into consideration that

spending was concentrated at the tertiary level in urban areas. Due to a lack of information that would permit the analysis of financing sources, the conclusion was perhaps reached that urban populations with a certain amount of resources, as opposed to populations with limited resources, made the most intensive use of hospital facilities financed with public funds.

In recent year, with a view to analyzing the sector's financial flows, the countries of the Region have joined in the world initiatives aimed at developing a useful methodology for designing health policies. Along this line, most countries have prepared national health accounts. The national health accounts are matrixes that make it possible to present, in an organized way, the tracking of financial resources from their integration in the sector to their final destination.

Although the development of the national health accounts has been an important contribution to the analyses of some areas—such as equity in financing—the systems of national health accounts should concentrate on the guarantee of care. Consequently, some elements of EPHF are in a category denominated "healthcare-related expenditures", described in the jargon of the United Nations System of National Accounts with the specification "below the line", in order to indicate that the category of expenditures is related to, but not an inherent part of, those accounts. In cases where expenditure on EPHF has been taken into account, it has been blurred as an administrative category.

The performance evaluation of EPHF in the Region—discussed in another chapter of this book—demonstrated that the countries generally reached a high level of performance in the most traditional functions, that is, those of public health. This conclusion underscores the need for restructuring the way in which public health is administered, so that health systems are adequately prepared to address health problems that arise world wide and to respond to the so-called "diseases of poverty" that affect a significant part of the population.

As previously stated in other chapters of the book, EPHF are primarily the responsibility of the health authorities in the sector. The fundamental task is to establish the operating rules of the health system and safeguard compliance to the rules. This role of the State is essential to guarantee equity in access and to ensure financing of care as well as the promotion of quality health services that ultimately lead to high levels of health in the general population and in each subgroup identified by either ethnicity, sex, age, and level of income.

The performance evaluation of EPHF confirmed the need to estimate both the level of resources allocated by the countries for that purpose and their sources of financing. Knowing the current level of expenditure and comparing it with the estimated cost required for adequate performance will make it possible to quantify the additional resources needed. At the same time, the data on financing sources will facilitate the determination of the additional sources required.

During the development and testing of the methodology provided in this chapter, the difficulties of the task were evident. Although there are several reasons for this with respect to setting limits on the analysis, the most important is the form and breadth of the information on budgets and expenditures presented. Another challenge arises because multiple institutions participate in the exercise of some EPHF.

This chapter outlines a preliminary methodological proposal for estimating the expenditure and financing of the EPHF.[1] The application of a methodology with these characteristics will provide data that have an inestimable potential usefulness in policy-making and public health practice. Some benefits of the proposal are indicated below:

- To improve the capacity for resource allocation—both in the immediate and in the long-term—for EPHF and, consequently, fro the increased the effectiveness of public spending.

- To improve knowledge of the manner in which the EPHF are executed and how the countries can move closer to the standard.

---

[1] In another chapter, a proposal is presented for estimating the cost of implementing the EPHF at a given level of performance.

- To contribute to the improvement of the public health infrastructure and performance of the EPHF.

- To improve the quality of health systems as a whole by increasing the regulatory capacity and performance of the health authorities.

- To record the allocation of resources to the EPHF in the budgetary statistics and, accordingly, in the national health accounts.

The evolution of the concepts related to EPHF and attempts to quantify society's efforts to produce them can be classified into three major initiatives:

- The PAHO "Public Health in the Americas" initiative dealing basically with the methodology for estimating the performance of EPHF in the countries of the region and their subsequent execution.

- The World Bank strategy, in which the institution proposes to utilize the tools of public health to improve the health of the population and help reduce poverty, expanding the content and quality of its health projects portfolio.

- The studies conducted in some states and counties of the United States to estimate the expenditure and financing of the essential functions defined by them.

Although this chapter presents some proposals on how to incorporate EPHF into the studies of financing by means of the national health accounts, the greater challenge remains to move beyond health services delivery to a broader study area that encompasses all the components of expenditure and financing sources for public health programs and, where possible, each of the EPHF in particular or, at least, all of them as a whole.

2. Estimates of Public Health Expenditure in the United States

For the last decade, the United States has shown interest in EPHF and how to estimate the quantity of resources assigned to them. As early as 1993, they recommended the need for structural health sector reforms to modify the allocation of resources in order to improve the health system and prevent diseases. For this, it was necessary to know the amount devoted to financing public health.

Naturally, the first step was to define the essential public health functions or services. The lack of a common language confused the political debate during the process of discussion of health sector reform in the United States. The task of structuring that common language was commissioned to the Public Health Association. We have already mentioned that these functions or services were defined through a participatory process, in which numerous agencies[2] contributed and which resulted in the definition of ten essential services, with their respective programmatic lines of action included and not included, that would facilitate the process of resource estimation.

In the mid-1990s, the Office of Planning and Evaluation of the Department of Health and Human Services recommended conducting a study on the possibility of collecting periodic information with regard to health services infrastructure, including expenditure and financing. Although the criteria were still provisional and therefore did not allow systematic and comparable information systems on the subject to be established, the work demonstrated the great potential for that area of study to respond to and to determine the important political issues concerning the effect of the public health services infrastructure on the operation and results of the health system.

An initial estimate of the state expenditure devoted to disease prevention indicated that only 1% of the national budget was allocated to public health programs. Although the study recognized the impossibility of establishing the appropriate amount, the results demonstrated the need for strengthening the public health services infrastructure so that it can react adequately in the future to possible outbreaks of epidemics. Three pilot studies of state and local expenditure were carried out, utilizing the Public Health Association's frame of reference on the ten essential services.

The first study, conducted by the Public Health Foundation in 1996, presented results from nine states. The second study, based on the previous one,

was conducted in three local jurisdictions and concluded in March 1998. The third and most recent study was performed by the Maryland state health agency and included all its local jurisdictions. The following table summarizes the three studies.

With respect to the results obtained, there is a clear disparity in the funds allocated to public health, ranging from US$ 30 to US$ 394. These disparities are attributable to the different institutional organizations and different political priorities, but also to incoherence in the definitions.

All the studies presented their results by grouping the functions into personal public health services—regarded as clinical services for individuals—and population-based public health services, considered measures to promote health and prevent disease in large population groups. As expected, the bulk of the expenditure is concentrated in the former, as demonstrated in table 2.

The results of the three studies indicate the need to delve even further into the definition of the functions, so that it becomes very clear "what is included and what is excluded", in order to make it possible to compare across different jurisdictions. Large differences were evident in the various types of institutional organization, with the consequent variations with respect to public responsibility.

It is recommended that these studies continue to be conducted repeatedly, both in the same location as the pilot studies and in new localities. In this way, the methodology can continue to be evaluated and improved in order to achieve valid, reliable, and comparable results.

---

[2] Some of the agencies participating in the Public Health Functions Steering Committee are: American Public Health Association, Association of Schools of Public Health, Association of State and Territorial Health Officials, National Association of County and City Health Officials, National Association of State Alcohol and Drug Abuse Directors, National Association of State Mental Health Program Directors, Public Health Foundation, Partnership for Prevention, Agency for Healthcare Research and Quality, Center for Disease Control and Prevention, Food and Drug Administration, Health Resources and Services Administration, Indian Health Services, National Institutes of Health, Mental Health Services Administration, and Office of the Assistant Secretary for Health Substance Abuse.

Table 1 Characteristics of U.S. studies on public health expenditure

Study year(s) and associations	Study objectives	Responses	Conclusions
1995–1996 PHF	• To create instruments that facilitate the estimation of expenditure allocated to the EPHF, in order to make comparisons among the various regions • To transfer the results to the national area • To evaluate the strengths and weaknesses of the instruments	9 States–AZ, IA, IL, LA, NY, OR, RI, TX, WA	1. Public spending in health can be measured and tracked through the EPHF 2. The local health institutions should be directly involved in the process of measuring the expenditure
1997–1998 NACCHO NALBOH PHF	• To enhance and adapt the local measurement instruments • To conduct studies on experiences of the institutions involved in the project • To make recommendations for developing a standard methodology and enhancing the instruments	3 local health inst. Onondaga, NY TriCounty, WA Columbus, OH	1. The process is safe and the results are very valuable 2. Despite differences in methodology and preparation, the results were acceptable 3. The guidelines and rules with regard to decision-making should be strengthened in order to obtain better parameters for comparison 4. The improved instruments should be tested at the national level
1998–1999 ASTHO NACCHO NALBOH PHF	• To check the measurement instruments (to improve definitions and rules for decision-making; to provide examples) • To compile the expenditures of all health institutions at the regional level, utilizing the improved instruments • To evaluate the safety, reliability, and comparability of the information • To evaluate the essential service paradigms, such as education and communication instruments	Health Department of Maryland, and the 24 local health departments of MD	1. The process can produce reliable estimates, usable as a guide for establishing policies 2. There should be more emphasis on awareness of the benefits derived from the entire project 3. The process can fit into the categories established by the health budgets

Other recommendations include the need for educating public agencies, health institutions, and students of public health with regard to the essential functions. It is also necessary to coordinate the work of institutions that develop instruments for performance measurement of public health functions.

3. The EPHF in the National Health Accounts

The national health accounts are a consistent set of matrixes that describe the financial flows within the health sector in a given year. They differ from the accounts that measure the national product and income, in that they are not intended to measure the value added but rather the financial resources transferred among the different institutions within the sector. The methodology utilized is entirely compatible with the United Nations System of National Accounts.

The national health accounts report on the origin of funds, their distribution among the different institutions involved, and the use of resources pertaining to areas of interest for establishing public health policies. The national health accounts are the most appropriate instrument for analyzing the health expenditure of any country, although the area corresponding to public health is still not very developed.

Many countries have not yet prepared national health accounts, but most are in process of doing so. The current methodological framework for estimating the expenditure and financing of the EPHF does not require that the national health accounts already exist in countries to which it will be applied. However, because it utilizes the principles and classifications of the national heath accounts, the results of this research can be applied to the national health accounts that are prepared in the future.

Table 2 Expenditure on health services per inhabitant, according to studies conducted on the EPHF

Study (date)	Site	Expenditure per inhabitant		
		Personal health services (total in%)	Population-based health services (total in%)	Total essential health services
Study in some states of the United States (1995–1996)	Arizona	US$ 73 (66%)	US$ 38 (34%)	US$ 111
	Iowa	US$ 29 (57%)	US$ 22 (43%)	US$ 51
	Louisiana	US$ 52 (61%)	US$ 34 (39%)	US$ 68
	New York	US$ 168 (77%)	US$ 51 (23%)	US$ 219
	Oregon	US$ 91 (63%)	US$ 53 (37%)	US$ 144
	Rhode Island	US$ 78 (55%)	US$ 65 (45%)	US$ 143
	Texas	US$ 56 (64%)	US$ 32 (36%)	US$ 88
	Washington	US$ 72 (53%)	US$ 64 (47%)	US$ 136
Study in LHD Local Health Depts. (1997–1998)	Columbus	US$ 24 (49%)	US$ 25 (51%)	US$ 49
	Onondaga	US$ 9 (19%)	US$ 42 (81%)	US$ 51
	TriCounty	US$ 2 (4%)	US$ 35 (96%)	US$ 37
Study in Maryland (1998–1999)	Maryland (Total)	US$ 170 (73%)	US$ 62 (27%)	US$ 232
	Local	US$ 54 (53%)	US$ 48 (47%)	US$ 102
	State	US$ 116 (89%)	US$ 14 (11%)	US$ 130

To analyze the national health accounts as a basic instrument for estimating expenditure on EPHF, the classifications in the document *A system of health accounts* were reviewed. This document, the basic manual for classifying allocations corresponding to the health sector, was prepared by the Organization for Economic Cooperation and Development (OECD), published originally in 2000 and revised in 2002. Furthermore, the latest version of the Producers' Guide—still in draft form—was studied; this Guide is being developed through a joint initiative by the PAHO, the WHO, the World Bank, and the U.S. Agency for International Development (USAID), through the project Partnerships for Health Reform (PHR).

The 1993 United Nations Manual on the System of National Accounts and the IMF Manual on Government Finance Statistics were also reviewed. It should be noted that the OECD manual on health accounts was written based on the United Nations and IMF classifications, as well

as other international classifications (those of private industry, for example). Hence, it is compatible with the systems of national accounts throughout the world.

The area of fundamental interest in the health accounts is "health care." It is limited to what is referred to as "disease prevention, improvement of sanitary programs, treatment, rehabilitation, and long-term care." Health care refers to the personal services provided directly whereas the population-based services are commonly called "public health." These services are the improvement of sanitary programs, regulatory standards, the tasks aimed at disease prevention, and the administration of the system.

3.1 Functional Classification

The functional classification of the OECD manual on health accounts specifies the functions within the health sector listed in table 3.

Current health expenditure refers to the set of economic contributions devoted to functions HC.1 to HC.7. *Total health expenditure* is obtained by adding to this the health-related function HC.R.1, representing the capital investment in the sector. The other related functions may or may not be added—according to the policy of each country—but are presented separately in order to allow them to be compared on an international level.

The public health functions are contained basically in category HC.6. Some of them fit into HC.7, referring to government administration. Others are included in some of the health-related functions, that is, HC.R. As shown in Chapter 6, the WHO made an initial attempt to individualize the nine essential functions identified. Its conclusions appear in the table of the OECD manual on health accounts. However, the functions are not the same as those analyzed in this document because as we have stated, these are the result of a process of

Table 3 Functional classification of the health accounts system

ICHA Code	Functional classification
HC.1	**Curative care**
HC.1.1	Inpatient curative care
HC.1.2	Day cases of curative care
HC.1.3	Outpatient curative care
HC.1.4	Services of curative home care
HC.2	**Rehabilitative care**
HC.2.1	Inpatient rehabilitative care
HC.2.2	Day cases of rehabilitative care
HC.2.3	Outpatient rehabilitative care
HC.2.4	Services of rehabilitative home care
HC.3	**Long-term nursing care**
HC.3.1	Inpatient long-term nursing care
HC.3.2	Day cases of long-term nursing care
HC.3.3	Long-term nursing care: home care
HC.4	**Auxiliary health care**
HC.4.1	Clinical laboratory
HC.4.2	Diagnostic imaging
HC.4.3	Patient transport and emergency rescue
HC.4.9	All other miscellaneous ancillary services
HC.5	**Medical goods dispensed to ambulatory care patients**
HC.5.1	Pharmaceuticals and other medical non-durables
HC.5.2	Therapeutic appliances and other medical durables
HC.6	**Prevention and public health**
HC.6.1	Maternal and child health; family planning and counseling
HC.6.2	School health services
HC.6.3	Prevention of communicable diseases
HC.6.4	Prevention of noncommunicable diseases
HC.6.5	Occupational health care
HC.6.9	All other miscellaneous public health services
HC.7	**Health administration and health insurance**
HC.7.1	General government administration of health
HC.7.2	Health administration and health insurance: private
HC.R	**Health-related functions**
HC.R.1	Capital formation of health care provider institutions
HC.R.2	Education and training of health personnel
HC.R.3	Research and development in health
HC.R.4	Food, hygiene, and drinking water control
HC.R.5	Environmental health
HC.R.6	Administration and provision of social services in kind to assist the ill or disabled
HC.R.7	Administration and provision of health-related cash-benefits

debate and consensus in the region over the last three years.

3.2 Preliminary Functional Classification of the EPHF

A preliminary attempt to classify EPHF is outlined below, solely to provide an idea of the allotments under which most of the actions of each EPHF will probably evolve. Without detailing the most important activities of each EPHF, this classification can only be provisional. Nevertheless, when the field investigation that clarifies which tasks are performed for each function is conducted—and the activities that the health authorities should undertake in order to carry out these functions are optimally defined—the classification should be reviewed.

It should be pointed out that the classification in the OECD manual does not coincide with the description of the EPHF. For example, the manual specifically mentions environmental health and occupational health as public health functions, neither of which are among EPHF, while it explicitly excludes reducing the impact of emergencies and disasters as part of health expenditures. It also mixes population-based measures with personal measures and with normative and regulatory tasks. For example, one of the public health functions in the manual is "prevention of communicable diseases", HC.6.3. Epidemiological surveillance and the population-based improvement of health programs would have to be included within this category, even though they are typical functions of the health authorities and therefore part of the steering role tasks. But numerous personal measures, such as advice at the primary level on the need to boil water in order to prevent diarrhea, immunization, or tuberculosis surveillance, are also the responsibility of the health authorities, although not an essential responsibility within the steering role.

Profound reflection is clearly indispensable at the international level on what information is of interest in the field of public health, which are the basic activities that permit the health authority to perform fully its steering role function, how those activities can be measured, and how they can be monitored over the course of time. The consensus reached in this area will orient the future modification of public health-related categories, within the system of

Table 4 Preliminary classification of the EPHF according to the OECD manual on health accounts

Essential public health functions (EPHF)	ICHA Code (preliminary)
1. Monitoring, evaluation, and analysis of health status	HC6.9/ HC7.1
2. Public health surveillance, research, and control of risks and threats in public health	HC6.3/ HC6.4/ HC7.1
3. Health promotion	HC7.1/ HC6.3/ HC6.4
4. Social participation in health	HC7.1/ HC6.9
5. Development of policies and institutional capacity for planning and management in public health	HC7.1
6. Strengthening of institutional capacity for regulation and enforcement in public health	HC7.1
7. Evaluation and promotion of equitable access to necessary health services	HC7.1
8. Human resources development and training in public health	HC.R.2
9. Quality assurance and improvement in personal and population-based health services	HC.R.3
10. Research in public health	HC.R.3
11. Reducing the impact of emergencies and disasters on health	—

health accounts. Meanwhile, it will be necessary to adapt to the existing classification, prepare the necessary explanations, and, if possible, slightly expand the classification criteria.

We should point out that the OECD manual on health accounts is a "work in progress;" the first version has just been published. In light of its implementation at the international level and the information needs of the different countries, it will be modified and adapted to match reality. The classification has been carried out mainly using two digits. In most cases, a more accurate way of breaking down the classification is still being researched. In this regard, the results of this work and the studies that are conducted in several countries to estimate the expenditure and financing of EPHF, will contribute valuable information that will stimulate thought about how to address the classification of public health tasks in the national health accounts.

It is important to consider that the majority of countries are only now beginning to develop national health accounts. Only very few of them consider this an institutionalized and ongoing activity. The reality is that national health accounts are generally done at various intervals as a sporadic study. Application of the OECD manual classification—that serves as the international model—is still an incipient initiative. For this reason, it is unlikely that the currently-existing national health accounts can be used to study the expenditure and financing of EPHF, although it is advisable that the studies dealing with the subject follow their methodology. The classifications of the system of health accounts and the matrix of the structure proposed—both by the national health accounts and the aforementioned Producers' Guide—will be very useful in understanding the movement of financial flows earmarked for the implementation of the EPHF.

3.3 Classification of Sources of Financing and Financing Agents

A different focus on the classification of sources of financing and financing agents exists between the systems in the OECD manual on health accounts and the Producers' Guide. The former calls "sources of financing" what the latter calls "financing agents." The Producers' Guide indicates that the national health accounts should be broken down into three categories: the flow of financing among sources, the financing agents, and how financing is to be utilized. The "sources" are the same as in the national product and income account system, namely:

- the government, at its various levels (central government, local governments, decentralized institutions, public corporations, social security funds)

- households

- corporations

- the rest of the world

As a last resort, the sources would be households and the rest of the world, since the government takes money from households in the form of taxes and other contributions. With regard to corporations, they could well consider their health expenditures part of the cost of labor and, ultimately, this would also benefit households. However, by convention and given the importance of what they represent, a distinction is made among the four sources. The rest of the world refers to the resources that enter a country to finance health by various means, such as donations, loans, and the net balance of expenditures by people who travel for health reasons, both inside and outside the country.

In the case of EPHF, the bulk of financing will come from the government, although in some countries international cooperation plays an important role in public health measures. Elements of personal health such as immunization can also receive financing from households in the form of recovery rates or fees.

In short, the resources assigned to health are mobilized through these sources. The "financing agents", in turn, are those that allocate the funds, in other words, that purchase and pay for the services. These are the entities that normally operate in the health sector: ministries, social security institutes, nongovernmental organizations, and others. The international classification for financing agents is presented in the following table.

In accordance with the purpose of this study, we will utilize the Producers' Guide approach, which separates the sources from the financing agents.

4. Challenges for Estimating Expenditure and Financing for the EPHF

As seen in the previous section, it is recommended that the methodology of the national health accounts proposed by the OECD manual on health accounts and the Producers' Guide be followed for the matrix approach and adapted to the needs of the essential public health functions. The following paragraphs present the expected format with the basic tables resulting from the field investigations executed in each country.

4.1 Review of the national health accounts Figures

The first task imposed is the review of the national health accounts. We have already noted that many countries still do not have them, and even those that do, have not always been able to break down their expenditures as they should, or else they lack a frame of reference to help them indicate the importance of identifying one allotment or another.

This instrument will make it possible to know the total government spending on all public health works, although the expenditure is not differentiated by type. For example, the Dominican Republic's national health accounts show the following categories in which EPHF could be found in table 6.

This table reveals surprising information that should motivate the health authorities to conduct more in-depth research and even rethink their priorities. It should be noted that spending on the improvement of sanitary programs and preventive care receives only 1.3% of the total assigned by the health authorities to the health of the public sector. The private sector allocates a considerably higher amount for those activities. How can that difference be explained? A true explanation is that Dominican families pay an important portion of the cost of preventive services out-of-pocket, either due to mistrust of public services or for other reasons.

Another explanation could be that public hospitals dispense certain primary-level services. This does actually occur and the problem stems from the fact that the accounting system does not differentiate the expenditure by level of care within public hospitals. As a result, the practice can lead to classification errors in the national health accounts, because—based on the statistics for budgetary spending—it is not possible to discern the expenditures corresponding to preventive services dispensed in the public hospitals. The anomaly requires specific research that has not yet been carried out in the country.

The allocations that would most likely include EPHF are the following:

Table 5   Classification of financing agents

ICHA Code	Financing agents
HF.1	**General government**
HF.1.1	Public administration, excluding social security
HF.1.1.1	Central government
HF.1.1.2	State/provincial government
HF.1.1.3	Local/municipal government
HF.1.2	Social security administrations
HF.2	**Private sector**
HF.2.1	Private social insurance
HF.2.2	Private insurance companies
HF.2.3	Private household out-of-pocket expenditure
HF.2.4	Nonprofit institutions
HF.2.5	Corporations (other than medical insurance)
HF.3	**Rest of the world**

Table 6 The Dominican Republic: health expenditure by function, 1996

Functions	Public sector	%	Private sector	Rest of the world	Total	%
Total	3,154.2	100.0	8,643.4	121.0	11,918.7	100.0
Improvement of preventive care programs	39.9	1.3	695.5		735.1	6.2
Curative care	1,520.3	48.2	4,009.6	121.0	5,650.9	47.4
Research and human resources development	4.5	0.1	5.4		9.8	0.1
Regulation	386.6	12.3	0.2		386.8	3.2
Production and purchase of inputs	885.7	28.1	220.3		1,106.0	9.3
Administration	301.8	9.6	2,989.4		3,291.2	27.6
Facilities	15.5	0.4	723.3		738.8	6.2

Source: Banco Central, Cuentas Nacionales de Salud del Sector Público, 1996 (cited in: Rathe, M. Salud y equidad).

- Improvement of health and preventive care programs

- Research and human resources development

- Regulation

- Administration

These allocations total RD $ 1,215.2 million for 1996, equivalent to 38.5% of the public sector health expenditure. That would be the "ceiling" for EPHF that year.

It should be pointed out that 1996 was the only year in which the Dominican Republic—with PAHO's support and the support of the PHR project—prepared complete national health accounts following the methodology developed by Harvard University. At that time, neither the OECD manual on health accounts nor the Producers' Guide existed. Accordingly, the functional classification utilized does not follow the international model used today.

In subsequent years, the Central Bank continued to repeat the national health accounts of the public sector using the same methodology as in 1996. Research on the private sector was never repeated.

In the Dominican case, these figures are approximate. We could have more complete and detailed information in the countries that have already applied the new methodology, albeit with the limitations previously indicated regarding to the functional classification in which public health activities are included.

A more recent example is that of the national health accounts of Nicaragua, where preventive services constituted 7% of the total health expenditure during the period 1977–1999. This amount, however, reflects only the spending on health care services at the primary level—the so-called SILAIS—and does not include the tasks related to EPHF. These cannot be identified in the national health accounts of Nicaragua since they are included within the Ministry of Health's administrative expenditures. Something similar would occur if we reviewed the national health accounts of any other country. The lack of specificity regarding EPHF, or the difficulty in separating the regulatory tasks from services are dependent on the methodology used in the functional classification of the health accounts.

As we will see further on, the national health accounts also show—in general terms—the financing sources of the

health authorities, a first step toward a detailed analysis of this aspect. Although the activities to which they are allocated are not clearly specified, the identification of the financing sources is the first step toward a more thorough study.

After performing an initial analysis of the overall figures, it will be necessary to address the work of estimating the expenditure and financing of each one of the EPHF. The task requires knowledge of the institutional organization for the implementation of each EPHF.

4.2 Government Budget Statistics

Since the figures of the national health accounts are not broken down as they should be, it is also necessary to review the budgetary spending statistics. The majority of the countries in Latin America budget by program without a uniform classification of these programs. In all cases, it is necessary to thoroughly analyze the systems of budgetary spending and to talk with the technicians who classify the expenditures. Accordingly, the work will necessarily deal with the area of each institution or department linked with the EPHF in question in order to obtain the required information first-hand.

Table 7 Identification of programs, subprograms, and activities related to EPHF 2 in the Dominican Republic

Public Health Function 2	Program	Subprogram	Activity
Public health surveillance, research, and control of risks and threats to public health	Program 1: High-level administration		
Principal institutions or departments involved:			
General Bureau of Epidemiology	Program 2: Coordination, standards, and control of health programs	Subprogram 1: Health services	Activity 4: Control of communicable and noncommunicable diseases
Provincial Health Bureaus	Program 3: Operational services	Subprograms 1 to 8 (services to the regions)	Activity 1 in each subprogram (intermediate coordination, supervision, and control services)
Dr. Defilló Laboratory	Program 2: Coordination, standards, and control of health programs	Subprogram 1: Health services	Activity 2: Laboratory and blood bank department
Laboratory department and provincial public health laboratory network	Program 2: Coordination, standards, and control of health programs	Subprogram 1: Health services	Activity 2: Laboratory and blood bank department
Bureau of the Environment	Program 2: Coordination, standards, and control of health programs	Subprogram 3: Environmental services	Activity 1: Bureau of services for protection of the environment Activity 2: Sanitation and environmental control
Expanded Program on Immunization–EPI (SESPAS)			
Maternal and child department (SESPAS)	Program 2: Coordination, standards, and control of health programs	Subprogram 1: Health services	Activity 3: Health services for the mother and child, nutrition
General Bureau for Control of AIDS and STI (DIGECIT)			
National Institute of Drinking Water and Sewerage (INAPA)	Program 5: Financing to institutions		Activity 1
Center for Control of Tropical Diseases (CENCET)	Program 5: Financing to institutions		Activity 3
Other			

By way of example, table 7 shows some of the programs identified in the case of the Dominican Republic. But an additional problem exists, concerning the separation between the planning and preparation of the budget, and its subsequent execution. The departments that prepare the budget are usually not the same as those that record its execution. The guidelines for budgetary execution follow the national methodology for preparing reports on this subject and in the process, a great deal of the information related to the health programs is lost. It is a problem that affects the entire government, not just the health sector.

As can be observed, in the case of the Dominican Republic, information provided by the budgets at the level of the central government or even by the Ministry of Public Health itself, is still not broken down precisely. To estimate the expenditure and financing of the EPHF, primary information must be collected. In summary:

- Identify the institutional organization for executing the EPHF in question.

- Analyze the budget of each institution or department.

- Separate the entity's EPHF-related tasks from other activities.

- Estimate the level of effort made in performing the EPHF.

- Identify the sources of financing.

- Add the values and present the results in a coherent manner.

The realization of this work obviously requires the unconditional support of the health authorities. It is essential to visit the authorities of the ministry, explain the work to be conducted, and gain their cooperation. We also suggest using the advisory services of an expert in the selected EPHF who is very familiar with its execution and the institutions and key people involved. In order to facilitate the fieldwork, we also recommend organizing an introductory

workshop and a plan of visits to the institutions or departments, in order to estimate the effort required by both the PAHO staff and the technicians from local institutions and departments.

4.3 Example of Institutional Organization to Execute the EPHF

We have already indicated that one of the first tasks in studying EPHF should be to decipher which institutional organization in the country is devoted to the EPHF in question. By way of illustration, in the case of EPHF 2—public health surveillance—the entities involved are detailed in the next table. It should be clarified that the column headed "activities related to EPHF 2" refers exclusively to those cited by the Annual Report of SESPAS for the year 2000. A more thorough field investigation needs to be performed in order to discern the basic programmatic lines related to the corresponding EPHF.

The table 8 shows the complexity of the work involved in estimating the expenditure and financing of the EPHF, since it requires the investigation of the different participating entities from a new perspective. The work is worthwhile as it helps coordinate the activities of all of the entities under the steering role of the health authorities.

5. Methodological guidelines for estimating expenditure and financing

This section presents the preliminary methodological criteria for estimating the expenditure and financing of essential public health functions. These crite-

ria will be utilized subsequently in the pilot study to be conducted in the Dominican Republic. Once completed, we will have a set of more consistent and complete guidelines, which will serve as a basis for the studies that case are conducted in various countries of the region.

We begin the section by offering research findings, that is, the basic tables obtained for EPHF, with the aim of estimating their expenditure and financing. These tables are based on those proposed by the OECD manual on health accounts and the Producers' Guide, but have been adapted to the need for understanding the financial flows of EPHF. After presenting the tables, we will offer some guidelines on how to analyze the work and analyze the results.

The scope of the exercise is limited to the expenditure made by the health authorities, that is, to research the expenditure of public funds. In turn, financing can come from both the public treasury (through various means or types of taxes) and the private sector (corporations and households) and the rest of the world (loans and donations).

Below we provide an initial approximation of the data collection design tools and some of the intermediate results of the process. We will then offer some ideas on how to address the field work in practice. Subsequently, we will provide some guidelines for data collection and results analysis.

5.1 Results Pursued

As we have already indicated, the proposed format for the final tables is preliminary. It will improve as it is compared against reality once the specific

Table 8 Example of entities that participate in the exercise of EPHF 2 in the Dominican Republic

Entities	Type of entity	Activities related to EPHF 2
General Bureau of Epidemiology (SESPAS)	General bureau of the central government, within the framework of SESPAS	• Investigation of outbreaks (patients with fever, vaccine-preventable diseases, meningococcemia, vital statistics, maternal and child mortality, etc.) • Investigation of isolated cases and patterns of outbreaks • Workshops and training • Participation in congresses and international meetings • Participation in national and international courses • Support for epidemiological surveillance at the international level • Support for vaccination campaigns • Evaluation of the epidemiological surveillance systems • Regulations
National Center for Control of Tropical Diseases (CENCET)	Decentralized agency of SESPAS	• Entomological surveillance and control of bilharziasis, malaria, dengue, and filariasis, and diagnosis of parasites.
Dr. Defilló National Laboratory	Decentralized agency of SESPAS	• Epidemiological surveillance: • Microbiology (bacilloscopy and parasitology) • Virology • National reference laboratory
General Bureau of the Environment (SESPAS)	General bureau of the central government, within the framework of SESPAS	• Environmental surveillance
Expanded Program on Immunization (SESPAS)		• Surveillance of eruptive febrile outbreaks and flaccid paralysis
Tuberculosis Program (SESPAS)		• Tuberculosis surveillance
Nutrition Program (SESPAS)		• Nutrition monitoring
Rabies Control Center (SESPAS)		• Rabies surveillance
Maternal and Child Bureau (SESPAS)		• Vital statistics
Provincial Health Bureaus (SESPAS)	Provincial Bureaus	• There are eight public health regions and 29 provinces, each with its own area of epidemiology. The provincial health bureaus play a key role in the detection, alert, and control of diseases. The type of surveillance performed in the country is basically of infectious diseases and syndromes.
Laboratory department of SESPAS	Department of SESPAS	• Coordinates the regional public health laboratory network
General Bureau for Control of AIDS and STI (DIGECIT)	General bureau of the central government, within the framework of SESPAS	• Surveillance of sexually transmitted diseases

Table 8 *(continued)*

Entities	Type of entity	Activities related to EPHF 2
Department of Infectious Diseases of the Robert Reid Cabral Hospital	Department in a hospital	• Surveillance of infectious diseases
Dermatological Institute	NGO with public funding in conjunction with CENCET	• Leprosy surveillance and control
National Institute of Drinking Water (INAPA)	Autonomous State Entity	• Monitoring of water quality

Source: SESPAS, Annual Report 2000.

data for the different countries is compiled. In addition, the table formats will be improved by incorporating expert opinion on both public health and on national health accounts. We refer to these tables (5 and 6).

In certain countries, it is customary to finance some public health activities with taxes or special contributions. It would be of interest to know this information in detail. In these cases, an auxiliary table, such as 5 and 6, could break down the origin of the public funds.

5.2 Design of Instruments

With the purpose of obtaining budgetary information related to EPHF, we have designed a set of instruments using the basic data described below.

Tool 1: General Information on EPHF

The purpose of this tool is to define each EPHF, the performance evaluation indicators, and the standards for each. Many of the technicians who will be involved in the work of financial data collection in the entities of the ministry of health have not been involved with the process of performance measurement and are therefore unfamiliar with it.

Tool 2 : Questionnaire to Estimate the Expenditure and Financing of the EPHF

The purpose of this tool is to identify the tasks carried out by the institution—whether related or unrelated to EPHF—in order to separate those that are not. At the same time, we intend to define as best as possible the programmatic activities that the entity considers part of the EPHF in question, in order to link them to performance indicators.

Tool 3: Estimate of the Required Labor Allocation

With this tool, we intend to estimate the time devoted by the entity's personnel to each of the EPHF. We begin with the list of personnel, annual wages, and the estimated time devoted to each EPHF, administrative tasks, and other tasks outside EPHF.

Tool 4: Budget Executed for Each Program by Financing Source

This spreadsheet will detail the programs and activities classified by financ-

ing source, as they are normally designated in the preparation of institutional budgets. We hope to obtain this information directly from the various departmental budgets. We will incorporate the information obtained relating to EPHF within the programs, based on the use of the tools mentioned above.

Tool 5: Budget Prepared according to Expenditure Allocation

Here we will indicate the expenditure made as it is normally calculated in preparing the budget, but without distinguishing the EPHF to which it corresponds.

All these instruments will be field-tested. In the implementation phase of the pilot plan for the Dominican Republic, it will be necessary to speak with the technicians who participate in the execution of EPHF 2 and 9. The strong and weak points of the plan will be detected as well as its usefulness and ability to adapt to real needs arising during the process. The information obtained for each institution or department should then be added to the function requirements to allow structuring of the final tables.

5.3 Data Collection

Since EPHF are carried out by various institutions, and since their content is still not very clear with regard to programmatic activities, the research requires the participation of the technicians involved in them.

The first task therefore is to determine the institutional agency involved in accomplishing each of the EPHF, in order to later organize a workshop in which the basic activities that define each EPHF are decided by consensus. The task could be completed in a single day with working groups on EPHF or in several separate workshops, one for each of the EPHF. This first workshop is also intended to describe the research, the importance of the results, and the most advisable instruments for data collection.

A simultaneous review of the public budgets should be performed, preferably using the budget preparation report for the most recent year. In general or at least, in the Dominican Republic, the published report does not clearly separate programs and activities, nor does it offer information on certain departments individually. Consequently, it will be necessary to obtain the tables detailing allocations or request a special printout from the budget department of the Ministry of Health.

These data will make it possible to meet the preliminary requirements of instruments 2 and 3. We will thus know what the activities and programs are as they are currently described by the Ministry, the corresponding sources of financing and the classification for each expenditure allocation. The next step will be to identify EPHF within the classification of programs and activities. During that phase, the attention of the researchers

should be focused on obtaining the cooperation of each entity's technicians and an estimate of the effort required. This means ascertaining how many people work in the corresponding function, the type of personnel involved, their wages, and the amount of time they devote to it. It also means determining whether the collaboration of each institution, technical assistance visits, and the organization of discussion workshops (general or for each EPHF) will be necessary.

The next task, which is the responsibility of the researchers, is to break down the activities of the EPHF and other functions and then attribute the administrative expenditures, gather figures, code by health account classification, and present the results.

5.4 Addition of Data

In order to be able to complete the final tables that will represent the findings, it will be necessary to create a group of tables devoted to each of the EPHF indicating the institutional agency that deals with them. The information reflected in those tables will be provided by the data collection instruments.

As such, each institution or department should prepare a table similar to the final tables. Subsequently, all the data will be aggregated to provide the information corresponding to each of the EPHF.

5.5 Presentation of Results

The explanation in the previous paragraph indicates that this research requires intensive fieldwork and should be performed in close collaboration with the agencies responsible for carrying out the EPHF.

Once all the information is gathered, it should be processed to generate the final tables. The next stage is the analysis of the figures and presentation of results.

We suggest that the final study report be structured according to the following chapters and sections: I. Status of public health in the country; II. General institutional organization and organization of each of the particular EPHF; III. Expenditure and financing of the EPHF: 1. Difference between expenditure on EPHF and expenditure on public health programs; 2. Quantity of resources mobilized; 3. Proportion relative to the total public health expenditure; 4. Proportion relative to public expenditure in health; 5. Other indicators of interest (proportion relative to the total expenditure, GDP, expenditure per capita, etc.); 6. Analysis of financing sources; IV. Analysis of expenditure and financing for each function: EPHF 1 to 11; and V. Conclusions and recommendations.

6. Essential public health functions: costs and budget

6.1 Objective and Basis for the Proposed Approach

The objective of this section is to attempt to contribute to the current methodology for costing and budgeting of EPHF and the measurement processes carried out in more than 41 countries of the Region of the Americas with the aim of identifying their outcomes and providing the conceptual tools for determining their cost.[3]

---

[3] PAHO/WHO, CDC, CLAISS. (2001). Instrument for Performance Measurement of Essential Public Health Functions. Public Health in the Americas Initiative.

To this end, an Input-Output approach was adopted, with a view to developing the analysis and definition of products, as well as their disaggregation into sub-products, activities, sub-activities, and inputs.

Unlike the contents related to the Expenditure and Financing of EPHF[4] that quantify current expenditure, this section on Costs and Budget seeks to determine the cost of the products required to achieve the optimal performance of each of the functions so that they can subsequently be integrated into a Budget Process.

It is important to note that we will concentrate on the concept of operating expenditures of the EPHF and the process of determining the cost of the activities financed by the operating budget, while, broadly speaking, the infrastructure required (capacity building) relates to the Investment budget, which will be discussed in the corresponding chapter of Institutional Strengthening of the EPHF.[5]

Finally, it is appropriate to clarify that the costs of EPHF have not yet been determined. This is probably due to the lack of regional consensus on the basic activities that should be included in each function in order for the objectives of the function to be completely achieved.

This represents an important stumbling block but also an exciting challenge for

[4] Rathe, Magdalena. OPS. (2002) Estimación del gasto y financiamiento de las Funciones Esenciales de Salud Publica (FESP): Un marco de referencia.
[5] Alvarado, Félix, OPS/OMS (2002). Fortalecimiento Institucional para el Desempeño de las Funciones Esenciales de Salud Pública. Lineamientos para Planes Nacionales de Acción.

those who recognize the strategic value of the knowledge of costs and budget preparation as management tools. Progress in this regard is of the utmost value to our countries, even more when considering that many discussions inexorably refer to the efficient allocation of the limited economic resources available.

6.2 Definition of Products, Subproducts, and Activities. Methodological Framework

In order to begin looking at measuring the costs of carrying out EPHF, they should be analyzed in detail to determine their outcomes as measurable consequences that make possible the recognition of their effectiveness and performance. Based on the analysis conducted and as previously indicated, the need to identify the products, subproducts, activities, and inputs that enable the performance of each of the EPHF should be determined.

In this regard, we will define *subproducts* as those goods or services required for the performance of EPHF. These are partial or detailed in nature and differ in their limited scope or in their specificity. *Products,* on the other hand, are those goods or services that in many cases are comprised of a set of subproducts.

Activities are those occurrences necessary for the effective performance of the EPHF, that result in the specific and general effects characteristic of each of them. Finally, the resources applied in exercising EPHF are called *inputs.*

It is important to note that these resources can be grouped or defined in various ways, depending on the executing organization or the characteristics of the input-output ratio utilized in each case.

The definition of products, subproducts, and activities elaborated below makes it possible to perform quantifications and physical measurements that provide the basis of information necessary for determining the cost of performing EPHF. In addition to differentiating products and subproducts, it has been deemed necessary to extend the breakdown in order to determine the operational elements involved in the exercise of EPHF.

It is worth noting that the activities described for each of the EPHF are in some cases specific for achieving the product desired for a particular function, and in other instances are common to more than one or all of the functions.

The following is an example of the differentiation between different types of activity:

- The activity entitled "establishing and coordinating a laboratory network" is specific to achieving subproduct 1 of Product 2 of EPHF 2.

- The activity entitled "advising and giving technical support at the subnational levels" is common to all of the EPHF.

This differentiation between common and specific activities will permit a more accurate estimation of costs.

The following are some examples of the separation of functions into products, subproducts, and activities:

Example 1

EPHF 2: Public health surveillance, research, and control of risks and threats to public health.

With regard to the purpose of this function, that is, the continuous monitoring of health to ensure that if events should occur (epidemics, outbreaks of disease), the adequate information is available immediately to facilitate the process of decision-making, the predominant *product* should be the formation and development of an Active System for Epidemiological Surveillance and Control of Communicable and Noncommunicable Diseases.

The *subproducts* necessary to achieve this product could be defined as follows:

- The existence of surveillance systems at the subnational levels that are active and coordinated with the national level.

- Creation of a warning system to monitor the communicable diseases prevalent in the country.

- The same monitoring system for non-communicable diseases.

- Structures and processes that detect and monitor the environmental factors that affect communicable and noncommunicable pathologies.

Among other *activities* that should be carried out in order to arrive at the product through the various subproducts could be:

- Prepare instruments (standardized guidelines) to permit the gathering of information for epidemiological surveillance.

- Develop a training process for all personnel involved in the collection and analysis of information.

- Implement an adequate epidemiological surveillance network.

- Systematize and standardize the process of decision-making.

- Evaluate and monitor the quality of the system for its improvement and adaptation.

Example 2

EPHF 5: Development of policies and institutional capacity for planning and management in public health.

The major *product* of this function is the establishment of a health policy. For its creation, we would first need essentially *two subproducts*:

The first would be the definition of the sanitary objectives pursued and the other, the monitoring and evaluation of the degree of achievement of these objectives.

To this end, we should define the following activities, among others:

- Update the legal instruments that facilitate the development of policies.

- Establish participatory forums that make it possible to achieve consensus on the policies.

- Establish indicators and utilize them in evaluating and implementing the policies.

Example 3

EPHF 9: Quality assurance and improvement in personal and population-based health services.

The purpose in this case is to improve the quality of Health Services and to be able to guarantee this quality improvement to the population. A *product* linked to this function could be the development of a program for evaluating and improving the quality of Health Services. One of the *subproducts* that contributes to the achievement of this product could be the production of regulations on the structure and processes of the Health Services. Another could be the preparation and use of indicators to evaluate the quality of services.

The following are among the *activities* that could be carried out:

- Implement the production of regulations on the structure and processes of the Health Services.

- Promote the development of quality in the Health Services.

- Monitor and evaluate quality through the use of indicators.

- Continuously train personnel.

7. Analysis of the Input-Output Ratio for EPHF with regard to the Optimal Regional Standard

In previous works associated with the definition and improvement of the EPHF in the Americas, the level or standard of optimal performance has been defined as that which can be achieved under the most favorable conditions and in a reasonable amount of time by all countries of the region.

This definition and its utilization to measure the levels of performance in each country require a complete knowledge of the resources and institutional processes of the countries involved. Furthermore, the exact definition of "most favorable conditions" and "reasonable time frames" cannot be formulated with absolute objectivity in view of the fact that the elements for consideration include subjective or debatable aspects.

Based on the above, the optimal level of performance is an amount that, while it should be adapted to the current and potential status of the countries of the region, should be conceived as a fair incentive for continuous improvement. If the level defined as optimal were very easy to attain, it would be ineffective as an incentive, but if it were excessively demanding, it would discourage efforts at improvement.

7.1 Bases

As mentioned earlier, in order to move ahead with the projects of health sector reform in which most countries of the region are involved, PAHO has implemented the "Public Health in the Americas" initiative. Within this framework, PAHO has defined EPHF through a participatory process at the continental level. At a later stage and based on the development of an appropriate instrument, the performance of countries in the achievement of EPHF was measured.

It is now necessary to move ahead in determining three fundamental aspects:

1. Financing currently allocated to the execution of EPHF by countries.

2. Financing necessary for developing EPHF that are operating deficiently or are nonexistent (an investment necessary for the development of institutional capacity and infrastruc-

ture to enable the performance of EPHF).

3. Financing necessary for the functioning and operation of EPHF.

We will focus on the analysis of the last of the aspects cited. In this regard, it is important to distinguish between:

- the expenditures aimed at developing and/or strengthening the capacity for performance of a given EPHF, that is, the investment budget necessary for the design, installation, and testing of new competencies within the sector, and

- the expenditures associated with those actions that should be carried out on an ongoing basis if the sustainability of the capacity to perform EPHF is to be ensured.

Thus, the first set of expenditures corresponds to actions that are carried out once and the second refers to activities that are performed repeatedly over time.

This distinction should also be recognized in the financing modality included in the budget for the execution of these activities; in the first case, the investment budget can come from an external source. On the other hand, in the second case, financing from an internal source should be ensured so as to guarantee recurrent expenditure and sustainability. The national interest in achieving optimal performance of EPHF should result in the support for the recurrent expenditure required.

In sum, this section will concentrate on the analysis of operational costs related to the products and activities defined for each EPHF.

This study has dealt only with determining the cost of recurrent activities with the aim of constructing the operational costs of EPHF. On the other hand, the determination of investment costs related to institutional capacity (Infrastructure, Resource Supply, etc.) is included in the development plans of the project "Institutional Strengthening for Performance of EPHF." In the first case, the costs would be assimilated into Short-Term Costs, while the second would introduce elements of Long-Term Costs.

7.2 Analysis of the EPHF, their Products and Costs

To identify the recurrent expenditures associated with the performance of EPHF, that is, the primary responsibility to which the institutions involved in their performance should dedicate themselves, they should be analyzed as participants in an input-output ratio. Table 9[6] presents a schematic representation of the problem areas associated with determining the cost of EPHF. In it, the national level has been differentiated from the subnational level, although their participation is similar with regard to the input-output ratios characteristic of each EPHF, and therefore, we will concern ourselves mainly with the analysis of the national level in this study.

The table describes the relationships and actions that must first be dealt with when determining the expenditures associated with the performance of EPHF, and second, it describes expenditures needed for their sustainability. Therefore, the time

[6] Prepared based on the work: Ginestar, Angel y colaboradores. (1990). Costos Educacionales para la gerencia universitaria. INAP – UN de Cuyo – CICAP – OEA. EDIUNC. Mendoza, Argentina.

period for which the analysis will be conducted must be specified.

As previously noted, at this stage of the analysis we will concern ourselves only with developing a methodology aimed at determining the production function and its associated costs at the national level, leaving the subnational level aside for the moment.

By disaggregating each of the EPHF into products, subproducts, activities, and sub-activities, it will be possible to identify the inputs necessary for the performance of each activity, to allocate costs, and to qualify them as fixed and variable, direct and indirect, as pertains to the analysis. Table 10, presented below, reports the sequence described thus far.[7]

7.3 Identification of the Principal Cost Categories of EPHF

In order to determine both the categories of costs that make up the different input-output ratios characteristic of each EPHF, and the proportion of their participation in it, an institutional analysis of the performance and expenditures associated with them must be carried out. This analysis will enable us to know:

- the institutional organization linked to the products that comprise each of the EPHF at the relevant level

- the activities and sub-activities carried out by each area within the framework of the particular input-output ratio of a given subproduct

[7] Prepared based on the work: Ginestar, Angel y colaboradores. (1990). Costos Educacionales para la gerencia universitaria. INAP – UN de Cuyo – CICAP – OEA. EDIUNC. Mendoza, Argentina.

Table 9 Problem areas associated with determining the cost of the EPHF

Performance of the EPHF at the national level

The objective of the NHA is to improve public health practice at the national and subnational levels

Performance of the EPHF at the subnational level

The agencies responsible for the benefits or actions involved in each function and the needs or demands that must be met should be identified, along with quantifiable indicators of the actions specified

Identification of the products and subproducts necessary to satisfy needs in a given period

Identify for whom and why each function will be performed in a given time

At the different levels and identifying responsibilities, propose what human and material resources will be used to perform the function in a given time

Identify and characterize the beneficiaries of the products and subproducts that comprise the EPHF

Identify the production functions associated with the products and subproducts that comprise the EPHF (expenditures, costs, supply relationships)

Agree on criteria among the different levels to compare objectives with requirements and decide what and how much to do, based on the availability of resources

Determine the product and subproduct amounts for each EPHF and the resources required to define goals for a certain period (utilizing agreed-upon quantifiable indicators–optimization)

Each responsible entity executes the specified actions as planned (projected and budgeted)

Compare objectives and goals with the results obtained to determine the degree of fulfillment

- the specific allocation of resources (human and material) in each area within the framework of the input-output ratio of a given subproduct

Given the work-intensive nature of most of the EPHF, a central aspect of this determination will be to establish the allocation of human resources necessary for their adequate performance.

Nevertheless, there are functions that can require a wide variety of inputs, and this study therefore adopts a broad clas-

Table 10 Determination of function cost

The total expenditure on the activity is determined by its duration and frequency and the levels at which it will be carried out.

The total expenditure on a subproduct is determined by the expenditure on the activities. It is made up of

The total expenditure on a product is determined by the expenditure on the subproduct. It is made up of

The total expenditure of a function is based on the expenditures for the subproducts and products that comprise it.

Direct expenditures	
National level	Subnational level
Year J	

↓

Activity

↓

Subproduct

↓

Product

↓

Function

appropriate for further study in the next stages of development of the methodology. The first are capital expenditures, considered primarily "one-time expenditures" that can be carried out within the framework of the project "Institutional Strengthening for Performance of the EPHF."

Secondly, we have also not included the expenditures corresponding to the "Charge for depreciation of the productive capacity assignable to the activity", since the current development of budgetary accounts generally hinders their determination (the countries of the region in which progress has been made in this area are limited).

8. Cost Analysis for EPHF in order to achieve Optimal Regional Performance Level

The different input-output ratios characteristic of each of the EPHF are affected by a set of factors, among which are the characteristics of political organization at the national level (unitary or federal), the different levels of decentralization with regard to the NHA, the assignment of the EPHF to the various agencies (ministries, decentralized bodies, etc.), and the modalities of production adopted by each of them for the performance of EPHF (labor-intensive or capital-intensive technologies).

The inputs that make up each of these input-output ratios have been previously characterized and can be summarized as Human Resources, Goods, and Services. Computer equipment (hardware) and applications (software) will play a prominent role as part of the technology associated with the performance of each EPHF. On this basis, the

sification of the possible inputs that would comprise the various input-output ratios and the budgetary imputation of the expenditures associated with them. Table 11 presents the categorization adopted for the expenditures.

7.4 Cost analysis

In accordance with the above, this proposal for determining the cost of EPHF is based on the attempt to specify the different input-output ratios characteristic of each EPHF in terms of their products, subproducts, and activities.

Table 12 presented below shows the expected sequence for determining the cost of EPHF and explains the development of the methodology used thus far.[8]

There are two types of expenditures that are key to the determination of costs but have not been included in the table and whose treatment is considered

---

[8] Prepared based on the work: Ginestar, Angel y colaboradores. (1990). Costos Educacionales para la gerencia universitaria. INAP – UN de Cuyo – CICAP – OEA. EDIUNC. Mendoza, Argentina.

Table 11 Budgetary categorization of expenditures

EXPENDITURES	ITEMS	CATEGORIES	SUBCATEGORIES	
CURRENT EXPENDITURE	Personnel	Permanent	Top-level	
			High-level	
			Administrative	
			Professional	
			Teaching	
			Technical	
			Worker	
		Temporary	Contracted	
			Monthly	
			Daily	
	Non-personnel goods and services	Goods	Medical and pharmaceutical products	
			Materials and supplies	
			Medical and sanitary equipment	
		Services	Publicity and advertising	
			Communications	
			Other	
CAPITAL EXPENDITURE	Capital goods	Hospital equipment		
		Technical and scientific instruments		
		Computer equipment		
		Vehicles and vessels		
		Real property		
		Other acquisitions		
	Construction	Construction public buildings		
		Infrastructure works		
		Other works		
	Maintenance of preexisting goods	Rehabilitation and repair of public buildings		

different input-output ratios characteristic of each EPHF will present different alternative combinations of these inputs to produce the activities, subproducts, and products, according to the technology adopted in each country.

On the other hand, it should be considered when carrying out the work that the composition of the activities, subproducts and products that comprise each EPHF can vary among countries, depending on their degree of institutional development and the availability of resources. Thus, the application of the cost methodology of the EPHF will

require adjustments for the characteristics of each country in terms of the aforementioned considerations.

With regard to the performance indicators as described in the Guide, it should be noted that some of these *indicators* are for *results,* others for *processes,* and still others for *institutional capacity.* The determination of the cost of EPHF and of these indicators as a part of them is based on associating the indicators with products and activities. To the extent that these indicators affect more than one product of the EPHF, the activities go from being specific to being com-

mon activities, distributed among the products they affect. The determination of the cost of the different input-output ratios is made possible as a result of the relationship between products/subproducts and the indicator/standard for the optimal regional achievement of the performance measurement instrument.

9. Conclusions and Recommendations

The methodological framework for estimating the expenditure and financing of EPHF presented in this chapter is a first broaching of the subject. It is based on the literature related to EPHF, the national health accounts methodology, and the experience of the United States in its attempt at this type of exercise. In the design of the methodology, the principal reference points are taken from the Dominican Republic, where a preliminary collection of data was carried out. It is highly probable that there are fundamental differences in both the scope and methods of estimation in other countries, particularly larger countries that are organized according to a federal model.

It should be noted that consensus has never been reached among the countries to determine the cost of and break down of the basic activities that each of the EPHF should perform for the complete achievement of all its components. The instrument currently utilized to measure the performance of EPHF focuses only on results and assumes a given institutional organization and some given methods of performing EPHF that, until now, have not been specified.

Accordingly, the work to estimate the expenditure for EPHF and their sources of financing requires the reconstructing of the way in which each of them is

Table 12   Sequence to be followed to finance the EPHF's

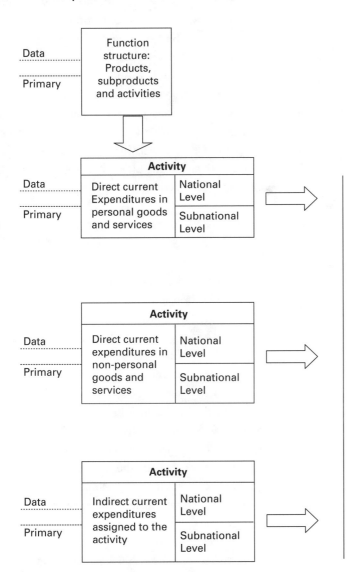
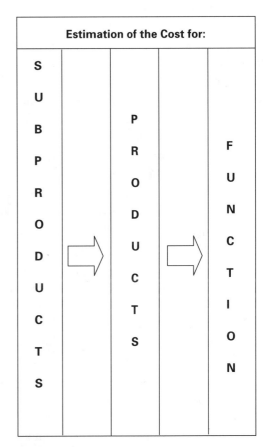

achieved, in those countries which apply the methodology. The lessons learned from their practical application will lead to the necessary changes, both in scope and in the procedure as well as in the presentation of results. For that reason, this methodological framework will not be completed until it has been applied in several countries. It will be verified by way of a pilot plan so that the practical viability of the methodological proposals and the differences with regard to the internal organization of each country, as well as the budgetary and statistical systems are considered. This way, the instrument will be transformed as it progresses through a process of successive applications.

In almost all countries, the health authorities are responsible for implementing most of the activities included within the EPHF. Nevertheless, there exists a growing sector of nonprofit institutions dealing particularly with the improvement of health, research, human resources education, and the tasks related to emergencies and disasters. Some of these functions could also be executed by the for-profit private sector, as in the case of private universities or the pharmaceutical industry. In this case, it would be of interest to determine which of these tasks corresponding to the steering role function of the health authorities are nevertheless delegated to private institutions.

In carrying out the work, it is important to consider that the content of the competencies included in each of the EPHF can vary a great deal from one country to another given the different levels of development and characteristics specific to each. There can be a significant factor of subjectivity that hinders the adoption of a uniform methodology involving the calculation of expenditures whether they are realistic or ideal.

The subject addressed in this chapter is completely new. For the first time, an attempt is being made to adapt the national health accounts to EPHF. The analysis performed shows that the functional classification of the national health accounts does not take into account public health functions, although it may be very exhaustive with respect to the care of disease. If we want health systems to be oriented further toward the promotion of health and the prevention of disease, it is indispensable that we be able to monitor changes in the allocation of resources to the tasks of public health, with respect to programs, essential functions, and services. It is necessary to be able to determine the lines of action; first, with regard to the budget, and second, with respect to the national health accounts.

The task implies reviewing the definition of health in the national accounts and, accordingly, the classification of functions. In order to do so, it is necessary to perform an in-depth and broad analysis of the function of public health and its importance in achieving the ultimate objective of every health system: to improve the health of the population. One of the principal advantages of the system of health accounts is the possibility of setting priorities in the allocation of resources devoted to those tasks and their monitoring over time.

Achieving that possibility is fundamental to the development of the health system. The current trend in reform proposals is to separate the functions of the steering role, financing, and services delivery. The lack of foresight in defining the sources of funds that make the steering role of the health system, within which the public health activities and functions are framed, operate, can lead the countries to a crisis in this area with consequent danger to the population.

Furthermore, it is well known that the market does not allocate health sector resources as it should, and that State intervention is necessary to correct market failures. Hence, the function of the State is described as the production of public goods and goods of social interest, that are part of the public health function. These include the capacity needed for the regulation of the entire health system—including the essential functions—and the decisive capacity for the performance of the steering role function. The health systems require that these activities be reflected in the public accounts and that it be possible to identify them clearly in the budgets to subsequently transfer them to the health accounts.

This issue leads us to the need for addressing an additional problem: the separation between the planning and preparation of budgets, on the one hand, and their subsequent application, on the other. It is a generalized problem in the financial administration of the State, but it is important that it be pointed out here.

This chapter also presented the elements of the Methodological Framework for determining the Cost and Budget of EPHF based on their optimal performance levels. This framework was addressed from an Input-Output approach in order to subsequently develop a budgeting and management-by-results process. The purpose of this methodology is to move toward the determination of the cost of EPHF and integrate management-by-results into the budget processes through identification of the products in their current state and the setting of goals to achieve their optimal performance (analysis of gaps).

To this end, it is suggested that each country implement the Methodological Framework for determining the Cost and Budget, adapting it to the national reality and to the health sector. The application of this Framework in each country should consider the general political characteristics (unitary or federal countries), the conditions of Health System organization (different degrees of decentralization), the staffing of public agency personnel and others (labor-intensive production relationship), with regard to the man-hours required for the products of each of the EPHF. On the other hand, the price vectors to establish the cost of inputs and products will be readjusted on the basis of the conditions and variability for each country.

It should be noted that the Methodological Framework for determining the Cost and Budget offers the possibility of its joint application with the respective frameworks for Expenditure and Financing and Institutional Strengthening of EPHF, which will make it possible to connect aspects of the operating budget with those of the budgets for Investments and National Accounts, contributing to an integral implementation of EPHF and completing the progress in measurement and characterization achieved thus far.

Finally, the development of the Methodological Framework for determining the Cost and Budget by country will facilitate an application of tools for management-by-results that are more advanced than in the case of the Analyses of Cost Effectiveness (for example: study of the cost effectiveness of Epidemiological Surveillance per population covered) or the introduction of systems of awards and penalties in the budget of EPHF (for example: Management Agreements based on goals for gaps in the performance of EPHF by the subnational levels).

Bibliography

Aiston E, Dickson K and Previsich N. Essential Functions in Canada's Public Health Care System, Decentralization, and Tools for Quality Assurance: Consistency through Change in the Canadian Health System. Washington, DC: Pan American Health Organization, Pan American Journal of Public Health, Vol.8, Nos. 1/2, July–August 2000.

Atchison, Barry, Kanarek and Gebbie, K. The Quest for an Accurate Accounting of Public Health Expenditures. Journal of Public Health Management and Practice; September 2000.

Barry, Centra, Pratt, Brown and Giordano, L. Where Do the Dollars Go? Measuring Local Public Health Expenditures. March 1998.

Claeson, Edward, Miller and Musgrove. Public Health and World Bank Operations, 1999–2001.

Eilbert K, et al. Measuring Expenditures for Essential Public Health Services. Washington, DC: Public Health Foundation; 1996.

Fondo Monetario Internacional. Manual de Estadísticas de las Finanzas Públicas. Washington, DC: FMI; 2001.

Ministerio de Salud (MINSA) de Nicaragua. Cuentas Nacionales de Salud. Informe 1997–1999. Managua; December 2001.

Molina R, Pinto M, et al. Gasto y financiamiento de salud: situación y tendencias. Organización Panamericana de la Salud. Revista Panamericana de Salud Pública, Vol.8, Nos. 1/2, July–August 2000.

Muñoz F, López Acuña D, et al. Las funciones esenciales de la salud pública: un tema emergente en las reformas del sector de la salud. Organización Panamericana de la Salud. Revista Panamericana de Salud Pública, Vol. 8, Nos. 1/2, July–August 2000.

Musgrove, P. Protecting Health in Latin America: What Should the State Do? (revised version, 19 October 2001—document prepared for CIPPEC).

Musgrove P. What is the Minimum a Doctor Should Know about Health Economics? Brazilian Journal of a Mother and Child Health; May-August 2001.

Oficina Nacional de Presupuesto. Informe de Ejecución Presupuestaria, año 200. Santo Domingo, República Dominicana; 2001.

Oficina Nacional de Presupuesto. Manual de Clasificaciones Presupuestarias. Santo Domingo, República Dominicana; 1990.

Organización de Cooperación y Desarrollo—Banco Interamericano de Desarrollo. Sistema de Cuentas de Salud. Washington, DC; 2002.

Organización Panamericana de la Salud—Organización Mundial de la Salud. La rectoría de los ministerios de salud en los procesos de reforma sectorial. Washington, DC; September 1997.

Pan-American Health Organization. Pan American Journal of Public Health. Washington, DC; July–August 2000.

Pan-American Health Organization and World Health Organization. Essential Public Health Functions. Washington, DC; September 2000.

Pan-American Health Organization, World Health Organization, Center for the Disease Control and Prevention, and Centro Latinoamericano de Investigación en Sistemas de Salud. Public Health in the Americas: Instrument for Performance Measurement of Essential Public Functions. Washington, DC; November 2001.

Rathe M. La reforma de salud y la seguridad social. Santo Domingo, RD: Pontificia Universidad Católica Madre y Maestra; 2002.

Rathe M. Salud y equidad: una mirada al financiamiento a la salud en la República Dominicana. Santo Domingo, RD: Macro Internacional; 2000.

United Nations, Comission of the European Communities, International Monetary Fund, Organisation for Economic Cooperation and Development and World Bank. System of National Accounts. Bruselas, New York, Paris, Washington, DC; 1993.

World Health Organization. The World Health Report 2000. Health Systems: Improving Performance.Geneva, Switzerland; 2000.

Barry, Mike; Bialek, Ron, MPP; Eilbert Kay W., MPH, MIM; Garufi, Marc, MPP. Public Health Foundation. (1996). Measuring Expenditures for Essential Public Health Services. Washington, D.C.

Barry, Mike; Bialek, Ron; Eilbert Kay W.; Garufi, Marc; Gebbie, Kristine; Maiese, Debbie; and Fox, C. Earl. (1997). Public Health Expenditures: developing Estimates for Improved Policy Making. Journal of Public Health Management and Practice.

Hewitt, Daniel y Van Rijckeghem, Caroline. (1996). Gastos salariales en los gobiernos centrales. Revista Internacional de Presupuesto Publico N° 32. ASIP.

HHS. Healthy People 2010. 2nd ed. With Understanding and Improving Health and Objectives for Improving Health. 2 vols. Washington, DC: U.S. Government Printing Office, November 2000.

Bobadilla, J.L.; Cowley P., Musgrove, P. & Saxenian, H. (1994). Design, content and financing of an essential national package of health services. WHS. Bulletin of the World Health Organization.

Sorensen, James E. y Grove, Hugh D. (1988). Uso de los análisis de costo-resultado y costo-efectividad para el mejoramiento de la administración y la contabilidad del programa. "Administración de Hospitales. Fundamentos y

Evaluación del servicio hospitalario". Capítulo 13. Ed. Trillas.

Lic. Salvo Horveilleur, Lucía. Republica Dominicana. (2002) Reunión Subregional de Seguimiento a las Funciones Esenciales de Salud Publica.

OPS/HSD, CDC, CLAISS. (2001). La Practica de la Salud Publica en Centroamérica y Republica Dominicana. Medición del desempeño de las Funciones Esenciales de Salud Publica. Informe a la XVII Reunión del Sector Salud de Centroamérica y la republica Dominicana.

OPS/OMS (Organización Panamericana de la Salud / Organización Mundial de la Salud), CDC (Centers for Disease Control), CLAISS (Centro Latinoamericano de Investigaciones en Sistemas de Salud). (2001). Guía para la Aplicación del Instrumento de Medición del Desempeño de las Funciones Esenciales de Salud Publica. Iniciativa "Salud Publica en las Américas", Medición del desempeño de las Funciones Esenciales de Salud Publica. Washington, D.C.

OPS/OMS, CDC, CLAISS. (2001). Informe Ejecutivo de la Medición de las Desempeño de las Funciones Esenciales de Salud Publica ejercidas por la Autoridad Sanitaria en los países de Centroamérica y Republica Dominicana. Iniciativa "La Salud Publica en las Américas". Nicaragua.

OPS/OMS, Ministerio de Salud de la Republica Argentina. (2001) Medición del Desempeño de las Funciones Esenciales de Salud Publica Ejercidas por la Autoridad Sanitaria en la Republica Argentina. Resultados del Taller de Aplicación del instrumento llevado a cabo en Buenos Aires, Argentina, November 2001.

OPS/OMS. (2002) Fortalecimiento Institucional para el Desempeño de las Funciones Esenciales de Salud Publica. Lineamientos para Planes Nacionales de Acción.

OPS/OMS. Dr. Pedro E. Brito. (2002). Lineamientos Metodológicos: Desarrollo de la Fuerza de Trabajo para el Desempeño de las Funciones esenciales de Salud Publica. Reunión Subregional sobre Funciones Esenciales de Salud Publica, Santo Domingo.

Berrueta Colombo, Oscar. (1995). La eficacia del proceso presupuestario. Revista ASIP N° 29.

García Balderrama, Teresa; Calzado Cejas, Yolanda. (1997). Metodología de evaluación de la eficiencia en las entidades publicas. Revista Internacional de Presupuesto Publico N° 35. ASIP.

U.S. Department of Health and Human Services (HHS). (1991). Healthy People 2000: National Health Promotion and Disease Prevention Objectives. Washington, DC: HHS, Public Health Service (PHS).

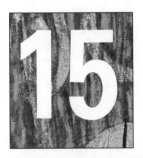

Development of the Public Health Workforce

1. Introduction

In addition to being a concerted action to renew the concept of public health (that will allow the adoption of new approaches, practices and training modalities) and an effort to empirically approach public health practice in Latin America—according to existing conditions—The "Public Health in the Americas" initiative is also an opportunity to redefine education in public health and in its practice contribute to the development of institutional capacity and workforce competence for those working in the field, who in Latin America are known as "sanitaristas".

Reorienting education in public health, using as a frame of reference the essential public health functions is a project that was begun in 1998 by the Human Resources Development Program in the Division of Health Systems and Services Development of the Pan American Health Organization, during the 2nd

Pan American Conference on Education in Public Health held in Mexico City, on "*Sector Reform and Essential Public Health Functions: challenges for human resources development*". This project is a joint effort with the Latin American and Caribbean Association for Public Health Education (ALAESP) as well as with other institutions in the Region. During this meeting, the academic institutions explicitly acknowledged their meager prominence in the processes of transformation of developing health systems in almost all of the countries in the Region. In addition, two significant gaps in the political agenda of health sector reforms were highlighted: the little attention given to the functions and participation of public health institutions during these processes (resulting in serious consequences for collective health) and the absence of topics related to human resources.

During the conference, aspects related to the demands of health sector reform

and essential public health functions were analyzed and debated with regard to education in public health; the influence of academic institutions in these reforms; the proposal of future strategies for the development of public health education. To overcome specific deficiencies in public health education, a proposal was made, within a programmatic framework, for academic institutions to develop five training areas that will contribute to the improvement and strengthening of the essential public health functions: political articulation; pedagogic and educational training; research and technology development; technical cooperation; and management capacity of academic institutions.

The "Public Health in the Americas" initiative, sponsored by the Pan-American Health Organization (PAHO)/World Health Organization (WHO), was an important step in keeping with the efforts begun in 1998 for changing education in public health. In the XIX

ALAESP Conference held in Cuba in July 2000, agreements were formalized and strategies and procedures were more precisely outlined. Schools committed more firmly to their essential functions as a principal political and programmatic reference in educational participation. From then on, various joint work plans have been carried out by PAHO and ALAESP. Today, ALAESP represents more than fifty teaching institutions dedicated primarily to graduate education in public health.

Nonetheless, there is still work to be done at the undergraduate level in terms of public health education in the health fields, as well as in continuing education of the public health workforce. In order to meet the professional development needs of public health staff in charge of everyday activities, programs and tasks, PAHO has formed a consortium with eleven academic and technical cooperation institutions in the Americas and Europe to develop the Virtual Campus in Public Health Initiative which was launched in July this year. This Initiative will be further addressed later in the chapter.

Progress in the development of a conceptual framework, evidence derived from the performance measurement of the essential functions in the countries of the Region, and results from a number of diagnostic studies on the state of graduate education in public health (done in Central and South America) show troublesome results urging us to double our efforts in taking concrete measures in the field of education in public health. As expected, the results of performance measurement of the essential public health functions—one of them being essential function 8—(Human Resource

Figura 1 Programatic proposal for the development of the public health workforce

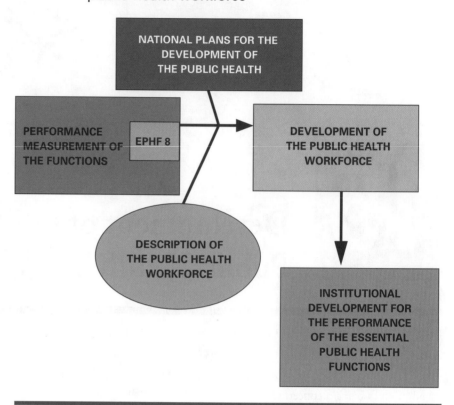

Development and Training in Public Health) irrefutably show a low level of performance, albeit with national and sub-regional differences. The formulation and implementation of plans to develop and boost public health practice in the member state countries requires an important pillar: education of the workforce which will allow the consolidation of the institutional capacity of the public health infrastructure.

The figure above shows the logic behind the programmatic proposal for the "Development of the Public health workforce". It is based on discussions and conclusions drawn from various national meetings and the sub-regional conference for Central America, Haiti, Cuba and Puerto Rico, held in April 2002.

This paper provides the conceptual, methodological and programmatic elements for preparing plans for the development of the public health workforce (highlighting PAHO/WHO's programmatic responsibility in educational and professional development), with the goal of contributing to the improvement of institutional capacity at the national level in the performance of the essential public health functions.

With this in mind, some general lines of action for the formulation of human resources development measures will be proposed (one of the key components of national and sub regional plans) and with time, design a feasible regional project that will allow for the development of public health based on the measurement of the essential public health functions.

2. Essential Function 8

As previously mentioned, EPHF 8 (Development of Human Resources and Training in Public Health) shows a low performance level with a mean of 0.40 for the Region. Despite the fact that all five indicators performed poorly, some point out deficiencies that deserve further comment given their importance for the development of plans that will improve the national capacity to offer public health services.

2.1 Description of the public health workforce profile

Although the countries report that the basic characteristics of the workforce are evaluated, only half define staff needs for performing public health activities that include an estimate of necessary personnel or the required profile. This situation makes it difficult for the health authorities to intervene in an effective manner should they decide to enhance the performance of the workforce or guide the development of personnel whether they be within or outside the health authorities' realm of action. The weakest areas are the lack of availability of information as well as lack of criteria to determine needs for future growth.

2.2 Improving the quality of the workforce

Most of the countries of the Region are weak in the area of workforce management in the field of public health. Despite the existence of criteria to evaluate staff credentials, these criteria are not met at the time of hiring. Neither re-cruitment strategies nor retention of these workers is evaluated. In general, there is a lack of an incentives system to promote professional development and the retention of the best performing employees. As is the case with the workforce, there are serious problems with the performance evaluation of staff and the availability of appropriate systems of remuneration and recognition.

In many countries that have implemented institutional development projects or investment projects in support of health sector reform, with external financing, it is necessary to highlight the anomaly in the structure of the executing or coordinating units. These units are usually created by outsourcing consultants hired for a limited time whose remuneration is significantly higher than that of the staff in the ministries of health. In many cases, the personnel of such units do not belong to the permanent units of the ministry, enter into collusion with the established programs, or duplicate efforts. This situation has generated much conflict and problems with regards to maximizing the performance of the hired consultants. In addition, this arrangement threatens the efforts of the national institutional capacity.

2.3 Continuing education and graduate training in public health

Most countries of the Region promote and create incentives for the participation of staff in continuing education (usually in accordance with the institutional needs of the moment) favoring formal agreements with academic institutions to facilitate training. This is done however, without adhering to the established policies and norms that en-sure continuing staff development, and without suitable systems for assessing the results or impact that these programs may have on the effect of educational plans. There are no criteria or norms for staff retention. It is evident the already mentioned lack of systems for assessing the performance of personnel and of incentives for public health workers.

These conditions have to do with the lack of coordination that has traditionally existed and continues to exist between academic institutions in the field of public health and the employing institutions of the public health workforce. This can be better exemplified by data in the U.S.A. where only 20% of the workforce has had the opportunity to receive some kind of formal education in public health. Although this case is not determinant, it draws attention to the limited communication between such institutions reflected—among other factors—in the almost non-existent offer of continuing education and public health programs by the schools, and their limited presence in most countries on debates held regarding the need for reforms.

2.4 Improving workforce to ensure culturally-appropriate delivery of services

Only a small proportion of the countries in the Region provide different communities with technical support and incentives to select and promote the incorporation of human resources according to their socio-cultural needs. And only half of these countries encourage the development of strategies to encourage the decentralized management of such human resources.

In this regard, it is essential to deal with and overcome these conditions in order to achieve efficiency in human resources development plans. From the previous considerations, it can be inferred that any measure to improve workforce performance should consider strategies for educational development and integrated management, generated and developed based on reliable information and the characteristics of the workforce.

As was mentioned in the meeting of Central America and the Caribbean region, there is a special condition of EPHF8 which must be taken into consideration: EPHF8 is not only one more function among the eleven defined functions, but rather, the one without which the other ten functions can be performed; that is, it is polyvalent with regard to the other ten essential functions. EPHF8 is strategic for the performance of the other essential functions which public health authorities must provide.

3. Public Health Workforce (PHWF)

In the initiative "Public Health in the Americas", public health workforce consists of all those health workers responsible for contributing—either directly or indirectly—to the performance of the essential public health functions, regardless of their profession and institution where they actually work. Given this wide definition, it is important, though challenging, to identify the various institutions which have responsibility in and contribute to the essential public health functions.

Recently, the condition of the public health workers has been emphasized as "**knowledgeable workers**". That is, they are workers who interpret and apply both knowledge and information to provide solutions with an added value regarding the problems of public health, and as part of their daily tasks, make recommendations in a continually changing environment. Thus, they require access to organizational conditions that will allow them to acquire theoretical and analytical concepts in addition to developing the practice of continuous education and to continue to be competent and productive throughout their lives. These conditions indicate a clear orientation of the educational proposals and management criteria that should be used for the public health workforce.

The definition of workforce that is used is similar to the one utilized in economics. In these cases, the definition of workforce in any economic activity is essentially based on socio-demographic and economic criteria. That is to say, it is about quantifying how many people are employed in a certain activity at a given moment, according to age, sex, educational level and established qualifications. This definition is thus limited, according to what they do rather than what they are or where they work.

As for public health which includes a wide field of practice and participation which goes beyond the limits of the health sector, the definition of the workforce cannot be limited to the people working in the public sector; it must also include all the State and civil organizations with responsibilities in public health. Therefore, the public health workforce is multi-professional, multi-sectoral, diverse and dispersed throughout a country. In the U.S., the PHWF is employed by a wide range of organizations with differing degrees of responsibility in public health practice: governmental public health organizations, other public sector organizations, health care organizations, volunteer organizations, community-based groups, academic institutions, etc.

Figure 2 attempts to show the various organizational groups where the PHWF is employed in the Region.

As can be noted in the performance measurement and according to the available reports, little is known in other countries about the public health workforce. This is a critical deficit since it determines an essential task yet to be done in planning workforce development. Nonetheless, it is important to mention that until recently even developed countries lacked such data.

For a number of years now, the United States has been conducting censuses of the public health workforce. These censuses have demonstrated, among other things, that public health nursing professionals are by far the largest group in this workforce (10.9%), estimated at 450,000 workers. Public health doctors represent a mere 1.3%. There is also a serious problem with supply and demand, and only a 20% of nurses have received formal education or training to perform their functions.

In most countries of the Region, the public health workforce had never been subject of analysis and least of all planning. It is necessary to acknowledge that there are serious problems with availability, quality and handling of information on human resources in health in the majority of the countries of the Region. However, these problems, little by little, are being overcome by the Human Resources Observatory initiative, already

Figure 2 Where does PHWF work?

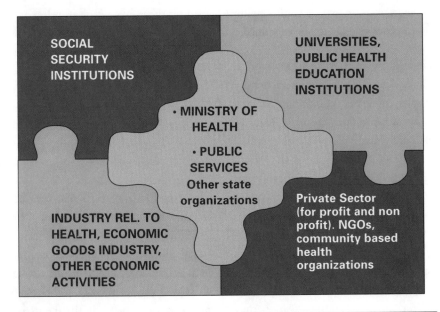

working in 16 countries in the Americas. The need to know the characteristics of the public health workforce within the initiative framework has to do with the objectives of human resources management, the improvement of distribution and accessibility, economic and gender equity, quality assurance, and the development of policies for the PHWF, among others. As previously mentioned, in order to quantitatively and qualitatively develop the public health workforce, it is necessary to fill the gaps in information and knowledge about that workforce.

There can never be too much emphasis placed on the diversity of the public health workforce. The essential functions are a responsibility of many occupational and professional categories throughout the structure of the health system: general and family doctors, public and primary health care nurses, nursing auxiliaries, sanitary engineers, health educators, promoters of sanitary measures, administrators, etc.

Within the public health workforce, there are those that are specifically public health workers but, there are also sanitary personnel that perform functions of health care and management in health services programs. Therefore, the description of the public health workforce should include this group of personnel that are not specifically identified as public health workers.

In order to define and set development strategies for the workforce, it is particularly important to take into account this situation, especially at the primary service level and basic levels of assistance, where the same individuals perform such public health services.

Possibly, due to a lack of an integral perspective, there is the mistaken idea that this workforce essentially consists of people who have attended school and who have completed graduate courses in public health or related disciplines. It would seem that no matter how important this negative factor is in qualitative

terms, it is not quantitatively nor functionally the main factor. It would also seem that, as is the case in the U.S., that most of the workforce has actually never taken a formal course in public health.

The PAHO-WHO Human Resources Observatory has developed a proposal to characterize the public health workforce. In this proposal, the Observatory regards the creation of a set of basic data to characterize the public health workforce as an essential element. To date this initiative has been working in 16 countries of the Region providing quality information to narrow the gap of existing information on human resources in most countries, as well as to provide information for decision making and to develop the bases for or to rebuild the deficient information systems.

The proposal of collecting basic data can be very useful for characterizing the public health workforce. Such data are collected by doing an exhaustive search of existing information not only regarding human resources in public health, but by also looking at other sources that generate or contain information such as various types of surveys. Whenever necessary, information from secondary sources can be complimented with ad hoc research of some of the variables that are not found in the primary sources.

Table 1 shows the proposal of basic data of the Observatory, adapted to meet the needs of the "Public Health in the Americas" Initiative, taken into consideration for the study of the main variables of the definition of the PHWF.

Further details about the selection of variables, indicators, availability and characteristics of sources can be found in the PAHO-WHO Human Resources Observatory website.

4. Development of the Public health workforce

4.1 A New Integrated Approach to Workforce Development

Unlike the usual approach which considers that the development of the workforce consists of only specific training activities, the approach used by the Pan-American Health Organization in its technical cooperation implies an integrated and complex approach (see figure 3) for workforce development in public health.

The concept of field is based on the idea that the workforce (in any area and also in public health) consists of people, agents who have developed a series of skills (based on knowledge, technologies, qualifications, values and specific attitudes of social service), which allows them to contribute to solving health problems (both collective and individual) of the population in a given institutional context. This contribution, specific to the development of health is an essential element that determines its social function. That is, it not a mere tech-

nical function but at the same time an important social function for the health of the population, which implies political decisions that should be examined.

The field in which these agents' work is mainly determined by the interactions of two key processes: education (acquired in social institutions created to educate such individuals) and work (or technical and social performance of the health agents) which takes place at the different levels of the health services systems. This complex interaction results in other important processes such as the functioning of the labor market, on the one hand, and professionalization processes on the other hand. In this latter process, the occupational groups—since they have and control certain knowledge—are structured as groups of autonomous power which, together with the society, are in conditions to impose regulations in the behavior of its members as well as to obtain special negotiation situations.

The proposed concept is that the development of the public health workforce implies political decisions and institutional interventions at various levels of the field. Table 2 matrix intends to provide a *modus operandi* of analysis to de-

termine the level of intervention and configure the bases of a development plan for the public health workforce. In the intersection of interventions and limits of the workforce, main areas and criteria are identified for the integral development of the public health workforce. These areas and criteria map out important topics which will differ in nature, magnitude and priority according to each country.

The main idea is that this matrix be applicable to any country, allowing the identification in the national institutional context, the main issues or problems to be faced, considering the characteristics of the health system, the results of the performance measurement, the priorities of the population, the institutional responsibilities and the availability of resources.

The main objective is to prepare and implement a **workforce development plan based on the competencies derived from the essential public health functions.** Such a plan must be supported by a clear resolve in development policies for the public health workforce and in guiding the improvement of public health practice, based on the following:

Figure 3 Development field of the public health workforce

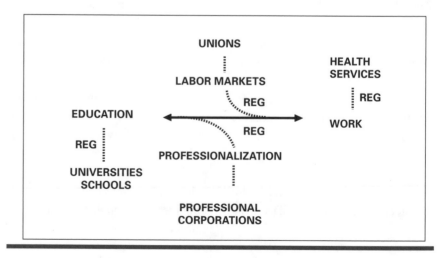

Table 2 Map of Issues for the Preparation of a Workforce Development Plan

Area Intervention	Education—Training of the PHWF	Work or performance of the PHWF	Labor market	Professionalization
Public health workforce development policy	It is a set of ideas and definitions that generate and shape efforts, considering the State and society, in order to create plans and institutional conditions to improve the contribution of the PHWF in the performance of essential public health functions (EPHF)			
Planning	Systematic prevision of the political conditions, institutional capacities and resources to meet the quantitative and qualitative needs of the workforce at a given time. Basically, it is the preparation of PHWF Development Plan. Efficiency in the placement of staff to improve its distribution			
Regulation	Accreditation of schools and programs. Quality strategies.	Regimens of work, modalities of hiring, labor protection	Regimens of remuneration and incentives Regulatory efficiency in the management and development of the workforce	Recertification? Organization and representation of the public health practitioners
Professional and technical education	Development of competency based in the EPHF in professional and technical careers	Orientation of training according to performance requirements	Structural and dynamic analysis of the labor markets for educational planning	Participation of professional agents in the definition of plans of curricula
Professional and technical Training and development	Participation of the public health academic institutions in the continuing education of the PHWF	Development of PHWF competencies based on EPHF Continuing education based on competencies.	Continuing education and development of employability	Participation of organizations of public health practitioners in continuing professional development
Management of the workforce	Use of continuing education as a strategy for the development of PHWF Access to continuing education as a condition of and definition of career development Non monetary incentives system	Management of individual and collective work relations Criteria and normative frameworks for selection, recruitment, induction, and assignment Management of the quality of productivity and performance	Design and implementation of incentives systems Distributive efficiency to revert the concentration of staff in urban areas	Participation in the definition of criteria for the professional career Assurance of good environment and working conditions

- Educational development of the workforce based on competencies

- Management of the public health workforce

- Regulation of educational and labor processes of PHWF

- Reorientation and improvement of the quality of both undergraduate and graduate education in public health based on the essential pubic health functions

Figure 4 illustrates what could be called the development cycle of the public health workforce.

4.2 Strategic Conditions for the Development of the Workforce

The national authorities which have approved the regional mandates to promote the "Public Health in the Americas" Initiative, have completed the performance measurement of the essen-

Figure 4   Development cycle of the public health workforce

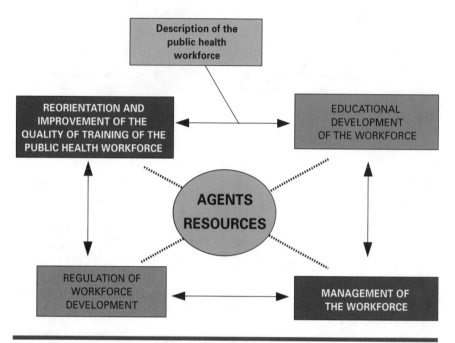

tial public health functions and have committed to preparing plans for the development of the public health workforce. Moreover, they have shown increasing concern in the face of the deterioration of public health practice in most of the countries as well as political will to change such conditions. Such political resolve should be highlighted since it is one of the basic conditions to bring about change.

Political resolve should be reflected not only in the mobilization of will and resources of the public sector, but it should also be reflected in the various institutions which, together with the State and society—are responsible for providing public health services and employees. Communication with institutions that provide public health education is essential. The improvement of public health depends on sensitization, awareness of the issues and commitment to finding solutions. The participation and involvement of academic institutions that pro-

vide public health education and training is extremely important. Without their involvement it is not possible to develop and implement plans for improving the competencies of the public health workforce.

As leaders of the Initiative, health authorities need to take measures to end the lack of communication and "divorce" that exists between the academic institutions, health service and state institutions, responsible for public health, in order to join efforts and resources for the development of the national sanitary capacity. Gradually the foundation will be set and conditions met for the development of an integrated educational system for public health. This system will be the primary infrastructure for workforce development, central to strengthening the national capacity in public health. As mentioned in the Santo Domingo Conference, the Central America experience shows that there are conditions for joining efforts

and consolidating collaboration. One of the goals of this initiative and specifically of the proposal outlined here is that it should contribute to the progressive development of the integrated education systems in the countries of the subregions.

Special attention should be given to the components of training that are part of almost all of the investment or institutional development projects in many countries in the Region to support processes of health sector reform. It is important to evaluate these experiences since a considerable amount of money has been invested. Thousands of workers have been trained in various areas of public health management. Such training has followed the logic of the respective projects and goals frequently without any previous agreement or general orientation of the institution or health system. In general, there has been little coordination between projects that share the same target population, objectives and areas of work. When properly coordinated, these projects have been and may continue to be an important source of institutional and financial resources which can be mobilized to develop the public health workforce.

5. Educational Development based on Competence

5.1 Continuing Education for Performance based on Competence

The objective of this measure is to improve the performance of the workforce currently working in the health system and related areas, through educational strategies and plans. The educational plans will be developed with the goal

Figure 5 Function of work performance

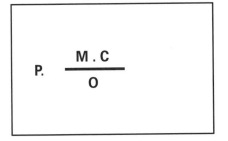

of forming competent staff. The plans must also be useful and valuable for undergraduate and graduate education in health, and in particular public health.

This approach is based on the concept that the performance of individuals as part of the workforce is a complex function whose main factors are self-motivation and professional competence, as well as institutional and organizational factors reflected in management, availability of resources and working conditions.

Where:

P is workforce performance

M is motivation

C is the workforce competence and

O are the obstacles (regulatory, managerial, organizational, etc.)

The focus of competence allows the development of educational plans and measure for workforce management from the point of view of requirements, problems and challenges of work, that is, from the point of view of performance that, for the "Public health in the Americas" Initiative means within the practice of the essential public health functions. One of the main features of this strategy is that this practice be interdisciplinary since it implies the coming together of various occupations and professions.

A second consideration in favor of the focus on competence approach is the changing and complex nature of the health systems, which continuously generates new challenges for continuing education and training of staff. Such challenges go beyond the fundamentally biomedical contents and focus by which the majority of health technicians and professionals are trained.

Dealing with these challenges requires a different approach, both theoretical and methodological, for the education of the workforce, both in training and the development and maintenance of the performance of quality functions, and maintenance and improvement of competence. The educational focus based on competence is part of a new approach of education in health called **Continuing Education in Health** by the Pan American Health Organization and a good part of the Region. It is characterized by the following components:

5.1.1 Learning at work place

Continuing education has emphasized "work" as the space where educational demands and needs are defined. The educational potential of the work situation, the analysis of daily problems at work and the orientation of the educational process towards the transformation of the social and technical practices of the worker make the work place a special place to develop learning. "Needs and problems are evaluated and continuing education strategies and processes are proposed so that they can integrate individual, institutional and social issues, besides taking into consideration the affective and intellectual aspects, strengthening thus the professional and social commitment of the worker."

Cognitive Constructivism

Cognitive constructivism states that the subject—the health worker—actively organizes the knowledge, integrating and reinterpreting the information and experiences received during the learning process. In order to achieve this, he/she uses previous experiences, comprehension skills, exchange of information and opinions that take place in various contexts. When learning, the immediate context (both work and social) plays an important role since the learning process has a meaning, thus, an impact and effect when it takes place in a context in which aptitudes and newly acquired knowledge can be used effectively. At this point a link with a motivation to learn is produced, stemming from a desire to understand and structure meanings to what is learned. All knowledge has to be "somewhere" in the learner's mind to have significance (that is, it should "make sense"). Otherwise, learning will be mechanical and an exercise of memorization. Moreover, it will lack the basic conditions of constructivist learning. Such conditions are: reflection, decision-making skills during the learning process and the ability to solve practical problems.

Adult learning

The technical basis of continuing education includes principles of adult education such as:

- Linking acquired knowledge with actual problems, thus generating a problem pedagogy

- A close relationship between learning, life and work

- Responsibility in learning and managing personal educational development

- Active participation in the process

- Cooperation in the design of learning processes

- Assessment of the usefulness of knowledge according to parameters of efficacy, based on personal experience and the ability to use the knowledge to solve practical problems

In other words, the health agent (the adult in the learning situation) is considered the architect of his/her practice. Learning is based on work and other vital experiences. This means that in the case of adult education, learning based on experience is essential. Experience is the foundation and starting point for the development of concepts and for seeking out the comprehension of concepts and theories. With this focus, the learning cycle begins thus with experience, continues with reflection and leads to action based on experience or practice, which gives way for a new experience and a new cycle of reflection-action.

5.1.2 Meta-cognitive strategies: learning to learn

In continuing constructivist education, organizing knowledge based on previous experience and knowledge is as important as the development of meta-cognitive strategies of each person. Meta-cognition is the process of thinking how to think. That is, it is a self analysis of one's personal cognitive process which allows one to regulate one's own learning process. It implies awareness of mental processes that the learner develops when learning a certain concept: what

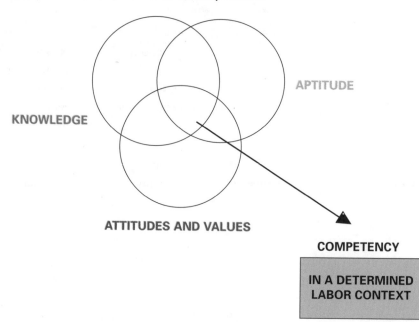

Figure 6   Concept of work competence

type of relationships are established, what reasoning process is used (induction, deduction, comparison, etc), what is his/her ability to recognize difficult learning aspects, where and how to begin to overcome them, how long it will take to achieve, etc. Reflection on these processes will lead the learner to search for help when he/she needs it and will allow him/her opportunities for learning increasingly more complex cognitive processes. This is what is commonly called "learning to learn".

Focus on what is understood as "work competence"

"Work competence" can be simply defined as: a person is competent in the work environment if he/she is able to use his/her knowledge practically. In other words, competence is evaluated by what a person knows, if he/she can put it into practice and why he/she does it in an given work context, with the in-

teraction of knowledge, aptitudes, attitudes, and work values put into action to achieve meaningful results in a given work context. The above figure shows a way to represent the meaning of the word "competence".

In complex adaptation systems (characterized by low levels of agreement and high degrees of uncertainty) such as health services organizations and health sector institutions, it is well known that a basic condition for good workforce performance is a clear definition of the organization's mission and organizational results. But, the achievement of such results requires a precise definition of the competence of the staff and an assurance of certain subjective conditions (intellectual strategies such as "learning to learn", a essential condition) and objective conditions (institutional), that allow the worker to adapt to change, acquire new knowledge and continuously improve performance. In specialized English literature, this concept is known as *capability*.

The identification of competence requires a frame of reference determined by a taxonomy of competence that converts "essential functions" into orientating elements of educational programming. With regards to the Initiative, PAHO's Human Resources Development Program consulted with experts and conducted a bibliographical review in order to reach a taxonomy which would functionally allow the step to be taken from "essential functions" to "competence." That is how the following taxonomic approach arose:

Basic competence

Competence which provides the fundamental understanding of what is public health and what is its purpose. All public health workers must master it.

Transversal competence

It provides the staff with both general and specific knowledge, aptitudes and skills in areas which allow the performance of one or more essential functions. It must be mastered by various categories of public health professionals and technicians according to their corresponding responsibilities.

Technical Competence

It is the technical knowledge, aptitudes and necessary skills to fulfill an essential function, program, or specific area of application. It is based on the previous two categories. Work teams in charge of a specific essential function, must master it.

That is to say, the satisfactory performance of one or more essential functions

is based on mastering the three categories of competence.

When essential functions are analyzed in regard to educational requirements to assess competence (knowledge, aptitude, attitudes, and values), the **fields of competence** are classified in the following manner in order to determine specific performance measures for public health workers (table 3).

Planning the development of institutional and personal capacities, like the ones proposed for the appropriate performance of the essential public health functions, is based on, in addition to the foresight of the quantitative needs of the various workforce categories, on a clear definition of work competence of the staff and the organizational conditions for their performance.

As previously stated, one of the basic components of the plan will be the educational development of the workforce based on competence. The implementation of this plan implies a complex process stretching from the conversion of the essential functions into competence, according to a given taxonomy, to the definition of the necessary knowledge, aptitudes and attitudes for effective performance, passing through the identification of elements of competence and the definition of performance criteria. Figure 7 reflects this process.

A necessary condition of the educational focus based on competence is that no objectives, strategies nor educational activities can be programmed without the participation of those who perform the function and demonstrate their competence. That is, without the participation of the workers. They are the ones who

Table 3 Fields of competence in public health practice

- Values and professional ethics
- Analysis and evaluation
- Adaptability and maintenance of competence
- Management of relations with the external environment
- Technical command specific to an essential function
- Communication
- Management skills
- Formulation, analysis and assessment of policies
- Management of the development of institutional capacities

provide the elements of work and performance that currently exist. Therefore, a basic premise is that the development of educational programs—from the phase of the identification of educational needs to the management of such practices—is a participatory experience between educators and workers, who will be the learning agents and at the same time the objective of the program.

a) Analysis of performance problems of the essential public health functions

It is the identification phase of learning needs. It aims to identify the performance problems of the essential public health functions in the specific contexts where they are applied by systematically desegregating the functions by the decisions and actions necessary to fulfill them.

As previously stated, it requires the participation of those responsible in practice for the performance of a function. The definition of participants will depend of the each function and on the

Figure 7 Process of educational programming based on competence

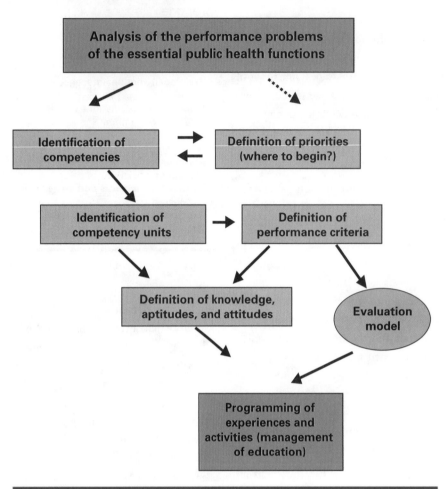

importance of the decisions that will be implied (executives at strategic political level, managers of programs and units, staff at the managerial or operational level). The result is a set of performance problems that will be considered in the future in a list of learning needs.

b) Definition of Priorities

It is a political decision that must be undertaken by those who direct the process of workforce development. This means that the function or problem that will begin the process will be determined according to the characteristics of the political process of the sector, the health needs of the population, the ob-

jectives of the change of the health system and the ability to insist on a certain public health function. The result is a critical path indicating a sequence to be followed which identifies the target workforce group that will be prioritized in the educational process.

c) Identification of competence

It is a process by which with the participation of educators and public health workers, problems with the performance of essential public health functions are identified as well as the learning needs according the previously established competence criteria. That means, it points out the learning needs in re-

gard to competence; it determines ex-pected performance and whenever necessary, the performance level considered as most desirable. From this expected performance, a level of competence can be set. In other words, competence is the expected performance in a specific work context of the staff. In some cases, the ideal requirements are complex and it is necessary to divide them into com-petence units if they are to be useful to determine the learning content.

d) Definition of criteria for performance evaluation

Once the expected performance is defined, it is necessary to define the criteria by which the performance will be evaluated, by assessing competence. Those responsible for designing learning programs must approximate as much as possible a realistic work situation in order to define variables and indicators which will eventually compare actual performance with expected performance. In other words, whether competence has been reached and if this acquired competence is exercised appropriately.

Conclusions in this regard are quite important since **learning assessment criteria** depend on such conclusions. Considerable effort is required to define **the learning assessment model**.

e) Definition of knowledge, aptitudes and attitudes

This is the most familiar stage since it is performed daily. It involves choosing between various methodologies for continuing education which is most suitable to the process in progress and the programming of the learning content. This educational plan must systematically establish the necessary knowledge, aptitudes and attitudes to proceed to

Figure 8 Identification of the work competence

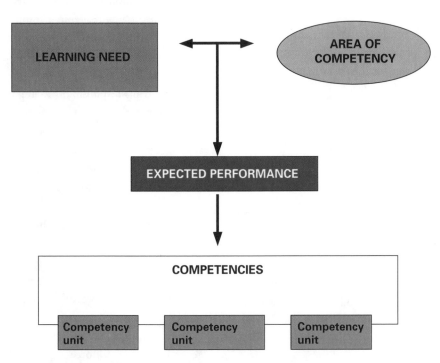

the stage of educational activities and experiences. It is during this stage that the taxonomy of basic, transversal and technical competence becomes quite useful, since it the most opportune moment to define the composition of the learning groups. The fundamental principal is that the learning groups be analogous to the working groups, which in education during actual service form part of the same team.

f) Educational evaluation

It is a permanent process in the educational cycle that from the perspective of the Human Resources Development Program should be follow the Kirkpatrick principles and take into account the four levels of evaluation, in particular level III (performance) and IV (impact).

On the one hand, it is based on a frame of reference that defines learning needs identified by the performance problems of the essential public health functions, and on the other hand, in the definition of performance criteria. In the current educational framework the Human Resources Development Program has created set of evaluation tools to provide technical support to ongoing training programs and projects in the Region.

5.2 An Education System for Public Health

The massive requests from various countries in the Region for workforce training to guarantee adequate performance standards, forces us to think of an educational infrastructure of national reach. It is necessary to develop a public health education system articulating with academic, employer, service and professional institutions, to jointly contribute to the development of the public health workforce.

Traditionally there has been a division between academic institutions of public health and institutions that employ the public health workforce. The same occurs in other areas of human resources development in public health. The associations of public health workers, which are not very developed in the Region, have been absent, with few exceptions, from the national debates on health sector reform.

Nonetheless, ever since PAHO and WHO began technical cooperation to stimulate the understanding and use of essential public health functions, as a response to the challenges of health sector reform, academic institutions and employing bodies have demonstrated a common interest and concern. As previously mentioned, the Latin America and Caribbean Association of the Public Health Education (ALAESP) has supported the essential public health functions proposal, regarding them as general guidelines for curricula development of public health graduate programs as well as for institutional development. Cuba is organizing an integrated public health education system utilizing the essential public health functions as a frame of reference for educational development that is based on competence. Through the family health strategy, Brazil is testing new and promising forms of integration between universities and municipalities, responsible for local health systems, within the framework for improving basic health care services. It will be necessary to evaluate and disseminate these experiences as good and correct practice.

5.3 Distance learning

The enormous need for education for the development of the public health workforce coupled with the increasing access to information technology in the countries of the Region, encourages the development of strategies for distance learning as one of the most important development plans.

The emergence of a world connected by computers, satellites and telecommunication technology represented by the Internet, the *world wide web* and the configuration of corporative nets (intranet) have changed the working and learning conditions of many workers, among them those in the field of public health. The increasing use of modern information and communication technology in distance learning allows not only the development of programs based on educational theories but also the improvement of education outcomes, the transformation of practice and accessibility for workers, who until recently did not have this access due precisely to work. Current circumstances make this modality become a fundamental strategy in the educational development of the workforce.

The Pan American Health Organization with the Cataluña Open University and ten leading academic institutions in public health education and international cooperation, are currently developing the "Virtual Campus in Public Health", whose goal is to stimulate the development of competencies demanded by the essential public health functions. At present, there are very few academic institutions that are not attempting to make the leap to education based on information networks. It is a strategic necessity to get these academic institutions to commit to offering distance learning to the public health workforce.

The Virtual Campus offers an effective wide reaching means to incorporate distance learning in workforce develop-

ment plans. The main objectives of the Virtual Campus are:

• Contribute to the development of professional and institutional competence for the performance of essential public health functions.

• Promote access to knowledge and information for the public health staff in the Region, for better decision making.

• Promote exchanges between professionals and public health institutions (education and health) for institutional learning purposes.

Figure 9 shows the general services and educational and informational programs offered by the Virtual Campus.

6. Management of the public health workforce

The development of the public health workforce also requires the conscience and sustained efforts of the health authorities as well as each of the employing entities to improve institutional, administrative and material conditions of the workforce where the work is carried out daily in exchange for a fee. Workforce management has been a grey area in health systems and services, limited to the administrative and formalist treatment of the tasks of personnel.

The means of work regulation (which decide, among other things, contracts and salaries) have changed very quickly in countries of the Region as a consequence of the changes in the economy, the State and in public administration. This far-reaching process has generated changes in the management of the general health workforce and in particular the public health workforce. The situation analysis and trends of workforce

management show an accumulation of management models, with some traces of flexibility which make up a complex framework that can be characterized as follows.

In transferring responsibilities and resources for workforce management, the processes of decentralization of health systems have been a determinant force for the transformation of management into a strategic and complex function that to be operative urgently requires qualified personnel, quality information and special tools.

Although there is a lack of specific and reliable information regarding the public health workforce, there is no reason to indicate that it may differ from the general health workforce in terms of salaries, professional career, etc. This is particularly true if one considers the deterioration of the infrastructure and institutional capacity of public health as reflected in the results of the performance measurement of the essential public health functions.

As established in the base document of the CS43.R6 resolution of the PAHO/WHO 43rd Directing Council (2001), both regional and national concerted efforts are required to strengthen the institutional capacity for the management of human resources, including processes and measures affecting the public health workforce. The following measures can be highlighted:

Short, medium and long term planning of the public health workforce

This function implies not only the quantitative estimate of needs (as has been done traditionally) but rather in the determination of competencies and

Figure 9   Services offered by the Virtual Campus in Public health

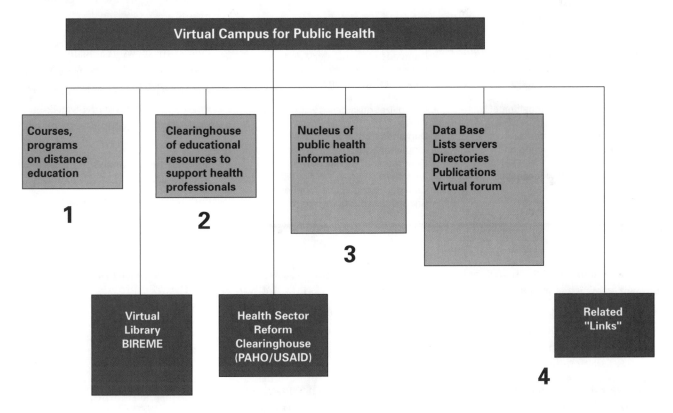

1 Continuing education for in-service personnel, responsible for management of services and programs, and leaders of the sector, in the various decision-making levels
2 Methodologies, technologies and educational instruments to strengthen public health education institutions.
3 Resources of information: newsletters, information, news, summaries, links to other web sites.
4 Example: Public Health Foundation, ALAESP, ASPHER, APHA, ASPH, etc.

workforce profiles. There is an essential interaction with the educational development programming based on professional competence. It is therefore a function of quantitative and qualitative foresight of **management based on professionalism.**

Qualitative improvement in selection, recruitment and retention of the workforce (staff supply)

This has been one of the weakest functions in the area of staff administration and has become an essential condition in the current context of increasing complexity and flexibility in work relations. It is probably in this function

where the greatest effort should be made in terms of modernization, changes in focus, procedures and tools.

Performance management

Management based on competence redefines criteria for programming, organizing and evaluating the work of the staff. It entails that, new forms of work organization to obtain higher levels of productivity and quality should be redefined based on the expected performance of the essential functions. In this regard, it is necessary to include the promotion of work teams, the application of adequate incentives, new modalities of performance evaluation and the

updating of retribution and acknowledgment systems.

Management of work relations

This function—which has generally dealt with the regulations regarding work life without taking into consideration the improvement of the development of staff administration—is strategic in the current context of reforms and deregulations. It entails participatory management, negotiated and concerted with union agents with regard to individual work relations (principally contract and salary) and collective work relations (representation, union, strike, negotiation, career). Likely changes and

Table 4 Problems with human resources management in health

Former problems
- Lack of balance in the availability of staff
- Inadequate geographical distribution of resources (inequity)
- Imbalance in the composition of health staff
- Weak information systems
- Low integration of training and services
- Low salaries and few incentives

New problems resulting from reforms
- Demands of productivity and performance quality
- Descentralization and disgregation of functions
- Flexibilization-precarización of the work
- Demands from new modes of regulation
- Generation of production-related incentives
- Changes in the educational offer
- Challenges of training for reform

chances to achieve better system performances are based on effective management of work relations, and consequently on a better performance of the essential public health functions.

Management of the continuing education of the workforce

In regular conditions, continuing staff education—the professional development by educational means—is one more function, although strategic, of workforce management. Given the urgent needs arising from the performance of essential function 8, certain conditions to meet the requirements of workforce development planning must be taken into account.

Safety conditions and work environment

It is another of the less developed functions which needs to be promoted due to the particular conditions and risks that public health workers are exposed to.

This functional framework for the development of the institutional capacity for workforce management—in regards to regulation of work processes and

educational development—serves as a guide to point out some of the demands that those teams responsible for essential function 8 must take into account.

The strategic approach of adopting the competence focus is to attain an integrated management of educational development and workforce performance. Moreover, it is important to emphasize that when speaking of work force development we are not talking about only training, but also the interaction and the integrated effect of education (both

training and continuing education), management, workforce regulation and its processes.

Figure 10 shows the main regulating mechanisms of the workforce development processes and can be used to characterize certain normative aspects in the field of public health.

Without further analysis of each one of the mechanisms, perhaps the most important ones with regards to the current changes in the Region are:

Accreditation of educational programs and institutions

The main objective is the development and application of quality criteria of educational processes and infrastructure which will guarantee a quality standard (predetermined and accepted) for the benefit of the students, the employing institutions, and the population benefiting from these services.

Incentives for staff performance

They are instruments for regulation and management. They encourage the in-

Figure 10 Main Regulatory Mechanisms

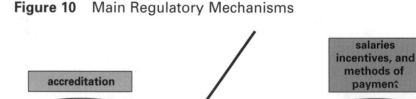

300

corporation of people into the public health workforce, their commitment to the function performed, and improvement of daily performance.

In this case, it is not only improving salaries (which are usually low) nor establishing a monetary policy of incentives (widely spread and encouraged in many reform processes, which many times results in questionable outcomes), to improve performance and commitment to the employer. It mainly entails of offering adequate conditions for personal and professional development. In this case, since it is dealing with a special worker, requiring ongoing acquisition of knowledge, the opportunities for educational development are important.

7. Reorientation and improvement of the quality of undergraduate and graduate education in public health

Defining the profile, evaluating and developing a competent worker for the performance of the essential public health functions is a task that has been defined as a frame of reference for graduate education in numerous academic institutions that are part of the ALAESP. This association develops joint activities with PAHO with the aim of increasing the quality of graduate education by promoting the use of suitable quality criteria in the processes of program and institution accreditation. This frame of reference also considered valid for the reorientation and strengthening of undergraduate education in various health professions, especially in medicine and nursing.

In regard to graduate studies in public health and related programs, PAHO and the ALAESP are promoting a strategy of institutional and associate alliances in the area of quality management, taking into account the needs of both students and teachers. These lines of action are mainly geared towards:

Invert the old pedagogic model **by adopting new ideas and promoting debates in both undergraduate and graduate studies.**

Promote and support the education sector to define or redefine a *quality focus* in public health, centered on objectives of changes in the health systems and based on agreements with various sectors that participate in public health education.

Table 5 summarizes these lines of action.

As for undergraduate health studies, it is necessary to acknowledge that public health has not been a topic of discussion in the past years, despite being regarded a priority area during the 70's and 80's. The progressive decrease of public health content and similar disciplines in schools of medicine around the region is well known.

Over the past six years, both the PAHO and WHO have evaluated the impact of health sector reforms in medical practice and nursing to identify new trends and reorient undergraduate education accordingly. Below is a summary of these trends:

- Demand of generalized profiles: universal expansion of proposals and models of practice in general and family medicine.

- Increasing regulation of specializations: recertification.

- Competence requirements regarding health promotion.

- Performance requirements using a medical focus based on reality.

- Increasing practice based on controlled care

- Clinical decisions based on criteria of cost and efficacy

Along with these trends, most of the health professions maintain an unsustainable concept in the current professional education: segregation between clinical and public health. The vanguard experiences in medical education propose that the 21st Century health professional have the appropriate competence, clearly demonstrating a break from the traditional profiles. In the case of medical doctors, it is considered that he/she must be competent as a professional providing integral care, responsible for adopting decisions, sharing information, community leader, health promoter, service manager, gatekeeper and manager of resources. It is also regarded that he/she must be able to work in a team, be a good clinician, take into consideration human relations, etc. All these conditions require a profound redefinition of the educational model and the incorporation of experiences in the learning environment.

In most cases, schools of health sciences require, among others, a substantial change in the disciplinary models of professional programs that allow an integral focus to the human being. This objective requires a new definition of health which goes beyond the biomedical definition,

Table 5 Lines of action to improve the quality of graduate public health education (PAHO-ALAESP)

Interventions	Educational programs	Teaching environment	Student environment
Improvement and strengthening of public health graduate degrees	Invert the tendency of simple information transmission and the weakness in knowledge production (research)	• Continuing education and selective sharing of information for educators Definition of areas of research and creation of conditions to permit the research. • Strengthening the tutoring capacity • Promotion of learning and problem resolution among interdisciplinary groups • Take advantage of the potential for the intellectual production of the student • Development of spaces for debate and discussion on Sanitary policies	• Review of selection criteria (profiles and requirements according to the quality approach and the institutional mission) • Application of an androgenic model: learning contracts, group learning, flexible curricula, integration of information and disciplines for learning based on problem solving • Early definition of thesis and graduate papers, permanent tutoring • Educational experience in services and institutions: New service-education links • Services
Proposal of initiatives for the promotion of quality in public health education	Promotion of the integration of disciplines and knowledge: Reorganization based on usefulness in resolving priority problems in the social and health systems. Incorporation of epistemological approaches and debates favoring this integration	Wide spread debates on essential public health functions, sector reforms, quality of education, quality management • Promotion of the participation of public health graduates in the creation of a quality focus • Organization of forums for the exchange of educational theoretical advances, sanitary changes, quality focuses, quality management models, etc. • Organization of work groups on priority topics of sanitary debate • Development of a critical mass of educational agents in quality managment	

Source: PAHO-ALESP. Quality of Public Health Education: an Imminent Challenge. from the Special Consultative Meeting in. Santiago de Chile, November 2001.

proposes the training of proto-clinical specialists with training that supports general practice and stimulates a new relation with services (beyond the formalities of the traditional articulation of service-education)

Among these redefinitions a new balance and a new relationship between clinical and public health is proposed. This change can be functional by means of a deep analysis of the essential public health functions and the educational stance taken in regard to those functions. As a general guide, in organizing the health care system, the improvement of the analysis capacity of health conditions, the community's health demands and ways of applying con-

Figure 11 Necessary change in Public Health Education

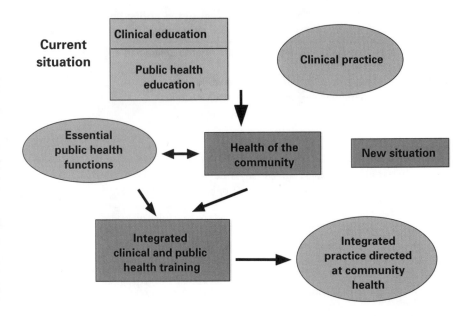

clusions must be taken into account. Figure 11 illustrates these necessary changes.

8. An integral look at technical cooperation for workforce development

In the present chapter approaches and proposals by the PAHO-WHO have been systematically presented to contribute to defining policies and public health workforce development plans as an important component in the improvement of national institutional capacities in the performance of the essential public health functions. This section provides a synthesized, but complete matrix of PAHO and WHO's possible areas of cooperation in the field of human resources development. See table 6.

8.1 Perspective of regional collaboration

Throughout this chapter, various approaches, orientations and useful suggestions for the preparation of national plans for the development of the public health workforce have been presented. As a tool for development a plan, it is not necessary to develop a special model. One can adopt the proposal developed in Chapter 13 on "Public Health Infrastructure", in a way that will be coherent with proposals of other plans.

Nevertheless, it would be pertinent to propose the formulation of the **purpose of the workforce development component** of the plan that should make reference to the accomplishment within a certain time frame of :

> . . . a competent and self motivated workforce to perform essential public health functions with quality and efficiency.

Since the Human Resources Development Program's technical cooperation is of regional reach, it is desirable to propose strategies of regional support in the

development and implementation of national plans for workforce development.

8.1.1 Active collaboration among countries

This strategy is fundamental for putting into practice the Pan-American principle of public health. It is imperative that the countries complement efforts to develop the workforce in each country. Complementation is very evident and has great potential. This has been demonstrated in the experience with Central America, the work of ALESP and the multinational participation of the Region in national and international public health events.

8.1.2 Strengthening of human resources policies in general and particularly those of the public health workforce

If the increasing trends of work flexibility and deregulation of higher education are taken into account, it is necessary, now more than ever, to have definitions of human resources policies in general and in particular for human resources development. Policies indicate change and set frameworks for educational development, planning and changes in regulation and workforce management.

9. Strengthening workforce management

Human resources management has always been a politically weak and underdeveloped function. If education based on work competence is proposed, it is impossible to develop the public health workforce in the different countries without transforming management in a strategic function of public health.

Table 6 PAHO-WHO Contribution to the development of public health workforce

Programmatic proposals	Contribution to the development of the public health workforce for the performance of essential functions
Human Resources Observatory in Health International network for the production of evidence in support to the development of policies in human resources	• Production of information and knowledge in order to define and execute policies of workforce development • Production of basic data to characterize the workforce • Strengthening of human resources information systems • Production of information for workforce planning
Continuing education New educational model based on adult education for ongoing education and professional development	• Methodologies and tools for educational programming based on work competence • Tools for the management of education based on competencies • Development of institutional capacities for ongoing education
Virtual Campus of Public Health Virtual educational environment for distance education in public health, guided by essential public health functions.	• Production of distance educational services and materials for continuing education of the public health workforce and development of institutional capacities • On-line courses and materials defined by competencies and according to the needs for the performance of essential functions • Coordinating center of educational and informational resources for public health practice • Access to education and information in English, Portuguese and Spanish
Development of management of quality in public health education Program to support academic public health institutions in the development of a quality focus as well as the strengthening of institutional capacities in the management of quality of public health education	• Development of frames of reference, tools and techniques for the educational and programmatic renovation and transformation of graduate studies in public health and health sciences careers • Development of a quality focus in public health education and appropriate regulating (accrediting) tools • Through an alliance of institutions, guarantee the spread of information and management of up to date pertinent knowledge for public health education • Promotion of the frame of reference of essential public health functions
Human resources management Support plan for the development of institutional capacities in the countries for the development of a new focus and practice in the management of human resource in health	• Service training in human resources management to improve the management of the public health workforce • Tools for short and medium term programming of the public health workforce • Adequate tools for the change and improvement of the functions and procedures for recruitment, selection, assignment and performance evaluation • Tools for the management of productivity and quality of workforce performance • Guarantee of workforce educational opportunities based on a competencies • Technical support for the improvement of the quality of the work life and work conditions

10. Intensive use of the existing capacity; coordination and complementation of resources

One of the most important lessons of cooperation—that accompanies educational projects in health sector reforms—has been to establish the transformation of the educational practices and training management in almost all the countries. This transformation allows the shaping of reforms according to advances consolidated in many national institutions (The Observatory Series 3, 2002). On the other hand, in many countries, there was a duplication of efforts, lack of coordination, waste of resources and excessive measures taken for similar objectives of the population. In these conditions, it is even more nec- essary to coordinate initiatives and join efforts.

11. Promotion, spreading and incorporation of correct practices and successful educational modalities

The past years have been very rich in both national and international educational development experiences inside and outside of the health sector. Therefore, it is important to take advantage of the good and successful practices that have been developed and to learn from these.

12. Guarantee the availability of tools and methodologies

The active dissemination and training of tools and methodologies developed and tested over the last years in education, planning, regulation and management of the public health workforce as well as in other fields, is a strategy that should be used in inter country collaboration.

13. Strategies for the creation of subregional programs in support of national efforts

This strategy revisits an initiative developed and reclaimed during the meeting of the Central American countries, Haiti, Cuba and Puerto Rico, which took place in the Dominican Republic March 15–16, 2002. There is much ac-

cumulated experience from sub regional initiatives across the Region that can be useful for promoting the development of the public health workforce.

Bibliography

Byrne N. y M Rozental. Tendencias actuales de la educación médica y propuesta de orientación para la educación médica en América Latina. Educación Médica y Salud, Vol. 28, No. 1: 53–93, 1994.

CDC/ATSDER. Taskforce on Public Health Workforce Development. www.pphppo.cdc.gov/taskforce.

Davini M.C. y M. A. Clasen Roschke. Conocimiento significativo: el diseño de un proyecto de educación permanente en salud. Educación de Personal de Salud. Serie de Desarrollo de Recursos Humanos 100. Washington, D.C., 1994.

Fraser S.W. y Greenhalgh. Complexity Science: Coping with Complexity: Educating for Capability. BMJ 2001; 323: 799– 803.

HRSA. The Public Health Workforce Enumeration. 2000.

Kirkpatrick D.L. Evaluating Training Programs. The Four Levels, Berrett-Kochler Publishers. San Francisco, 1994.

Kolb D.A. Experiential Learning: Experience as the Source of Learning and Development. Englewood Cliffs, N. J. Prentice–Hall, 1984.

OPS-CINTERFOR. Competencia work. Manual de conceptos, métodos y aplicaciones en el sector salud. Montevideo, 2002.

Organización Panamericana de la Salud. Desafíos para la educación en salud pública: La reforma sectorial y las funciones esenciales de la salud pública. Washington, D.C., OPS, 2000.

Organización Panamericana de la Salud. Desafíos para la educación en salud pública: Nuevas perspectivas para las Américas, Washington D.C., OPS, 2001.

Organización Panamericana de la Salud. Manual de promotion de la educación en servicios. PALTEX, 2002.

Organización Panamericana de la Salud. Observatorio de Recursos Humanos de Salud: Conjunto de datos básicos, 1999.

Public Health Leadership Society—Principle for Enumeration. 2000.

Rogers C.R. Freedom to Learn: A view of What Education Might Become. Westerville, Ohio, Merrill, 1969.

US.DDHHS.PHS.HRSA. Bureau of Health Profession. Sixth Report to the President and Congress on the Status of Health Personnel in the United States, June 1998.

Wislow, CD y W.L. Bramer. Future Work: Putting Knowledge to work in the Knowledge Economy. New York. Free Press, 1994.

16 International Cooperation for Improving Public Health Practice

1. Cooperation for Development and Strengthening of Steering Capacity in the Health Authority

PAHO has made a commitment to its member countries to support the processes aimed at transforming their health sectors, commonly known as health reform. This means working intensely with the countries to devise options for the health sector that represent real progress toward equitable access to health services by the peoples of our Hemisphere.

At the first hemispheric summit in Miami, the heads of State and government of the countries of the Americas were very clear about the need to forge ahead with health sector reform processes that would ensure equitable access to basic health services. Not to reform for reform's sake, but to reform with an awareness and a direction that imply improving the health of the people, promoting healthy environments and social practices, reaching out to the poorest, most excluded members of society, and eliminating the current inequities in the health situation, access to services, and sectoral financing.

On that occasion in December 1994, the leaders of our member countries recommended that a hemispheric forum be convened to discuss progress and the challenges confronting health sector reform processes in the Region. It was held in September 1995, in Washington, D.C., within the framework of PAHO's Directing Council, comprised of all the ministers of health of the Americas. Also participating were representatives of the social security health institutions and other government sectors responsible for economic decision-making and development planning related to the sector. As requested by the heads of State and government, PAHO joined forces with several bilateral and multilateral cooperation agencies, along with the principal international financing institutions, to sponsor a hemispheric meeting to discuss the status of health sector reforms.

The heads of State and government also issued a mandate to PAHO in Miami in 1994 to launch a process for monitoring and evaluating health sector reform in the countries of the Region. Today, backed by the member countries, this framework is an ongoing process that is making it possible to study the course that the reforms have taken and lay the foundation for the adjustments and changes in direction required—changes that will ensure that the transformations in the sector have a truly positive impact on the delivery of health services, making them accessible to the people who need them the most.

The deliberations held and the mandates subsequently signed by the ministers of health of the Americas at the meetings of PAHO's Governing Bodies in 1997 and 2001 underscore the high priority given to strengthening the steering function of the health authorities at all levels of the State and to improving the performance of the essential public health functions pertaining to them. They also stress the need to intensify cooperation in this area, given the multiplicity of actions that these tasks require.

Within the framework of PAHO's strategic and programmatic orientations for the quadrenniums 1995–1998 and 1999–2002, the proposed Strategic Plan 2003–2007, and the technical cooperation activities to support the sectoral reform processes, an effort has been made to pay special attention to strengthening the health authority, developing its steering capacity, and improving the exercise of the EPHF as the basic lines of action for the institutional development of the sector.

To this end, regional and country programming efforts have centered on activities geared to:

a) preparing, disseminating, and promoting a conceptual and operational framework for the steering role of the ministries of health, within the new context of state modernization and sectoral reform;

b) providing technical guidance and support for the reorganization and institutional strengthening of the ministries of health of the member countries to enable them to serve as steering entities to confront the new sectoral realities;

c) preparing, disseminating, and promoting guidelines, methodologies, and specific instruments for consol-

idating the institutional development of the health authority in the countries of the Region, to enable them to fully discharge their responsibilities in management, regulation, exercise of the essential public health functions, coordination of health service delivery, oversight of insurance, and the compensatory redistribution of sectoral financing;

d) circulating information and sharing national experiences on the exercise of the steering role by the ministries of health and on institutional development for that purpose.

These activities were designed to help the health authorities in the Region to strengthen their steering capacity and intersectoral leadership through progress in the following areas:

• heightening their regulatory role, giving them the necessary flexibility to identify national and local problems and solve them, within the framework of decentralization;

• ensuring that social participation plays a key role in public health practice in our societies;

• ensuring effective promotion and use of mass communication for health purposes;

• strengthening public health practice;

• formulating and executing policies that promote greater equity in access, use, and financing of the health services, fostering social solidarity in the solution of health problems;

• preparing forecasts that will make it possible to formulate policies whose implementation and actions will lead

to economically sustainable and socially irreversible achievements;

• promoting policies that foster continuous quality improvement in the services to ensure the satisfaction of the population;

• utilizing research for decision-making and technological upgrading of the health system;

• utilizing health situation analysis to set policies that promote greater equity;

• promoting research in public health and health services to steer health policies in the direction of greater equity;

• evaluating popular satisfaction to monitor the impact of the policies on users of the services.

• developing the capacity to analyze the demands and conflicts arising from civil society and the responses provided, together with their impact on public health policy.

These tasks call for new professional capacity, extensive development of the corresponding legislative instruments, and a reorganization of the structure and operations of the ministries of health to enable them to perform their duties. In many cases, it is not just a matter of administrative reorganization, but of a profound reengineering that demands institutional strengthening, workforce development, and well-targeted investment. As part of its efforts to support health systems and services development and the sectoral reform processes in the countries of the Region, PAHO must give high priority in the coming years to cooperation activities that improve the health authority's exercise of the sectoral steering role by strengthening the institutional capacity for that purpose.

2. The Need for International Cooperation to Improve Public Health Practice

PAHO's Centennial, which commemorates a century of collaboration in health in the Americas, offers an unparalleled opportunity for international cooperation and joint action by all the countries of the Region to improve the health of our peoples. To this end, it is essential to intensify collaboration to strengthen the health authorities' steering role as the key to good performance of the EPHF and, thus, to the improvement of public health practice.

The EPHF performance measurement exercise in 41 countries and territories of the Americas, grounded in a renewed framework for action in public health and in the pressing need to strengthen the steering role of the health authorities (as discussed in the first three parts of the book), has yielded results whose immediate follow-up must be a major effort to promote institutional development and strengthen the infrastructure to improve public health practice in the Region.

As seen in the earlier chapters of this fourth and final part, the magnitude and complexity of the task at hand still demand conceptual, methodological, and instrumental action that transcends national borders and can benefit from joint efforts by countries and international cooperation agencies in health. This will make it possible to join forces, share information on successes and failures, identify opportunities for joint action, and create economies of scale to

advance more rapidly and staunchly in this effort.

Hence, the importance of gradually crafting a multifaceted international cooperation program or "agenda" in this field in terms of content and the necessary implementation processes. This is central for the future work of PAHO, both regional and in each member country. Notwithstanding, this program cannot be limited to the efforts of the Organization, since it transcends its sphere of action. Naturally, a program of this type must bring together other international actors in the field of health (bilateral, multilateral, international financing institutions, and private foundations). It must also involve subregional health groups and major actors within the countries—especially the health authorities and public health education and research institutes—whose assistance is required.

International cooperation, both technical and financial, must be characterized by a spirit of collaboration among countries and agencies to support the development and strengthening of public health in our countries and, ultimately, improve the health of our peoples. Thus, it is essential for the countries of the Hemisphere to maintain a dialogue and close collaboration with bilateral, multilateral, and private agencies, on the one hand, and with the development banks, on the other, to ensure the greatest possible convergence between technical and financial cooperation. This is especially important for the health sector reforms, which must define how our societies will meet the needs of individuals; for development of the health authorities' institutional capacity to exercise their steering role in the health system; and for strengthening the infrastructure needed to improve the per-

formance of the EPHF and thereby obtain substantial improvements in public health practice.

3. Toward the Definition of Priority Areas and Critical Processes to Guide International Cooperation

The wealth of experience garnered in the three years since the design and implementation of the Public Health in the Americas Initiative, the information yielded by the hemisphere-wide evaluation of the performance of the EPHF pertaining to the health authority in 41 countries and territories, and the commitment made and internalized by the supreme health authorities of the member countries to overcome the weaknesses and reinforce the strengths identified after the EPHF performance measurement have made it possible to determine a number of priority areas of action for international cooperation and certain critical processes that make them viable, create synergies among them, and establish economies of scale.

Very briefly, as a preliminary sketch, the priority areas for cooperation in this field in the coming years can be summarized as follows:

1) *The EPHF performance measurement instruments should continue to be refined and adapted* to changing concepts, realities, and technologies and to the institutional and organizational structure of public health in the Region. The progress to date should serve as the basis for further review and validation of the variables, indicators, and forms of measurement that will increasing the objectivity of the instrument and directly link it with decision-making

and resource allocation to develop the public health services infrastructure. The goal is for it to become a common tool for self-evaluation, the determination of investment needs, and the promotion of improvements in practice.

2) There is a growing *need to move forward with the development of subnational EPHF performance measurement instruments* for unitary and federal States alike. The instrument currently employed to measure the performance of the EPHF by the national health authority can be used at the intermediate (provinces, states, regions, etc.) and local levels (municipalities, counties, parishes) to increase the effectiveness of the process and the instruments, bringing the exercise closer to the particular operational realities and permit swifter corrective action. This should involve a certain degree of regional or subregional harmony, in order to identify common lines of action and generate economies of scale. It will be equally important to adapt the design of the instruments and the definition of the weighted variables in the subnational exercise to competencies by each country to the health authority at the different levels of the State (national, intermediate, and local).

3) Particularly important are *the development and refinement of methodologies and instruments for planning and strengthening the infrastructure, for promoting the institutional development of the health authority, and for procuring general improvements in public health practice*. This line of action must be consistent with other national processes for planning and the design of sectoral investment to

ensure that it does not end up as a parallel, and to certain extent, vertical exercise that represents an opportunity cost for the rest of the organized development efforts of the sector. Chapter 13 outlines some of the key guidelines that must be considered to advance successfully in this endeavor, analyzing some of the obstacles and opportunities that arise along the way. The national EPHF performance measurement exercises serve as a reference point for defining intervention areas and resource needs for institutional strengthening. Nevertheless, as noted in points 1 and 2 above, as the effectiveness of the instrument improves and progress is made in EPHF performance measurement at the subnational level, the planning exercises and efforts to improve practice will become more relevant and draw ever closer to operational realities.

4) An area that is just beginning to be explored and uncovered, and whose methodologies, concepts, and applications require a much more detailed analysis, is the *development of analytical frameworks for financing, expenditure, cost-analysis, and budgeting of the EPHF*. Chapter 14 offers a very preliminary examination of the topic, suggests some initial approaches, identifies a series of relevant issues, and indicates the long road that must be traveled in this direction. Much of the work consists of improving the capacity to identify more precisely the sources of resources and items of expenditure related to the EPHF. Even more important, however, is defining the production functions of the various components of the EPHF to provide a solid foundation for cost-analysis. This will paint a clearer picture of

the magnitude of the resources necessary to sustain operations and make the necessary investments to enable the health authority to exercise its essential functions. The current levels of expenditure have a historic inertial dimension but are not based on a sound cost-analysis that would allow for adequate evaluation of the interventions from an economic and health standpoint and permit optimization of the types of institutional organization needed to exercise the EPHF.

5) Very little progress can be made in improving public health practice if adequate priority is not given to *institutional strengthening activities and building national, subregional, and regional capacities to develop the public health workforce*. Chapter 15 explores in detail the conceptual and instrumental aspects associated with this key element in infrastructure strengthening. It outlines a range of possibilities that should be discussed in each country to identify how much emphasis should be given to developing and upgrading the competencies of public health workers. Action in this area should be geared, on the one hand, to the staff currently working in the services who perform tasks related to the exercise of the EPHF, and on the other, to academic institutions devoted to training and public health research to give them greater relevance in the processes for improving public health practice. In this regard, innovative multi-institutional collaborative efforts, such as the Virtual Public Health and Health Management Campus, are critical for reaching large numbers of public health professionals through distance learning via the Internet and information re-

sources for professional development in public health.

6) Development of the concepts of social practices and essential health public functions, the progress made in EPHF performance measurement, and the growing interest in developing and implementing processes to improve public health practice—all stemming from the Public Health in the Americas Initiative—open the door and at the same time demand new opportunities for *conceptual debate, methodological development, and instrumental design for articulating the EPHF with the rest of the health system.* Areas that must be addressed include the link between the EPHF and primary health care, the impact of the EPHF on the reorientation of services using health promotion criteria, the link between the definition of health objectives and EPH performance measurement, the impact of the EPHF on policy-making, strategy design, and health planning, and, last but not least, the rethinking of traditional public health programs defined by category that imply substantive population-based interventions and personal care (immunization, vector control, prevention and control of communicable and noncommunicable diseases, occupational health, etc.) from the standpoint of the EPHF and the institutional development and infrastructure strengthening implicit in them.

With regard to the *critical processes* that can make the priority actions indicated above viable, the following should be noted:

1) It is important to make progress in *instituting EPHF performance evaluation as a periodic national exercise.* The challenge is to shift from self-evaluation sponsored by international cooperation to a permanent periodic activity, in which the exercise becomes an integral part of infrastructure development and the ongoing improvement of public health practice. This presupposes that EPHF performance measurement is viewed, with the adaptations that each country deems pertinent, as a component of the instrument panel that must be switched on to evaluate and improve health system performance; as an indicator and a spur to action that enable the health authority to keep its guard up to undertake a critical part of the activities that constitute its *raison d'être.*

2) Of similar importance will be the development of conceptual and instrumental aspects *to guarantee linkage between EPHF performance measurement, the formulation of national plans to improve practices and develop the public health workforce, and the establishment of national, subregional, and regional health objectives.* Increasingly, the countries of the Hemisphere are developing strategic plans for the sector and establishing medium- and long-term objectives in terms of health outcomes (reductions in mortality and morbidity, improvements in the quality of life, and elimination of threats to health), and of the intermediate processes necessary to meet the targets set for results (organization of health care, evaluation of system performance, intersectoral interventions, adequate execution of the EPHF). This is almost virgin territory in many countries in the Americas, but it is also fertile ground and can be turned into a cat-alyst for efforts to improve public health practice in the Hemisphere.

3) The experience acquired in the field of EPHF performance measurement and the actions to improve public health practice must be documented and circulated among stakeholders, both in the countries and internationally. Here, it would be very useful to *create an observatory or clearinghouse for the collection and dissemination of information and the lessons learned.* This center would record, analyze, compare, and lend added value to the available information, thus serving as an information and intelligence resource to support the countries' efforts in this field.

4) Closely allied with the previous point is the issue of *promoting and consolidating institutional networks for information exchange, as well as interagency coalitions that support EPHF performance evaluation and the improvement of public health practice.* To accomplish this, it will be essential to encourage the participation of national institutions that adopt the concepts and methodologies consolidated during the implementation of the Public Health in the Americas Initiative, disseminate them, and replicate them in their spheres of action, perfecting and developing them as far as possible and adapting them to the specific circumstances of the countries. Building this critical mass in the Region will promote a more intensive horizontal exchange and increase cooperation among countries in this field. However, for this type of effort to pay off, it will be necessary to maximize the collaboration of technical and financial cooperation agencies—

bilateral, multilateral, and private—so that their actions converge and heighten the countries' institutional capacity to take up the challenges outlined in this book.

5) The complement to the four critical processes mentioned above is *sustained advocacy and promotion in the countries and the international community to meet the challenges, explore the possibilities, and recognize the importance of public health.* The goal here is to improve the health of the population, contribute to a reduction in poverty, and reduce inequities in health and access to health care, to advance toward meeting the millennium development goals set by the United Nations system, affirm a culture of health and life, create healthy spaces, ensure universal access to health care and, ultimately, improve the quality of life and human security.

It is becoming increasingly clear in today's world that the work of public health and its material translation as the EPHF are a global public good. Thus, international cooperation in this field has become a priority. It demands special efforts to foster the development of convergent processes—within the countries and beyond national borders—to strengthen the infrastructure and contribute to institutional development leading to improvements in public health practice. If this occurs, we will have learned how to rethink our future and contribute to integral human development, which, as Amartya Sen would say, expands human freedom and dignity and permits full expression of the potentialities of individuals and societies. The Public Health in the Americas Initiative has sought to make a modest contribution to that effort, and this book, to place it on record.

APPENDICES

APPENDIX A

EPHF Performance Measurement Instrument

Introduction

Due to the fact that chapters 8, 9, and 10 of the book give a detailed description of the EPHF measurement instrument, the present annex has omitted that information to avoid duplications. The reader may refer to the chapters in section III to complement the contents of Appendix A.

The measurement exercise begins with the EPHF, explicitly defining each EPHF. Indicators are created, standards are determined, and a group of measures and sub-measures are applied that are described below.

EPHF 1: Monitoring, Evaluation and Analysis of Health Status

Definition

This function includes:
- Up-to-date evaluation of the country's health situation and trends including their determinants with special emphasis on identifying inequities in risks, threats, and access to services.

- Identification of the population's health needs including an assessment of health risks and the demand for health services.
- Management of vital statistics and the status of special groups or groups at greater risk.
- Assessment of the performance of health services.
- Identification of those nonsectoral resources that support health promotion and improvements in the quality of life.
- Development of technology, expertise and methodologies for management, analysis and communication of information to those responsible for public health (including key players from other sectors, health care providers and civil society).
- Identifying and establishing agencies that evaluate and accurately analyze the quality of collected data.

Indicators

1.1 Guidelines and Processes for Monitoring Health Status

Standard
The NHA:

- Has guidelines for measuring health status at all levels of the health system.
- Has a comprehensive and integrated national system for monitoring health status, focusing on identifying inequities.

- Has specific protocols that protect the confidentiality of personal data.
- Uses health status profiles to allocate resources and prioritize community health problems based on criteria of equity.
- Uses trending in health status parameters, correlations with risk factors, gender analysis and other relevant variables to monitor health status.

1.1.1 The NHA has developed guidelines for measuring and evaluating the health status of the population.

Have the guidelines or other instruments for monitoring health status:

1.1.1.1 Been developed for use by the health system at the national level?

1.1.1.2 Been developed for use by the health system at intermediate levels?

1.1.1.3 Been developed for use by the health system at local levels?

1.1.1.4 Described suitable methods for collecting data and selecting appropriate sources of information which provide that data?

1.1.1.5 Described the roles of the national and subnational levels in collecting data?

1.1.1.6 Given citizens and organized community groups access to information while at the same time protecting the right to privacy?

1.1.1.7 Included a process that continuously improves information systems to better meet user needs at both national and subnational levels (decisionmakers, program directors, etc.)?

If so, does the process:

1.1.1.7.1 Include uniform standards at all levels (national and subnational) of the information system?

1.1.1.7.2 Include procedures that provide information to national and international agencies that form part of the health system?

1.1.1.7.3 Include a periodic review of standards and procedures that evaluate their relevance in view of the technological advances and changes in health policy?

1.1.1.8 Described procedures for communicating information to the mass media and general public?

1.1.1.9 Protected the confidentiality of information through the use of specific protocols for accessing data?

1.1.1.10 Described the procedures to organize a health status profile that contains information on national health objectives?

1.1.2 The NHA identifies and annually updates the data collected in a country health status profile.

Does this profile include:

1.1.2.1 Social and demographic variables?

1.1.2.2 Mortality data?

1.1.2.3 Morbidity data?

1.1.2.4 Data on risk factors?

1.1.2.5 Information on lifestyles?

1.1.2.6 Data on environmental risks?

1.1.2.7 Data on access to personal health services?

1.1.2.8 Data on contact with population-based health services?

1.1.2.9 Data on utilization of population-based and personal health services?

1.1.2.10 Data on cultural barriers in accessing health care?

1.1.3 The NHA uses the health status profile.

Is the health profile used:

1.1.3.1 To monitor the health needs of the population?

1.1.3.2 To evaluate inequities in health conditions?

1.1.3.3 To monitor trends in health status?

1.1.3.4 To monitor changes in the prevalence of risk factors?

1.1.3.5 To monitor changes in utilization of health services?

1.1.3.6 To determine the adequacy and significance of reported data?

1.1.3.7 To identify the population's priorities and needs in terms of access to services, participation in health promotion activities, resource allocation, focusing on the elimination of inequities in access and improving health services?

1.1.3.8   To define national health objectives and goals?

1.1.3.9   To evaluate compliance with national health objectives and goals?

1.1.3.10   To improve the efficiency and quality of the health system in discharging the essential public health functions by the NHA?

1.1.3.11   Can you cite an example where this profile has been used?

1.1.4   The NHA disseminates information on the health status of the population.

Does the NHA:

1.1.4.1   Produce an annual report?

1.1.4.2   Disseminate this report and its information to interested parties?

1.1.4.3   Present this report to groups of key decisionmakers in the country?

1.1.4.4   Regularly organize seminars or other activities that explain and raise awareness of key decisionmakers about the implications of the information on the health status of the population contained in the annual report?

1.1.4.5   Provide data on trends in health outcomes, comparing them with standards and goals specifically mentioned in the profile?

1.1.4.6   Provide communities with a common set of measures that help them make comparisons, prioritize community health problems and determine allocation of resources?

1.1.4.7   Periodically solicit and evaluate suggestions that improve the content, presentation and dissemination of the health profile?

1.1.4.8   Regularly evaluate how the recipients of the health profile report use the information?

1.2 Evaluation of the Quality of Information

Standard

The NHA:

- Has objective instruments to evaluate the quality of the information generated by the different levels of the health system.
- Has protocols and standards for producing, analyzing and interpreting data so that the instruments used are compara-

ble throughout the country and allow international comparisons as accepted by the country.

- Continuously updates these instruments, protocols and standards in concordance with advances in technology and knowledge, as well as with local information needs.
- Collaborates with other national institutions in producing relevant data for monitoring health status so as to ensure the quality of the data.

1.2.1   The NHA has a unit that evaluates the quality of the information generated by the health system.

1.2.1.1   Is the unit outside the direct control of the NHA?

1.2.1.2   Does the unit conduct periodic audits of the information system that assesses the country's health status?

1.2.1.3   Does the unit suggest modifications to the system in areas recognized as being weak or in need of improvement?

1.2.1.4   Does the NHA take into consideration the suggestions made by the evaluation unit for improving the measurement of health status?

1.2.2   The NHA is part of an national coordinating agency for statistics.

Do the NHA and the national coordinating agency for statistics:

1.2.2.1   Meet at least once a year to propose modifications to the information systems to make these systems more compatible?

1.2.2.2   Take the proposed modifications into account to improve the NHK's information systems?

1.2.2.3   Propose specific measures to improve the quality and usefulness of information from the NHA?

1.2.2.4   Know the percentage of medically certified deaths known?

If so,

1.2.2.4.1   Does the NHA consider that this percentage makes the mortality data reliable?

1.3 Expert Support and Resources for Monitoring Health Status

Standard

The NHA:

- Has personnel skilled in the collection, evaluation, management, translation, interpretation, dissemination, and communication of health status data.
- Has developed specialized monitoring and evaluation capacities based on the characteristics of the country's health profile.
- Has access to expertise and resources necessary to convert data into useful information for individuals who influence health policy and also for community leaders and representatives involved in the planning of health activities.
- Has the above capacities at the different levels of the public health system within which the national level should have (or have access to) at least one professional with a doctorate in epidemiology.

1.3.1 The NHA uses or has access to personnel with training and expertise in epidemiology and statistics.

Does this personnel have expertise in the following areas:

1.3.1.1 Was this personnel trained in epidemiology at the Doctoral level?

1.3.1.2 Sampling methodologies for collecting qualitative and quantitative data?

1.3.1.3 Consolidating data from various sources?

1.3.1.4 Data analysis?

1.3.1.5 Interpreting results and formulating scientifically valid conclusions based on the data analyzed?

1.3.1.6 Translating data into clear and useful information to produce comprehensible and well-designed documents for different audiences?

1.3.1.7 Design and maintenance of disease registries (e.g. cancer registries)?

1.3.1.8 Communicating health information to decision makers and members of community organizations?

1.3.1.9 Research and quantitative analysis?

1.3.2 The intermediate levels of the NHA use or have access to personnel with training and expertise in epidemiology and statistics.

Does this personnel have training and expertise in the following areas:

1.3.2.1 Sampling schemes for data collection?

1.3.2.2 Consolidating data from various sources?

1.3.2.3 Data analysis?

1.3.2.4 Interpreting results and formulating scientifically valid conclusions based on data analyzed?

1.3.2.5 Translating data into clear and useful information?

1.3.2.6 Design and maintenance of disease registries (e.g., cancer registries)?

1.3.2.7 Communicating health information to the population?

1.3.2.8 Communicating health information to decisionmakers?

1.3.2.9 Was this personnel trained in public health at the Master's degree level?

1.4 Technical Support for Monitoring and Evaluating Health Status

Standard

The NHA:

- Has computer resources for monitoring and evaluating health status at all levels
- Is capable of sharing data from various sources and converting them to standard formats.
- Uses a high-speed computer network to link with other agencies and individuals in the national and international arena.
- Ensures that those at all levels of the public health system who access these computerized data systems and registries are trained in the proper use of these resources.

1.4.1 The NHA utilizes computer resources to monitor the health status of the country's population.
Does the NHA:

1.4.1.1 Utilize computer resources to monitor the health status of the country's population at the intermediate levels?

1.4.1.2 Utilize computer resources to monitor the health status of the population at the local level?

1.4.1.3 Have personnel trained in the use and basic maintenance of these computer resources?

1.4.1.4 Use a system that includes one or more computers with high-speed processors?

1.4.1.5 Have programs with commonly used utilities (word processors, spreadsheets, graphic design and presentation software)?

1.4.1.6 Have the capacity to convert data from various sources to standard formats?

1.4.1.7 Have a dedicated line and high-speed access to the Internet?

1.4.1.8 Have electronic communication with the subnational levels that generate and utilize information?

1.4.1.9 Have sufficient storage capacity to maintain the databases on the country's health profile?

1.4.1.10 Meet the design requirements for compiling vital statistics?

1.4.1.11 Have rapid access to specialized maintenance of the computer system?

1.4.1.12 Annually assess its need for upgrading its computer resources?

1.4.1.13 Can you give an example in which computer resources were used to monitor health status?

1.5 Technical Assistance and Support to the Subnational Levels of Public Health in Monitoring, Evaluating and Analysis of Health Status

Standard

The NHA:

- Collaborates with the subnational levels to ensure the timely collection, analysis and dissemination of data that support the development and evaluation of health policies.
- Offers mechanisms for training and practice to professional at the subnational levels in interpreting and using data.
- Supports the preparation and publication of community health profile and informs the entire jurisdiction of the availability of this support.

1.5.1 During the past 12 months, the NHA has provided technical assistance to one or more subnational levels in data collection and analysis.

1.5.1.1 Has the NHA advised the subnational levels on the design of instruments for collecting relevant health data?

1.5.1.2 Have all subnational levels been informed of the NHK's availability to advise them on data collection methodology?

1.5.1.3 Have the subnational levels been informed of the NHK's availability to advise them on methodology for the analysis of data collected locally?

1.5.1.4 During the past 12 months, has the NHA actually advised one or more subnational levels on the methodology to analyze data collected locally?

1.5.2 During the past 12 months, the NHA has constantly disseminated information periodically to users at the subnational levels.

1.5.2.1 Has feedback been sought from these users of this information?

1.5.2.2 Have these users been advised on how to interpret these analyses?

1.5.2.3 During the past 12 months, has the NHA advised those responsible for producing the community health profile at the subnational levels?

1.5.2.3.1 Have those responsible for publishing the community health profile been informed that provisions exist to advise them on this?

EPHF 2: Public Health Surveillance, Research, and Control of Risks and Threats to Public Health

Definition

This function includes:

- The capacity to conduct research and surveillance of epidemic outbreaks, patterns of communicable and noncommunicable disease, injury and exposure to toxic substances or environmental agents harmful to health.

- A public health services infrastructure designed to conduct population screenings, case-finding and general epidemiological research.

- Public health laboratories capable of conducting rapid screening and processing of a high volume of tests necessary for identifying and controlling emerging threats to health.

- The development of active programs for epidemiological surveillance and control of infectious diseases.

- The capacity to link with international networks to allow better management of health problems.

- Preparedness of the NHA to initiate a rapid response for the control of health problems or specific risks.

Indicators

2.1 Surveillance System to Identify Threats to Public Health

Standard

The NHA:

- Operates one or more, ideally integrated, public health surveillance systems[1] in collaboration with local and intermediate levels capable of identifying and analyzing threats to public health.

- Assumes leadership in defining the roles and responsibilities of the system's key personnel and in developing communication and epidemiological response networks that provide feedback to the subnational levels.

- Identifies public health threats and risk factors in the country.

- Is prepared to respond rapidly at all levels of the surveillance system to control the problems detected.

2.1.1. The NHA has a surveillance system in place with the capacity to detect risks and threats to health in a timely manner.

    2.1.1.1. Is the surveillance system capable of analyzing the nature and magnitude of the threats?

2.1.1.2. Is the surveillance system capable of monitoring threats and health hazards over time?

2.1.1.3. Is the surveillance system capable of monitoring changes in living conditions that call for a public health response?

2.1.1.4. Can the surveillance system identify those threats that call for a public health response?

2.1.1.5. Is the system integrated with surveillance systems at the subnational levels?

2.1.1.6. Does the surveillance system provide information for the production and dissemination of periodic bulletins?

2.1.1.7. Does the surveillance system process systematic feedback on its publications?

2.1.1.8. Have the threat response roles of key individuals in the surveillance system been defined at subnational levels (especially the local levels)?

2.1.1.9. Does the surveillance system regularly analyze trends in disease, threats and risk factors?

2.1.1.10. Does the surveillance system include information from other health surveillance systems (e.g. private insurers or service providers, NGOs, etc.)?

2.1.1.11. Is the surveillance system part of an international surveillance system?

2.1.1.12. Does the surveillance system include activities that describe the nature and implications of the information generated?

2.2 Capacities and Expertise in Public Health Surveillance

Standard

The NHA:

- Has sufficient epidemiological expertise[2] at the national and subnational levels to develop and disseminate written protocols that help identify and analyze priority problems and health risks.

---

[1]Having an integrated epidemiological surveillance system for various problems is the ideal, provided that the effectiveness of the surveillance systems already in place is not compromised by the integration process.

---

[2] In the case of small countries, this expertise can be concentrated at the international level.

- Has access to clinical and environmental services capable of conducting rapid population screening and environmental sampling.
- Conducts timely analyses of threats to health and health risks, using inputs from the above services, as well as other epidemiological surveillance systems at subnational levels (e.g. private insurance or private clinic data).
- Directly conducts or solicits research from other institutions on leading public health threats.

2.2.1. The NHA has sufficient expertise in public health surveillance to analyze threats and risks to public health.

Does this include expertise in:

2.2.1.1   The capacity to develop written protocols for identifying threats to public health?

2.2.1.2   Forensic medical services? (e.g. pathology, medico-legal, police laboratories, etc).

2.2.1.3   Management and use of geographic information systems?

If so,

2.2.1.3.1   Does the NHA have in use an active geographic information system?

2.2.1.4   Basic sanitation?

2.2.1.5   Environmental health and toxicology?

2.2.1.6   Analyzing and conducting demographic (population-based) research on infectious diseases?

2.2.1.7   Analyzing and conducting demographic (population-based) research on chronic diseases?

2.2.1.8   Analyzing and conducting demographic (population-based) research on injury?

2.2.1.9   Mental health?

2.2.1.10   Occupational health

2.2.1.11   Rapid epidemiological evaluation methods (aggregate sampling, detection of risk factors, rapid survey methods, etc.)?

2.2.1.12   Conducting rapid screening of at-risk populations or populations for which specific health problems have been reported?

2.2.1.13   Conducting rapid environmental sampling in response to reports of environmental health risks?

2.2.1.14   Designing new surveillance systems for emerging health problems?

2.2.2   The NHA regularly evaluates information generated by the public health surveillance system.

2.2.2.1   Does the NHA annually evaluate the quality of the information generated by the public health surveillance system?

2.2.2.2   Does the NHA annually evaluate the use of this information?

2.2.2.3   Has the NHA conducted or requested research that provides a greater understanding of problems representing threats to public health?

If so,

2.2.2.3.1   Can you give an example of such research conducted during the past 12 months?

2.2.2.4   Has the NHA used the results of this research to improve its epidemiological surveillance system?

2.3 Capacity of Public Health Laboratories

Standard

The NHA:

- Has a national public health laboratory network of growing complexity with the capacity to support epidemiological surveillance and research.
- Complies strictly with the norms and standards for accreditation and evaluation with respect to the public health laboratories' personnel, equipment, physical structure and security, exercising quality control over their procedures.
- Has the capacity to carry out all procedures for diagnosing diseases subject to compulsory notification and that require epidemiological surveillance.
- Ensures that network laboratories have the capacity to exchange information with other participating laboratories, standardizing their procedures with those of a national reference laboratory.
- Ensures that the national reference laboratory effectively coordinates with international reference laboratories.
- Ensures that the public health laboratory network has mechanisms in place to utilize information received from public and private laboratories to monitor diseases.

- Oversees strict compliance with the norms, accreditation standards, and protocols for handling, storing and transporting samples collected by public and private laboratories.
- Ensures a timely response by which laboratories are capable of analyzing clinical or environmental samples in epidemic outbreaks or changes in disease behavior.

2.3.1. The NHA has a laboratory network capable of supporting epidemiological surveillance and research.

2.3.1.1   Does the laboratory network have the capacity to identify the causative agents of all reportable diseases in the country?

2.3.1.2   Does the laboratory network maintain an up-to-date list of laboratories capable of performing specialized analyses that meet needs indicated by surveillance?

2.3.1.3   Does the laboratory network have strict protocols for the handling, transportation, and storage of samples collected by public or private laboratories?

2.3.1.4   Does the laboratory network have formal mechanisms for coordination and reference between the national public health laboratory network and one or more international laboratories of recognized excellence?

2.3.1.5   Does the laboratory network periodically evaluate the quality of the results from the network's reference laboratory by comparing them with results from an international reference laboratory?

2.3.1.6   Does the laboratory network have standardized procedures for obtaining information from private and public laboratories to monitor specific diseases?

   If so,

   2.3.1.6.1   Have some of these procedures been evaluated to determine their effectiveness in specific situations?

2.3.1.7   Is the laboratory network capable of meeting routine epidemiological surveillance needs?

2.3.1.8   Does the laboratory network have a mechanism that determines the degree of compli-

ance with regulations for certifying the quality of laboratories within the network?

If so, have these public health laboratories:

2.3.1.8.1   Complied strictly with the regulations governing certification of the quality of these laboratories within the network?

2.4 Capacity for Timely[3] and Effective Response to Control Public Health Problems

Standard

The NHA:

- Is capable of responding promptly and effectively at all its levels to control public health problems.
- Evaluates the capacity of its system to respond in a timely and effective manner.
- Ensures that the subnational levels have the human resources and infrastructure necessary for this response.
- Promotes ongoing evaluation of the intersectoral links necessary to respond at all levels.
- Ensures that organized action in response to public health threats is systematically evaluated, indicating deficiencies for subsequent correction.
- Ensures that constantly active mechanisms for communication between the various levels are in place.
- Ensures that appropriate, timely and educational public information for the control of public health problems is made available and disseminated.
- Ensures that the response of levels closest to the problem is automatic and does not require waiting on a national response or directives.

2.4.1. The NHA has the capacity to respond in a timely and effective manner to public health problems.

   Does the NHA:

   2.4.1.1   Have protocols and procedure manuals in line with surveillance information to provide a rapid response to health and environmental threats?

---

[3] "Timely" refers to acting within a time frame that permits effective public health intervention for each specific problem.

322

2.4.1.2 Define the responsibilities for personnel who maintain active communication between the different components of the surveillance system?

2.4.1.3 Promote in its procedural manuals and standards the importance of a rapid, autonomous response by the levels closest to the health problem?

2.4.1.4 Have formal mechanisms in place to recognize good performance by surveillance teams?

2.4.1.5 Have formal mechanisms in place to recognize good performance by teams responding to emergencies?

2.4.1.6 Has the NHA detected public health threats in a timely manner in the past 24 months?

If so,
2.4.1.6.1 Can you give an example of such a detection?

2.4.2 The NHA evaluates the response capacity of its surveillance system to each health emergency that it has had to confront.

Does the NHA:

2.4.2.1 Communicate the results of the system evaluation to all those who contribute information to the system in order to correct any deficiencies identified?

2.4.2.2 Oversee implementation of these corrective actions in order to improve response capacity?

2.5 Technical Assistance and Support for the Subnational Levels in Public Health Surveillance, Research, and Control of Risks and Threats to Public Health

Standard
The NHA:

- Guides and supports the subnational public health systems in identifying and analyzing public health threats.
- Informs subnational levels how to access the public health laboratory network.
- Provides guidelines, protocols, standards, consultations and training in the epidemiological methods to the subnational levels.

- Provides information on best practices in public health, including current research findings on the most effective methods of disease prevention and control.
- Ensures that communication systems between all levels are simple, expeditious and based on widely used software.

2.5.1 The NHA provides technical assistance and support to the subnational levels to develop their surveillance capacity.

Does the NHA:

2.5.1.1 Conduct an assessment of its needs for specialized personnel, training, equipment, maintenance of equipment and other needs for surveillance at the subnational levels?

If so,
2.5.1.1.1. Does it utilize this assessment to prioritize the contracting, training and investment in the epidemiological surveillance system?

2.5.1.2 Inform all subnational levels how to access the public health laboratory network?

2.5.1.3 Provide information and training to the subnational levels in critical areas to ensure the quality of the work of the subnational levels?

2.5.1.4 Advise the subnational levels how to respond to queries on what to do when faced with an emergency?

2.5.1.5 Define the responsibilities for personnel at subnational levels on how to communicate with those responsible for the central management of the surveillance system?

2.5.1.6 Inform the subnational levels of the availability of experts from the national level for collaboration in dealing with public health emergencies?

2.5.1.7 Have simple and effective standards for communication between the different levels of the surveillance system?

2.5.1.8 Disseminate information to the subnational levels on the current status of the diseases under constant surveillance?

2.5.1.9 Disseminate information to the subnational levels on "best practices" in disease control?

2.5.1.10 Disseminate guidelines to the subnational levels for developing plans to deal with public health emergencies?

2.5.1.11 Receive periodic and regular reports from the subnational levels on trends and disease behavior under constant surveillance?

EPHF 3: Health Promotion[4]

Definition

This function includes:

- The promotion of changes in lifestyle and environmental[5] conditions to facilitate the development of a "culture of health."
- The strengthening of intersectoral partnerships for more effective health promotion activities.
- Assessment of the impact of public policies on health.
- Educational and social communication activities aimed at promoting healthy conditions, lifestyles, behaviors and environments.
- Reorientation of the health services to develop models of care that encourage health promotion.

Indicators

3.1 Support for Health Promotion Activities, Development of Norms, and Interventions to Promote Healthy Behaviors and Environments

Standard

The NHA:

- Has a health promotion policy that is in accordance with relevant sectoral and extrasectoral actors.
- Implements health promotion strategies at all levels, both intra- and extra-sectoral, that respond to the health needs of the population.

- Assists local communities in creating incentives for the development of effective health promotion initiatives that are integrated with personal health care and other related extrasectoral programs.
- Promotes interventions and regulations that encourage healthy behaviors and environments.
- Creates incentives for the subnational levels to develop and implement health promotion and education activities accessible to the population.

3.1.1 The NHA has a written statement of its health promotion policy.

3.1.1.1 Does the NHA take into account the recommendations of international conferences in this area?[6]

3.1.1.2 Does the NHA take advantage of information technology to facilitate health promotion?

3.1.1.3 Has the NHA clearly defined its short- and long-term goals in health promotion?

If so, have these goals been established for:
3.1.1.3.1 The national level?
3.1.1.3.2 The intermediate levels?
3.1.1.3.3 The local level—for example, Healthy Cities or similar strategies?

3.1.2 The NHA has established an incentive system that encourages the participation of the subnational levels, private institutions, other public-sector institutions, and community organizations in health promotion activities.

Has the NHA:
3.1.2.1 Conducted an annual evaluation of this incentives system?

If so,
3.1.2.1.1 Are modifications to this system based on the results of the evaluation?

Does the NHA:
3.1.2.2 Have national recognitions for excellence in health promotion?

---

[4] This function encompasses the definition of the capacities specifically required to implement, from the perspective of the NHA, the components of health promotion defined in the Ottawa Charter and reaffirmed in the recent Global Conference on Health Promotion in Mexico. Since it has been considered necessary to define another essential function to cover social participation, this latter has concentrated on defining capacities that largely facilitate health promotion.

[5] In this context, the term environment encompasses a wider scope than just physical environment, but also includes social and cultural environment.

[6] That is, the global conferences in Ottawa, Jakarta, and Mexico, among other meetings on this topic.

3.1.2.3 Finance trainings, attendance at health promotion events, etc.

3.1.2.4 Provide funding for health promotion projects on a competitive basis?

3.1.2.5 Can you mention an example of an incentive provided in the past 12 months to a private institution?

3.1.2.6 Can you mention an example of an incentive provided in the past 12 months to a nonprofit, nongovernmental organization?

3.1.2.7 Can you mention an example of an incentive provided in the past 12 months to a community organization?

3.1.3 The NHA encourages the development of standards and interventions that promote healthy behaviors and environments.

3.1.3.1 Has the NHA identified a set of standards that promote healthy behaviors and environments?

3.1.3.2 Does the NHA annually plan the course to follow in preparing standards that promote healthy behaviors and environments?

3.1.3.3 Does the NHA have a policy designed that encourages the development of interventions promoting healthy behaviors and environments?

If so,

3.1.3.3.1 Can you mention an example of the above interventions that have implemented in the past 12 months?

3.1.3.3.2 Are the results of the interventions evaluated at least once a year?

3.1.3.3.3 Has the course of action ever been modified as a result of the evaluation?

3.2 Building Sectoral and Extrasectoral Partnerships for Health Promotion

<u>Standard</u>

The NHA:

- Ensures that activities carried out reinforce the actions of State institutions and are consistent with defined health priorities at subnational levels.
- Has the support of a broad-based action and advisory group that guides the process to improve health.
- Enters into partnerships with governmental and nongovernmental organizations that contribute to or benefit from the essential public health functions, creating incentives to promote the development of linkages at the subnational levels.
- Periodically reports on health priorities, actions to strengthen health promotion, public health policies and engages in advocacy for the establishment of those policies.
- Monitors and evaluates the health impact of extrasectoral public policies, taking corrective action based on the results of the evaluation.

3.2.1 The NHA has access to a coordinating unit[7] that brings together representatives from community organizations, the private sector, and other government sectors to plan initiatives for meeting health promotion targets.

3.2.1.1 Is there a plan of action with explicit responsibilities for individuals who belong to this coordinating unit?

If so,

3.2.1.1.1 Does the plan of action take into account the health status profile as well as the country's health needs?

3.2.1.1.2 Is health promotion evaluated periodically and are results of this evaluation communicated to members of the coordinating unit?

3.2.1.1.3 Does the plan of action describe corrective measures based on the results of the evaluation?

3.2.1.1.4 Is a report issued each year to key decisionmakers about the activities of the health promotion coordinating unit?

3.2.1.2 During the past 12 months, has the NHA carried out some national promotional ac-

---

[7] This coordinating unit may be located outside of the NHA.

tivity in conjunction with another organization or sector?

If so, has the NHA:

3.2.1.2.1 Evaluated the results of this intersectoral partnership?

3.2.1.2.2 Has it reported the results of this evaluation to its collaborators?

3.2.1.2.3 Taken corrective action to improve the results based on this evaluation?

3.2.2 The NHA has the capacity to measure the health impact of the public policies generated by other sectors.

3.2.2.1 Does it have access to personnel proficient in the use of multifactoral epidemiological analysis?

3.2.2.2 Are resources allocated to measure the health impact of public policies?

3.2.3 The NHA works to promote the development of healthy social and economic policies.

Does the NHA:

3.2.3.1 Identify and promote the definition and implementation of those policies having a greater probable impact on the health of individuals and the environment?

3.2.3.2 Monitor and assess the health impact of social and economic policies?

If so, can you cite an example of a health impact assessment conducted by the NHA with respect to:

3.2.3.2.1 Environmental policies?

3.2.3.2.2 Economic policies?

3.2.3.2.3 Social policies?

3.2.3.3 Advocate the strengthening of public policies in order to improve the population's health and environment?

If so, can you cite an example of advocacy conducted by the NHA with respect to:

3.2.3.3.1 Environmental policies?

3.2.3.3.2 Economic policies?

3.2.3.3.3 Social policies?

3.3 National Planning and Coordination of Information, Education, and Social Communication Strategies for Health Promotion

Standard

The NHA:

- Engages in a systematic effort to inform and educate the public to play on their role in improving health conditions.
- Collaborates with public and private, sectoral and extrasectoral agencies at various levels to carry out health promotion initiatives that ensure healthy lifestyles and behavior.
- Coordinates health promotion initiatives to ensure an integrated approach consistent with healthy lifestyles and behaviors.
- Supports the development of culturally and linguistically appropriate educational programs that target specific groups.
- Conducts health education campaigns through mass media, such as television, radio, and the press.
- Uses a variety of methods to disseminate health information to the entire population.
- Uses feedback from the population to annually evaluate the effectiveness and relevance of health promotion and education activities.

3.3.1 In the past 12 months, the NHA has developed and implemented a community education agenda that promotes initiatives to improve the health status of the population.

3.3.1.1 Was this agenda developed in collaboration with other public institutions?

3.3.1.2 Does this agenda include private institutions?

3.3.1.3 Does this agenda include input from the community?

3.3.1.4 Does this agenda include current scientific perspectives on communication in health?

3.3.1.5 Does this agenda include the most significant international recommendations on health promotion?

3.3.1.6 Does this agenda ensure nationwide consistency of health promotion activities?

3.3.1.7 Does this agenda include activities that make health promotion accessible to culturally diverse groups?

3.3.2 During the past 12 months, the NHA has conducted health promotion campaigns through the mass media.

Did the campaigns include:

3.3.2.1 The press?

3.3.2.2 Radio?

3.3.2.3 Television?

3.3.2.4 Internet?

3.3.2.5 Were campaign results evaluated through population surveys or focus groups?

If so, did this evaluation include:

3.3.2.5.1 Understanding of the messages?

3.3.2.5.2 Ability to access to the messages?

3.3.2.5.3 Results based on changes in knowledge of the population?

3.3.2.5.4 Results based on changes in behavior of the population?

3.3.2.5.5 Incorporation of the results in planning subsequent mass media campaigns?

3.3.3 The NHA has special systems in place for delivering information and educational materials to the population to promote health (e.g. information offices, websites, telephone hotlines, and other alternative media).

3.3.3.1 Does the NHA have a Web page for conveying useful health information?

If so,

3.3.3.1.1 Is utilization of this Web page evaluated periodically (at least every six months) by taking into account the number of hits and users' opinions?

3.3.3.2 Have the educational materials distributed in these media been updated in the past 12 months as a result of the evaluation?

3.3.3.3. Has the management of the information office (clearinghouse) and its usefulness been evaluated in the past 12 months?

3.3.3.4. Are the results periodically evaluated?

3.3.3.5. Does the NHA have a telephone hotline for conveying health promotion messages?

If so,

3.3.3.5.1 Is the use of the hotline evaluated at least every six months?

3.3.3.6 Does the NHA evaluate the usefulness of other alternative media in use?

3.4 Reorientation of the Health Services toward Health Promotion

Standard

The NHA:

- Promotes and facilitates dialogue and consensus among decisionmakers in order to maximize health promotion resources in providing health services.
- Has mechanisms in place that allocate resources to service providers, motivating them to adopt a health promotion approach.
- Reorients public health infrastructure to improve the performance of services from health promotion perspective.
- Includes health promotion criteria in the regulatory mechanisms governing certification and/or accreditation of health facilities, service provider networks, health professionals and health insurance plans.
- Emphasizes primary health care (PHC) and establishes programs through which providers assume responsibility for comprehensive community care.
- Strengthens the concept of health promotion in human resource development programs at all levels of the health system.
- Promotes consensus among experts on clinical guidelines that incorporate disease prevention and health promotion, as well as oversees their application.
- Encourages communication between service providers, communities and patients to make health care more effective and establishing joint responsibility for health care through specific commitments.

3.4.1. The NHA has discussed the importance of encouraging health promotion in the health services with other organizations and decisionmakers.

3.4.1.1 Has it provided evidence with respect to investing in promotion versus curative activities and the outcomes of such of activities?

3.4.1.2 Has it obtained a commitment from other organizations to support investments in health promotion activities in the delivery health services?

3.4.2 The NHA has developed strategies for reorienting health services using health promotion criteria.

    3.4.2.1.   Has the NHA established payment mechanisms to encourage health promotion in public insurance systems?

        If so, has the NHA

        3.4.2.1.1. Evaluated the results of these payment mechanisms in terms of fostering health promotion in health services?

    3.4.2.2   Has the NHA established payment mechanisms to foster health promotion in the private insurance systems?

        If so, has the NHA

        3.4.2.2.1 Evaluated the results of these payment mechanisms in terms of fostering health promotion in health services?

    3.4.2.3   Has the NHA drawn up a plan for developing public health infrastructure that encourages health promotion?

    3.4.2.4   Has the NHA drafted guidelines for the accreditation of health professionals that provide for training in health promotion?

    3.4.2.5   Has the NHA drafted guidelines for the accreditation of health facilities that provide for health promotion activities?

    3.4.2.6   Has the NHA encouraged health promotion interventions in the health insurance plans?

    3.4.2.7   Has the NHA promoted the use of clinical protocols validating effective practices in health promotion in personal health services?

        If so,

        3.4.2.7.1 Can you cite an example of such a protocol that is currently in use?

    3.4.2.8   Has the NHA promoted agreements that include a health promotion component and explicitly state the responsibilities of communities, patients and providers?

        If so,

    3.4.2.8.1 Can you cite an example that was achieved as a result of such an agreement?

3.4.3 The NHA has promoted the strengthening of primary health care (PHC).

Does the NHA:

    3.4.3.1   Promote population-based models of care for which health teams trained in health promotion are responsible?

    3.4.3.2   Promote incentives that encourage health teams to address health issues through health promotion?

    3.4.3.3   Provide health teams with the resources and authority needed to implement health promotion programs for target populations?

    3.4.3.4   Establish formal incentives in PHC to develop programs in health promotion that are geared towards communities and individuals?

3.4.4 Has the NHA strengthened its human resources development by using a health promotion approach?

Does the NHA:

    3.4.4.1   Encourage training centers related public health to include health promotion content in an effort to instill positive attitudes towards health promotion among students pursuing a career in health?

    3.4.4.2   Include a component on health promotion in continuing education programs for health personnel?

3.5 Technical Assistance and Support to the Subnational Levels to Strengthen Health Promotion Activities

Standard

The NHA:

- Has expertise in health promotion and shares this expertise with subnational levels.
- Ensures consistency of information with scientific evidence as well as adapting this information to the needs of the subnational levels.

- Encourages the subnational levels to make resources, facilities, and equipment available that maximize the impact of and access to health promotion and education in the country.

3.5.1 The NHA has the capacity and expertise to strengthen health promotion initiatives at the subnational levels.

Does the NHA have expertise in the following areas:

3.5.1.1. Health promotion at the workplace?

3.5.1.2. Health education?

3.5.1.3. Working with groups?

3.5.1.4. Social marketing?

3.5.1.5. Collaboration and advocacy with communication media?

3.5.1.6. Communication techniques?

3.5.1.7. Development of educational materials for health promotion suitable for various cultures?

If so,

3.5.1.7.1 Has an evaluation been conducted in the past 12 months of the education materials currently in use to determine whether they represent current knowledge and best practices for formulating health promotion messages?

3.5.1.7.2 Have the materials been evaluated to assess their cultural appropriateness for each country?

3.5.1.8 Have the subnational levels been informed of materials and expertise available at the national level and the willingness to support subnational efforts in health promotion?

3.5.1.9 Have the subnational levels received support in implementing specific health promotion activities in the past 12 months?

3.5.2 The NHA evaluates the need for health education specialists at the subnational levels.

3.5.2.1 Has the NHA prepared a plan to develop capacity in health education at the subnational level.

3.5.2.2 Has the NHA evaluated the results of the above plan and taken action based on the results of this evaluation?

3.5.2.3 Is there access to facilities and equipment that permit the development of educational materials?

If so, is there access to:

3.5.2.3.1 Graphic design software?

3.5.2.3.2 Professionals trained in the use of this technology?

3.5.2.4 Is there coordination between actors who have the capacity to implement health promotion activities?

If so,

3.5.2.4.1 Can you cite examples of coordinated action with these actors in the past year?

3.5.3 The NHA uses media and technologies at the national level to maximize the impact of health promotion and access to it in the country.

Are the following resources utilized:

3.5.3.1 Radio programs?

3.5.3.2 Community educational theater?

3.5.3.3 Television programs?

3.5.3.4 Video-conferencing?

3.5.3.5 Professionals trained in the use of these media?

EPHF 4:   Social Participation in Health

Definition

This function includes:

- Strengthening the power of civil society to change their lifestyles and play an active role in the development of healthy behaviors and environments in order to influence the decisions that affect their health and their access to adequate health services.

- Facilitating the participation of the community in decisions and actions with regard to programs for disease prevention and the diagnosis, treatment and restoration of health in order to improve the health status of the population and promote environments that foster healthy lifestyles.

Indicators

4.1 Empowering Civil Society for Decision-Making in Public Health

Standard
The NHA:

- Guarantees permanent mechanisms for consulting with the civil society to receive and respond to public opinion on those behaviors and environmental conditions that impact public health.
- Promotes the development of entities that protect the rights of persons as members of civil society, consumers and users of the health system.
- Reports, in a timely manner, to civil society, the health status of the population and the performance of public and private health services.

4.1.1   The NHA ensures the existence and operation of mechanisms for consulting citizens and obtaining community feedback on matters of public health.

    4.1.1.1   Has the NHA established formal entities to consult civil society?[8]

    If so, do these entities exist and operate:
    4.1.1.1.1   At the national level?
    4.1.1.1.2   At the intermediate level?
    4.1.1.1.3   At the local level?

    4.1.1.2   Does the NHA have other means for obtaining the opinion and feedback from civil society?

    If so, do these operate:
    4.1.1.2.1   At the national level?
    4.1.1.2.2   At the intermediate level?
    4.1.1.2.3   At the local level?

    4.1.1.3   Does the NHA have mechanisms in place allowing it to respond to the opinions given by civil society?

    If so, are these mechanisms in place:
    4.1.1.3.1   At the national level?
    4.1.1.3.2   At the intermediate level?
    4.1.1.3.3   At the local level?

---

[8] Examples of these entities are complaints offices, consultative health boards or commissions, and the health commissions of community organizations.

4.1.2   The country has an agency that acts as an ombudsman in matters related to health.

    4.1.2.1   Is this entity independent of the State?

    4.1.2.2   Is this entity empowered to take legal and/or public action to protect people and their right to health in relation to personal health care, both public and private?

    4.1.2.3   Is this entity empowered to take legal and/or public action to protect people and their right to health in relation to population-based health services?

    4.1.2.4   Does this entity have the capacity to engage in social and civic action in health on behalf of persons with limited resources and who are victims of discrimination?

4.1.3   The NHA reports to the public on the health situation and on the performance of personal and population-based health services.

    4.1.3.1   Is this report issued at least every two years?

    4.1.3.2   Are the report's findings distributed to communication media?

    4.1.3.3   Are the report's findings distributed to community groups?

    4.1.3.4   Are there formal channels available for the public to give feedback on the findings?

    4.1.3.5   Are changes in policy, resulting from deficiencies identified in the report, communicated to the public?

4.2 Strengthening of Social Participation in Health

Standard
The NHA:

- Promotes the building of partnerships in health at all levels.
- Develops and uses mechanisms at all levels to inform and educate civil society about their rights and responsibilities in health.
- Maintains an accessible information system containing a directory of organizations that work, or could potentially work, in public health initiatives, as well as provides access to information on "best practices" in social participation in health.

- Defines the objectives and goals of public health at the different levels in conjunction with the community, promoting the development of public health projects managed by civil society.
- Periodically evaluates its capacity to strengthen social participation in health and introduces in a timely manner changes recommended by these evaluations.

4.2.1 The NHA has established a policy that considers social participation the key to setting and meeting its goals and objectives in public health.

4.2.1.1 Does the NHA take into consideration social participation when defining its public health goals and objectives?

If so, is this social participation considered:
4.2.1.1.1. At the national level?
4.2.1.1.2. At the intermediate level?
4.2.1.1.3. At the local level?

4.2.1.2 Does the NHA take into account input provided by civil society through social participation in health?

4.2.1.3 Has the NHA established formal entities that strengthen social participation in health?

If so, do these entities operate:
4.2.1.3.1 At the national level?
4.2.1.3.2 At the intermediate level?
4.2.1.3.3 At the local level?

4.2.1.4 Does civil society participate in decision-making that affects the administration of health services?

If so, is this done:
4.2.1.4.1 At the national level?
4.2.1.4.2 At the intermediate level?
4.2.1.4.3 At the local level?

4.2.1.5 Can you cite an example in which a public health objective was defined through social participation?

4.2.1.6 Does the NHA have programs that inform and educate the public about its rights to health?

If so, are these programs:
4.2.1.6.1 At the national level?
4.2.1.6.2 At the intermediate level?
4.2.1.6.3 At the local level?

4.2.2 The NHA has staff trained to promote community participation in personal and population-based health programs.

If so, is this staff adequately trained in:
4.2.2.1 Methodologies that facilitate group participation?
4.2.2.2 Planning and coordination of community action in health?
4.2.2.3 Leadership, group work, and conflict resolution?
4.2.2.4 Development of strategies for social participation in health?
4.2.2.5 Building partnerships within the community?

4.2.3 The NHA encourages and promotes the development of best practice in social participation in health.

If so, does the NHA:
4.2.3.1 Have a directory of organizations that can collaborate in developing population-based and personal community health initiatives?
4.2.3.2 Disseminate information about successful social participation initiatives?
4.2.3.3 Allocate resources for the development of public health programs managed by civil society?

If so,
4.2.3.3.1 Can you mention a civil society group that has received such funding in the past year?

4.2.3.4 Does the NHA facilitate the organization of meetings, seminars, workshops and other venues to discuss community health issues?

If so, is this done:
4.2.3.4.1 At the national level?
4.2.3.4.2 At the intermediate level?
4.2.3.4.3 At the local level?

4.2.3.5 Does the NHA assist other organizations with the preparation of these meetings?

If so,
4.2.3.5.1 Can you recall at least one example of this type of meeting in the past year?

4.2.3.6 Is there access to adequate facilities–including meeting rooms, audiovisual equipment, and supplies—to convene a wide range of meetings for social participation in health?

If so, are these facilities available:
4.2.3.6.1 At the national level?
4.2.3.6.2 At the intermediate level?
4.2.3.6.3 At the local level?

4.2.4 The NHA evaluates its capacity to promote social participation in health.

4.2.4.1 Does it evaluate this capacity annually?
4.2.4.2 Are changes suggested by the findings of the evaluations incorporated into future strategies?
4.2.4.3 Are policy changes resulting from the evaluations communicated to partners in social participation?

4.3 Technical Assistance and Support to the Subnational Levels to Strengthen Social Participation in Health

Standard
The NHA:

- Provides assistance as needed to the subnational levels in developing and strengthening of mechanisms for participation in decision-making in health.
- Provides assistance as needed to the subnational levels in creating and maintaining partnerships with civil society and organized community groups.
- Supports the subnational authorities in building relationships with the community.
- Supports community leadership efforts to identify and utilize best practices in public health through partnerships.
- Uses evidence-based technical support to help the subnational levels improve their capacity to encourage social participation.
- Encourages the development of local community groups and provides technical support for this development process.

4.3.1 The NHA advises and supports the subnational levels in the development and strengthening of their social participation mechanisms for decision-making in public health.

Does this support include:
4.3.1.1 Providing Information to the subnational levels on experiences in this area?
4.3.1.2 Convening advisory groups and executive committees with a focus on social participation and partnership building?
4.3.1.3 Evaluating the results of social participation in health and partnership building within the community?
4.3.1.4 Creating formal bodies to consult civil society?
4.3.1.5 Designing systems to obtain public opinion in health?
4.3.1.6 Designing and implementing systems to respond to public opinion in health?
4.3.1.7 Designing public accountability mechanisms?[9]
4.3.1.8 Implementing effective mechanisms for conflict resolution in the community?
4.3.1.9 Building community networks?
4.3.1.10 Implementing intervention methods that promote community organization in health?
4.3.1.11 Supporting the organization of social participation activities at the local level?
4.3.1.12 Facilitating partnerships to improve community health?

EPHF 5: Development of Policies and Institutional Capacity for Planning and Management in Public Health

Definition

This function includes:

- The definition of national and subnational public health objectives which should be measurable and consistent with a values-based framework that favors equity.
- The development, monitoring and evaluation of policy decisions in public health through a participatory process.

---

[9] "Accountability" refers to the formal process whereby the NHA periodically conveys to the community the results of its activities and obtains its opinion to improve its performance in the future.

- The institutional capacity for the management of public health systems, including strategic planning with emphasis on building, implementing and evaluating initiatives designed to focus on health problems of the population.
- The development of competencies for evidence-based decision-making, planning and evaluation, leadership capacity and effective communication, organizational development and resource management.
- Capacity-building for securing international cooperation in public health.

Indicators

5.1 Definition of National and Subnational Health Objectives

<u>Standard</u>
The NHA:

- Defines national and subnational objectives to improve the health of the population, taking the most recent health profile into account.
- Identifies, in conjunction with key actors, health priorities that take into account the heterogeneity of the country, recommending measurable health objectives and proposing a joint effort to attain these objectives.
- Ensures the coherence of national and subnational health objectives.
- Identifies and develops indicators of improvement and measures of their success as part of an extensive and continuous plan to improve health status.
- Promotes and facilitates the development of partnerships with key groups involved in the financing, purchasing and delivery of health services.

5.1.1   The NHA heads a national health improvement process aimed at developing national and subnational health objectives.

    5.1.1.1   Does the NHA seek the input of key actors in identifying priorities at the national and subnational levels?

    5.1.1.2   Does the NHA develop a plan with national goals and objectives that is closely related to national health priorities for a defined period?
    If so,

5.1.1.2.1.   Are these health goals and objectives based on the current health status profile?

5.1.1.2.2.   Are these health goals and objectives based on previously defined health priorities?

5.1.1.2.3.   Are these health goals and objectives consistent with other national development objectives within the framework of social policy?

5.1.1.2.4.   Does adequate financing exist to execute plans and programs aimed at attaining the health goals and objectives?

5.1.1.2.5.   Does the NHA seek the input from community representatives in defining health goals and objectives?

5.1.1.2.6.   Does the NHA identify those individuals and organizations responsible for achieving the defined health goals and objectives?

5.1.1.2.7.   Does the NHA develop performance indicators that measure the level of achievement of the defined health goals and objectives?

    If so,
    5.1.1.2.7.1   Does this measurement process include indicators for each of the policies, activities and/or components of the plan?

5.1.1.2.8   Are other organizations that contribute to or benefit from improvements in the national health profile involved in the development of these indicators?

5.1.2   The NHA uses indicators to measure success in meeting health objectives.

5.1.2.1 Are these indicators monitored and evaluated through a participatory process?

If so, does this participatory process:
5.1.2.1.1 Include key actors involved in the financing of health care?
5.1.2.1.2 Include key actors involved in health care purchasing (management of health care financing)?
5.1.2.1.3 Include key actors involved in health care delivery?
5.1.2.1.4 Contribute to the implementation of a comprehensive national health policy?

5.1.3 The NHA evaluates current and potential partners to determine their degree of support and commitment to the development, implementation, and evaluation of the national efforts to improve health.

5.1.3.1 Is this partner evaluation process carried out in the public health sector?
5.1.3.2 Is this partner evaluation process carried out in the private health sector?
5.1.3.3 Do the results of the latest partner evaluation indicate that the partners are properly identified and suitably prepared to assume their responsibilities in the health improvement process at the national level?
5.1.3.4 Are the results of the partner evaluation used to develop partnerships with key actors in the private and public sectors?

5.2 Development, Monitoring and Evaluation of Public Health Policies

Standard
The NHA:

- Takes the lead in defining public health policies and involves the Executive and Legislative branches of government, key leaders and civil society in the process.
- Develops a pluralistic approach to inform and influence the genesis of sustainable national public health and regulatory policies in the country. ,

- Periodically monitors and evaluates the process to develop policy and takes the necessary action to show the potential impact of policies on the health of individuals.

5.2.1 The NHA assumes leadership in developing the national health policy agenda.

If so,
5.2.1.1 Is the above agenda consistent with the national objectives as defined by the NHA and its partners, and as described in Indicator 5.1.1?
5.2.1.2 Does the above agenda have the endorsement and approval of the highest level of the Executive branch?
5.2.1.3 Does the above agenda have the endorsement and approval of the Legislative branch?
5.2.1.4 Does the NHA request and take into account input from other key decisionmakers responsible for generating a health policy agenda?
5.2.1.5 Does the NHA request and take into account input from civil society to formulate a national health policy agenda?

5.2.2 The NHA coordinates social participation activities at the national level to help set the national health policy agenda.

If so, do these activities include:
5.2.2.1 Generating public health agreements and consensus in areas of national importance?
5.2.2.2 Facilitating for a the public discussion of concerns, testimonies and consensus-building on public health issues?
5.2.2.3 Communicating with national committees and advisory groups responsible for policy development?
5.2.2.4 Negotiating public health legislation that supports the defined national health policy agenda?
5.2.2.5 Sharing this national health policy agenda with other interested parties at the national or subnational levels?

If so, do these include:
5.2.2.5.1 Unions?

5.2.2.5.2 Professional associations?

5.2.2.5.3 Private groups?

5.2.2.5.4 Local health jurisdictions?

5.2.2.5.5 Consumer groups?

5.2.2.5.6 Community organizations?

5.2.2.5.7 Nongovernmental organizations?

5.2.2.6 Developing policies that translate into public health laws and regulations?

If so,

5.2.2.6.1 Can you cite a specific example of such a law or regulation drafted in the past year?

5.2.3 The NHA monitors and evaluates current public health policies in order to measure their impact.
Does the NHA:

5.2.3.1 Alert decisionmakers and civil society of the impact that may result from implementing public health policies?

5.2.3.2 Use this evaluation of current public health policies to define and implement health policies?

5.2.3.3 Have personnel with the necessary expertise to develop and implement evidence-based public health policies?

If so, does this expertise include:

5.2.3.3.1 Proposing public health policy?

5.2.3.3.2 Proposing public health legislation?

5.2.3.3.3 Convening of public fora to define public health policies?

5.2.3.3.4 Prioritizing public health policy issues?

5.3 Development of Institutional Capacity for the Management of Public Health Systems

<u>Standard</u>
The NHA:

5.3.1 Leadership and communication
- Ensures that its leadership is capable of moving the health system in the direction of a clearly articulated vision with clearly defined standards of excellence.

- Provides the resources and strategies necessary for attaining these standards of excellence.
- Has the necessary personnel skilled to effectively communicate the vision and implementation strategies through on a system-wide basis.

5.3.2 Evidence-based decision-making
- Has the necessary competencies and resources to collect, analyze and evaluate data from different sources to develop the capacity for evidence-based management, including support for planning, decision-making and evaluation of interventions.
- Facilitates access to pertinent data sources that support decision-making and ensure that these sources are used at the subnational levels
- Guarantees the systematic analysis of information about the results of its operations and has the necessary personnel with the capacity to conduct this analysis.
- Uses operations research on health systems to inform the decision-making process.

5.3.3 Strategic planning
- Has the institutional capacity to apply a strategic focus for health planning based on relevant and valid information.
- Generates and ensures the feasibility of strategic plans through measures that build partnerships with civil society geared to meeting health needs.
- Ensures that the necessary steps have been taken to coordinate planning and collaborative efforts with other agencies and civil society.
- Ensures coordination and consistency between the national and subnational planning levels of public health in implementing diverse strategies by the subnational levels.

5.3.4 Organizational development
- Establishes an organizational culture, process and structure that learns and operates through continuous feedback on the changes in the external environment.
- Facilitates the involvement of and access by institutional personnel and civil society in providing feedback to help solve public health problems.
- Has the necessary competencies in inter-institutional relations, conflict management, teamwork and organizational development to move the institution towards a clearly defined vision and provide a response based on standards of excellence.

5.3.5 Resource management

- Ensures the availability of resources necessary to develop skills indispensable to its operations including financial, technical and human resources that can be efficiently allocated based on changing priorities.
- Has the capacity to manage the resources needed to ensure efficiency, quality and equity in accessing health care.
- Empowers its personnel to strengthen the capacity of providers and managers at all levels of the health system in designing, implementing and effectively managing support systems to ensure an integrated health system.

5.3.1 The NHA is developing the institutional capacity to exercise leadership in health management.

    5.3.1.1 Is the necessary institutional capacity in place at the NHA that allows it to exercise its leadership in the public health system?

        If so, does this capacity include:

        5.3.1.1.1 Tools for consensus-building?

        5.3.1.1.2 Promoting intrasectoral collaboration?

        5.3.1.1.3 Conflict resolution methods?

        5.3.1.1.4 Expertise in communication?

        5.3.1.1.5 Mobilization of resources?

        5.3.1.1.6 Promoting intersectoral collaboration?

        Does the NHA:

        5.3.1.2 Use its leadership role to steer the public health system towards its objectives?

        5.3.1.3 Have the necessary skilled personnel to effectively communicate its vision and strategies on a system-wide basis?

5.3.2 The NHA is developing institutional capacity for evidence-based decision-making.

    Does the NHA:

    5.3.2.1 Have evidence-based managerial capacity for planning, decision-making and the evaluation of activities?

        If so, does the NHA:

    5.3.2.1.1 Possess the necessary capacity to collect, analyze, integrate and evaluate information from different sources?

    5.3.2.1.2 Have information systems that can process collected data and build a comprehensive database to be used in be used in the planning process?

        If so, does the database provide information on:

        5.3.2.1.2.1 Existing resources in the health sector?

        5.3.2.1.2.2 Cost analysis?

        5.3.2.1.2.3 Service output?

        5.3.2.1.2.4 Quality of services?

    5.3.2.1.3 Use information from different sources to improve decision-making in managing public health systems at all levels?

    5.3.2.1.4 Stimulate and facilitate the use of information on community health status in its decision-making?

    5.3.2.1.5 Have the qualified personnel to use this information for evidence-based decision-making?

        If so:

        5.3.2.1.5.1 Is this information presented in an coherent manner?

5.3.2.2 Use scientific methodologies for health systems research to inform the decision-making and evaluation processes?

5.3.2.3 Have supervisory and evaluation systems to ensure that goals and objectives are met?

5.3.2.4 Have clear, well-defined performance measurements that are an integral part of the health system?

    If so, do these performance measurements include:

    5.3.2.4.1 Systematic data collection and analysis?

5.3.2.4.2 Continuous improvement of health system performance?

5.3.2.4.3 Can you cite an example of such a performance measurement?

5.3.2.5 Does the NHA have the qualified personnel able to effectively communicate the results of its operations?

5.3.3 The NHA has the institutional capacity for strategic planning.

5.3.3.1 Does the NHA have personnel with the necessary expertise and capacity to define and implement strategic planning?

5.3.3.2 Does the NHA use strategic planning in its activities and operations?

If so,

5.3.3.2.1 Has the NHA carried out a strategic planning process in the past year?

If so, did the process:

5.3.3.2.1.1 Define the vision and mission of the NHA?

5.3.3.2.1.2 Analyze the strengths and weaknesses of the NHA?

5.3.3.2.1.3 Identify the threats to and opportunities for the NHA?

5.3.3.2.1.4 Define the objectives and strategies of the NHA?

5.3.3.2.1.5 Build partnerships to carry out its strategic plan?

5.3.3.2.1.6 Define tasks and responsibilities needed to carry out the process?

5.3.3.2.1.7 Undergo an iterative and systematic evaluation?

5.3.3.2.2 Does the NHA coordinate these planning and collaborative activities with other agencies?

5.3.4 The NHA has a permanent organizational development process.

Does the NHA:

5.3.4.1 Have a clear, shared organizational vision?

5.3.4.2 Ensure that it has the organizational culture, processes and structure to continually learn from changes in the external environment and to adequately respond to those changes?

If so, has the NHA:

5.3.4.2.1 Examined its organizational culture?

5.3.4.2.2 Conducted a performance assessment of its organizational development process?

If so,

5.3.4.2.2.1 Is this assessment used to respond to changes in the external environment?

Does the NHA:

5.3.4.3 Define standards of excellence?

If so, does the NHA:

5.3.4.3.1 Implement the necessary strategies to meet these standards?

5.3.4.3.2 Provide the necessary resources to meet these standards?

5.3.4.3.3 Facilitate the implementation of these standards in daily practice?

5.3.4.3.4 Have an organizational culture that facilitates empowerment of personnel for their ongoing development?

5.3.5 The NHA has the institutional capacity for managing resources.

5.3.5.1 Does the NHA have the institutional capacity to manage its resources?

If so,

5.3.5.1.1 Does it have the authority to reallocate its resources as priorities and needs change?

If so,

5.3.5.1.1.1 Can you cite specific examples of this reallocation in the last year?

5.3.5.1.1.2 Does the NHA use its capacity for resource management to ensure efficiency, quality and equity in the health services?

5.3.5.1.1.3 Does the NHA have trained staff in technology management who can offer advice on the selection and management of appropriate technologies?

5.4 Management of International Cooperation in Public Health

Standard
The NHA:

- Has the capacity and expertise necessary to negotiate with international agencies and institutions that collaborate in public health.
- Has the capacity to design and implement medium- to long-term cooperation programs, as well as projects of a more limited scope and duration.
- Has information systems in place that match national needs with the international cooperation ventures available and actively search for cooperation projects that make it possible to better address national health priorities.
- Is in a position to develop cooperative programs, inside or outside the Region, that can be systematically jointly evaluated.

5.4.1 The NHA has the capacity and resources to direct, negotiate and implement international cooperation in public health.

Does the NHA:

5.4.1.1 Have the necessary resources and technology to search databases of international cooperation opportunities that will enable it to better address national priorities in health?

5.4.1.2 Have knowledge of the policies, priorities, conditions and requirements of the various international cooperation agencies for the allocation of resources?

5.4.1.3 Have the necessary capacity to implement joint cooperation projects with countries inside and outside the Region?

If so, do this capacity include:
5.4.1.3.1 Joint cooperative programs with international agencies?

5.4.1.3.2 Specific and short-term joint cooperative projects?

5.4.1.3.3 Projects of cooperation between countries?

5.4.1.4 Guarantee that all cooperative projects are systematically and jointly evaluated with their respective international partners?

If so,
5.4.1.4.1 Does the NHA have professionals at all levels of the health system that are able to participate in this evaluation?

5.5 Technical Assistance and Support to the Subnational Levels for Policy Development, Planning, and Management in Public Health

Standard
The NHA:

- Advises and provides technical support to the subnational levels of public health on policy development, planning and management activities.
- Promotes and facilitates the use of planning processes at the subnational levels, as well as integrates planning with other community initiatives that impact public health.
- Ensures that its managerial capacity supports the development of public health at the subnational levels and advises those levels on management practices to ensure sustainable mechanisms for good communication.
- Establishes linkages with training institutions to improve the sustainable management capacity of personnel at the subnational levels.

5.5.1 The NHA advises and provides technical support to the subnational levels for policy development, planning, and the management of activities in public health.

Does this support include:

5.5.1.1 Training in methods for public health planning?

5.5.1.2 Training in methods for formulating public health policies?

5.5.1.3 Training in methods to ensure sustainable management?

If so, does the NHA:

5.5.1.3.1 Have training programs to promote sustainable management that strengthens the institutional capacity of the subnational levels?

5.5.1.3.2 Provide in-service training?

5.5.1.3.3 Provide formal continuing education?

5.5.1.3.4 Establish linkages with schools or organizations that offer training programs in sustainable management to strengthen institutional capacity at the subnational levels?

5.5.1.4 Advise on effective strategies to identify and address subnational priorities in health?

5.5.1.5 Have the necessary resources to assist subnational levels with strategic planning activities?

5.5.1.6 Facilitate the development of local health planning processes?

5.5.1.7 Promote the integration of local health planning process with other similar initiatives?

5.5.1.8 Strengthen the decentralization of management in public health?

5.5.1.9 Provide assistance to promote the continuous improvement of management at the subnational levels?

5.5.2 The NHA has the necessary systems in place to rapidly and accurately detect needs to improve management at the subnational levels.

Does the NHA have mechanisms and policies in place at all levels to:

5.5.2.1 Detect deficiencies in management capacity at the subnational levels?

5.5.2.2 Respond rapidly to deficiencies revealed at the subnational levels?

5.5.2.3 Can you cite a specific example of such a mechanism that has been implemented in the past two years?

EPHF 6: Strengthening of Institutional Capacity for Regulation and Enforcement in Public Health

Definition
This function includes:

- The institutional capacity to develop the regulatory and enforcement frameworks that protect public health and monitor compliance within these frameworks.
- The capacity to generate new laws and regulations aimed at improving public health, as well as promoting healthy environments.
- The protection of civil society in its use of health services.
- The execution of all of these activities to ensure full, proper, consistent and timely compliance with the regulatory and enforcement frameworks.

Indicators

6.1 Periodic Monitoring, Evaluation and Revision of the Regulatory Framework

Standard:
The NHA:

- Periodically reviews the current laws and regulations that protect public health and ensure healthy environments, based on the best national and international information available.
- Prepares and reviews laws and regulations proposed for future use.
- Proposes updates to the wording and content to ensure laws and regulations reflect current scientific knowledge in public health and correct any undesirable effects of the legislation.
- Requests information from lawmakers, legal experts and civil society, particularly subject to regulation or directly affected by the legislation under review.
- Monitors legislative proposals under discussion and advises lawmakers on them.

6.1.1 The NHA has expertise in drafting laws and regulations to protect public health.

Does this expertise include:

6.1.1.1 Its own legal counsel?

6.1.1.2 Legal counsel contracted externally for specific reviews?

6.1.1.3 Personnel familiar with legislative and regulatory procedures for the passage, amendment and rejection of laws and regulations in public health?

6.1.2 The NHA reviews the laws and regulations to protect the health and safety of the population.

Does the NHA:

6.1.2.1 Include draft legislation in the above review?

6.1.2.2 Consider whether the legislation is consistent with current scientific knowledge in public health?

6.1.2.3 Consider the positive and negative impact of these laws and regulations?

6.1.2.4 Complete the review in a timely manner?

6.1.2.5 Conduct this review periodically?

6.1.2.6 Involve other regulatory mechanisms in the above review?

6.1.3 The NHA seeks input for the evaluation of health laws and regulations.

Is this input sought from:

6.1.3.1 Key lawmakers who support the development of public health?

6.1.3.2 Legal advisors?

6.1.3.3 Other government agencies?

6.1.3.4 Civil society?

6.1.3.5 Representatives of community organizations?

6.1.3.6 Users' associations, interest groups, and other associations?

6.1.3.7 Individuals and organizations directly affected by these laws and regulations?

6.1.3.8 Interested international organizations?

6.1.4 The NHA spearheads initiatives to amend laws and regulations based on the results of the evaluation.

Does the NHA:

6.1.4.1 Offer advisory services and assistance to lawmakers for the drafting of the necessary legal revisions based on the results of the review?

6.1.4.2 Actively engage in advocacy to facilitate the necessary legal revisions that protect the health and safety of the population?

6.2 Enforcement of Laws and Regulations

Standard:
The NHA:

• Exercises oversight of public health activities within its jurisdiction to ensure the adherence to clearly written guidelines.

• Coordinates with other sectors to oversee activities that have impact on public health.

• Monitors oversight activities and procedures that correct abuses of authority or the failure to exercise authority if pressured by influential groups.

• Adopts a regulatory stance not only centered on education about public health law and the prevention of infractions, but also on the punishment of violators after the fact.

• Promotes the compliance of health regulations through educating and informing consumers and integrating enforcement activities at all levels of the health system.

• Implements a clear policy formulated to prevent corruption as a practice that can permeate enforcement and ensures its periodic monitoring by independent entities to correct irregularities.

6.2.1 The NHA has systematic processes in place to enforce the existing laws and regulations.

Does the NHA:

6.2.1.1 Have clear, written guidelines that support enforcement in public health?

6.2.1.2 Identify the personnel responsible for enforcement procedures?

6.2.1.3 Supervise the enforcement procedures that are utilized?

If so, does the NHA:

6.2.1.3.1 Seek to identify the abuse or misuse of its enforcement authority?

6.2.1.3.2 Monitor compliance with the enforcement guidelines?

6.2.1.4 Does the NHA act in a timely manner to correct the abuse or misuse of its authority?

6.2.1.5 Does the NHA have an incentive system in place for enforcement personnel to help ensure that they exercise their authority in an appropriate manner?

6.2.1.6 Does the NHA monitor the timeliness and efficiency of its enforcement procedures?

6.2.2 The NHA educates society about public health regulations and encourages compliance

Does the NHA:

6.2.2.1 Widely inform the public about the importance of compliance with health laws and regulations and the applicable procedures for doing so?

6.2.2.2 Have established procedures that inform those individuals and organizations affected by health laws and regulations?

6.2.2.3 Have an incentive system to foster compliance with laws and regulations?

If so,

6.2.2.3.1 Does this incentive system include recognition and certification of quality and certification with respect to compliance with laws and regulations?

6.2.3 The NHA develops and implements policies and plans for preventing corruption in the public health system.

Are these policies and plans:

6.2.3.1 Periodically evaluated by independent entities and adjusted when needed in accordance with the results of the evaluation?

6.2.3.2 Consistent with national priorities on the subject of corruption?

6.2.3.3 Considering measures needed to prevent the influence of external pressure groups on the NHA?

6.2.3.4 Capable of responding to corruption in the public health system by utilizing a penalty mechanism?

If so,

6.2.3.4.1 Is the existence of these penalty mechanisms made known to NHA personnel at all levels?

6.3 Knowledge, Skills, and Mechanisms for Reviewing, Improving and Enforcing Regulations

Standard
The NHA:

- Has a competent team of advisors who have thorough knowledge (both national and international) of regulatory procedures that govern the adoption, amendment, and rescinding of public health laws.
- Ensures that mechanisms and resources are available to enforce laws.
- Periodically evaluates national knowledge and competencies, as well as oversight and enforcement capacities in regards to public health laws and regulations.

6.3.1 The NHA has the institutional capacity to exercise its regulatory and enforcement functions.
Does the NHA:

6.3.1.1 Have a competent team of advisors to develop the regulatory framework and draft regulations?

6.3.1.2 Have the knowledge, skills and resources to exercise the regulatory function in public health?

If so, does the NHA:

6.3.1.2.1 Have sufficient human resources to exercise the regulatory function?

6.3.1.2.2 Have the institutional resources to draft the regulations?

6.3.1.2.3 Have adequate financial resources to exercise its regulatory and enforcement functions?

6.3.2 The NHA has procedures and resources to enforce the regulations.

Does the NHA:

6.3.2.1 Have an entity that exercises its enforcement function?

6.3.2.2 Have sufficient human resources for enforcement?

6.3.2.3 Have sufficient institutional resources to enforce regulations?

6.3.2.4 Have financial resources to carry out enforcement?

6.3.2.5 Provide orientation to enforcement personnel with regard to procedures they should follow?

If so,

6.3.2.5.1 Is orientation on the regulatory framework provided?

6.3.2.5.2 Does this orientation include setting priorities for enforcement in specific situations?

6.3.3 The NHA ensures the availability of training courses for enforcement personnel.

Does the NHA:

6.3.3.1 Train/orient new staff on enforcement?

6.3.3.2 Ensure the availability of training courses on enforcement?

6.3.3.3 Include in these courses content on best practices in enforcement?

6.3.3.4 Ensure that continuing education for enforcement personnel is offered on a regular basis?

6.3.3.5 Help its enforcement personnel develop interpersonal communication and personal safety skills (e.g., handling difficult situations and people)?

6.3.4 The NHA evaluates its capacity and expertise for drafting laws and regulations in public health.

6.3.4.1 Has the NHA made progress toward improving its capacity for reviewing and drafting laws and regulations based on the findings of the most recent evaluation?

6.3.4.2 Can you cite an example of such improvement in capacity for reviewing and drafting laws and regulations?

6.4 Support and Technical Assistance to the Subnational Levels of Public Health in Developing and Enforcing Laws and Regulations

Standard:
The NHA:

• Orientate and supports the subnational levels in how to best comply with current laws and regulations within their jurisdiction.

• Prepares protocols, answers questions and provides technical assistance and training to the subnational levels in best practices for enforcement procedures.

• Assists the subnational levels in difficult and complex enforcement activities.

• Periodically evaluates the technical assistance and support it provides to the subnational levels in regulation and enforcement.

• Introduces improvements based on the results of the above evaluations.

6.4.1 The NHA provides assistance to the subnational levels for drafting laws and regulations to protect public health.

Does the NHA:

6.4.1.1 Provide protocols to the subnational levels for the decentralized drafting of laws and regulations?

6.4.1.2 Offer advisory services to the subnational levels on the drafting of laws and regulations?

6.4.1.3 Provide training to the subnational levels in decentralized regulation?

6.4.1.4 Offer technical assistance to specialized personnel at the subnational levels for the drafting of complex laws and regulations?

6.4.2 The NHA offers orientation and support to the subnational levels to enforce the public health laws and regulations in their jurisdiction.

Does the NHA:

6.4.2.1 Furnish protocols to the subnational levels that describe best practices in enforcement?

6.4.2.2 Advise the subnational levels on implementing enforcement procedures?

6.4.2.3 Assist the subnational levels with training in enforcement procedures?

6.4.2.4 Assist specialized personnel at the subnational levels who handle complex enforcement activities?

6.4.2.5 Periodically evaluate the technical assistance it provides to the subnational levels on the enforcement of public health laws and regulations?

If so,

6.4.2.5.1 Does it use the findings of these evaluations to improve the quality of its technical assistance?

EPHF 7: Evaluation and Promotion of Equitable Access to Necessary Health Services

Definition:

This function includes:

- The promotion of equity of access by civil society to necessary health services.
- Actions designed to overcome barriers when accessing public health interventions and help link vulnerable groups to necessary health services (does not include the financing of health care).
- The monitoring and evaluation of access to necessary health services offered by public and/or private providers and using a multisectoral, multiethnic and multicultural approach to facilitate working with diverse agencies and institutions to reduce inequities in access to necessary health services.
- Close collaboration with governmental and nongovernmental agencies to promote equity able access to necessary health services.

Indicators:

7.1 Monitoring and Evaluation of Access to Necessary Health Services

Standard:

The NHA:

- Monitors and evaluates access to the personal and population-based health services delivered to the population of the jurisdiction at least once every two years.

- Conducts the evaluation in collaboration with subnational levels for the delivery of clinical care at all points entry to the health system.
- Determines the causes and effects of barriers to access, gathering information on the individuals affected by these barriers and identifies best practices to reduce those barriers and increase equity of access to necessary health services.
- Uses the results of this evaluation to promote equitable access to necessary health services for the population of the country.
- Collaborates with other agencies to ensure the monitoring of access to necessary health services by vulnerable or underserved population groups.

7.1.1 The NHA conducts a national evaluation of access to necessary population-based health services.

7.1.1.1 Do indicators exist to evaluate access?

7.1.1.2 Is the national evaluation based on a predefined package of population-based services accessible to the population?

7.1.1.3 Is information available from the subnational levels to implement the national evaluation?

7.1.1.4 Is the national evaluation conducted in collaboration with the subnational levels?

If so,

7.1.1.4.1 Is the national evaluation conducted in collaboration with the intermediate levels?

7.1.1.4.2 Is the national evaluation conducted in collaboration with the local levels?

7.1.1.4.3 Is the national evaluation conducted in collaboration with other governmental entities?

7.1.1.4.4 Is the national evaluation conducted in collaboration with other nongovernmental entities?

7.1.1.5 Is the national evaluation conducted at least every two years?

7.1.2 The NHA conducts a national evaluation of access to personal health services.

7.1.2.1 Is the national evaluation based on the definition of a predefined package of personal health services accessible to the population?

7.1.2.2 Does the national evaluation examine problems related to cost of services and the payment systems for these services?

7.1.2.3 Does the national evaluation examine the coverage of personal health services by public and private entities, insurance companies and other payers?

7.1.2.4 Does the national evaluation examine access by distance to the nearest health facility?

7.1.2.5 Is the national evaluation conducted at least every two years?

7.1.2.6 Is the national evaluation conducted in collaboration with the intermediate levels?

7.1.2.7 Is the national evaluation conducted in collaboration with the local levels?

7.1.2.8 Is the national evaluation conducted in collaboration with the personal health services delivery system?

7.1.2.9 Is the national evaluation conducted in collaboration with other governmental entities?

7.1.2.10 Is the national evaluation conducted in collaboration with other nongovernmental entities?

7.1.2.11 Is the national evaluation conducted in collaboration with social security health agencies to ensure the monitoring of access to personal health services by vulnerable or underserved[10] populations?

7.1.3 The NHA investigates and lifts barriers to access in the health services.

Has it identified barriers related to:

7.1.3.1 Age?
7.1.3.2 Gender?
7.1.3.3 Ethnicity?
7.1.3.4 Culture and beliefs?
7.1.3.5 Religion?
7.1.3.6 Language?
7.1.3.7 Literacy?

7.1.3.8 Residence?
7.1.3.9 Transportation?
7.1.3.10 Level of education?
7.1.3.11 Income?
7.1.3.12 Insurance coverage?
7.1.3.13 Nationality?
7.1.3.14 Sexual orientation?
7.1.3.15 Physical disability?
7.1.3.16 Mental disability?
7.1.3.17 Type of disease?

7.1.3.18 Does the evaluation utilize methodologies capable of detecting disparities (e.g. adequate disaggregation of data, sampling and surveys) aimed at population groups that the NHA wishes to target?

7.1.3.19 Does the evaluation identify best practices to reduce the barriers and enhance the equity of access to necessary health services?

If so,

7.1.3.19.1 Does the NHA disseminate information on best practices to all levels and recommend their use within the health services delivery systems?

7.1.4 The NHA uses the results of the evaluation to promote equity in access to essential health services.

7.1.4.1 Does the national evaluation include input from those affected by the barriers to access?

7.1.4.2 Does the NHA use the national evaluation to define conditions for accessing the necessary health services?

7.1.4.3 Does the NHA apply regulations that ensure these conditions for access to necessary health services by the population?

7.2 Knowledge, Skills and Mechanisms to Improve Access to Necessary Health Services by the Population

Standard:
The NHA:

• Works with subnational levels to communicate information to the population on personal and population-based health services, including their rights to health.

---

[10] This refers to situations in which people are assured health services coverage but nevertheless encounter barriers to receiving the health care they need.

- Encourages and supports initiatives to introduce innovative and proven methods of health services delivery (such as mobile care units, health fairs, health care campaigns and operations, and/or telemedicine) that improve access to necessary health services.
- Periodically evaluates its capacity to facilitate access to necessary health services by the population and makes improvements based on the results.

7.2.1 The NHA has specialized personnel in community outreach programs to increase the use of the health services.

Does it have personnel devoted to:

7.2.1.1 Identifying and tracking service utilization patterns?

7.2.1.2 Identifying problem cases in terms of barriers to access to necessary health services?

If so, does this personnel identify these problem cases
7.2.1.2.1 At the national level?
7.2.1.2.2 At the intermediate levels?
7.2.1.2.3 At the local levels?

7.2.2 The NHA has personnel capable of informing the public about access to the health services.

Does this personnel have competencies in:

7.2.2.1 Reducing linguistic and cultural barriers?

7.2.2.2 Targeting activities to vulnerable or underserved populations?

7.2.2.3 Informing providers about prevention programs?

7.2.2.4 Bringing services to high-risk populations?

7.2.2.5 Developing national early detection programs?

7.2.2.6 Helping vulnerable or underserved populations obtain necessary health services?

7.2.2.7 Introducing innovative methods of service delivery that promote access to necessary health services (e.g., mobile clinics, health fairs, etc.)?

7.2.2.8 Collaborating with social security agencies to ensure the monitoring of vulnerable or underserved populations?

7.2.3 The NHA periodically evaluates its expertise and capacity to provide mechanisms that offer the community greater access to personal and population-based health services.

7.2.3.1 Does the NHA improve its capacity to deliver necessary health services based on the results of this evaluation?

If so, does the NHA have personnel trained to evaluate this capacity:
7.2.3.1.1 At the national level?
7.2.3.1.2 At the intermediate levels?
7.2.3.1.3 At the local levels?

7.3. Advocacy and Action to Improve Access to Necessary Health Services

Standard:
The NHA:

- Delivers information to decisionmakers, key actors and the general public about specific barriers that impede access to necessary health services.
- Collaborates and forms partnerships with the other key actors within the health service delivery system, implementing programs that promote access to necessary health services.
- Advocates the adoption of laws and regulations that increases access by those most in need of necessary health services.
- Collaborates with universities and other training institutions to orientate human resource development, focusing on the knowledge and skills needed to improve access to necessary health services.
- Utilizes evidence-based information on public health to develop policies that improve access to necessary health services.
- Identifies gaps in the distribution of human resources available to underserved populations and develops remedial strategies.

7.3.1 The NHA engages in advocacy with other actors to improve access to necessary health services.

Does the NHA:

7.3.1.1 Inform key decisionmakers, representatives and the general public about barriers that impede access to necessary health services?

7.3.1.2 Advocates the adoption of policies, laws or regulations that increase access to necessary health services by vulnerable and underserved populations?

7.3.1.3 Establish and maintain formal relationships with other actors capable of addressing the problems of access to necessary health services?

7.3.1.4 Collaborate with universities and other training institutions in an effort to increase the availability of human resources in necessary health service delivery?

7.3.1.5 Recruit public health workers from all levels to enroll in continuing education programs that promote equitable access to necessary health services by the population?

7.3.2 The NHA takes direct action to improve access to necessary health services.

Does the NHA:

7.3.2.1 Coordinate national programs aimed at resolving problems in access to necessary health services?

7.3.2.2 Identify those areas that lack human resources and work towards correcting this deficiency?

7.3.2.3 Identify gaps in the human resources needed to deliver necessary health services to vulnerable or underserved populations?

7.3.2.4 Identify strategies to fill gaps in the distribution of these human resources?

7.3.2.5 Identify successful interventions that can increase access to necessary health services?

If so, does the NHA

7.3.2.5.1 Use this information on successful interventions to make informed policy decisions in this area?

7.3.2.6 Evaluate the effectiveness of interventions aimed at improving access to necessary health services?

7.3.2.7 Create incentives that encourage service providers to reduce disparities in equity of access to necessary health services?

If so, do these incentives target::

7.3.2.7.1 Population-based health services?
7.3.2.7.2 Personal health services?

7.3.2.8 Is there a system in place at the subnational level that assists communities in developing links to promote equitable access to the necessary health services?

7.4 Support and Technical Assistance to the Subnational Levels of Public Health to Promote Equitable Access to Necessary Health Services

Standard:
The NHA:

• Assists the subnational levels with identifying access needs of vulnerable and underserved populations matching needs to availability of health services.

• Supports the subnational levels in creating and disseminating public service announcements to inform the population about the availability of necessary health services.

• Assists the subnational levels in establishing innovative partnerships and coordinating with service providers to promote access to necessary health services.

• Supports the subnational levels in collaborating and coordinating with complementary programs designed to attract vulnerable or underserved populations to necessary health services.

7.4.1 The NHA assists the subnational levels in promoting equitable access to necessary health services.

Does the NHA assist the subnational levels in:

7.4.1.1 Defining a basic package of personal and population-based health services that should be available to the population?

If so, does the NHA assist the subnational levels in:

7.4.1.1.1 Coordinating the roles and responsibilities of service providers in the delivery of this basic package of necessary health services?

7.4.1.1.2 Creating and disseminating public service announcements that inform the population, particularly vulnerable or underserved populations, about the availability of this basic package of necessary health services?

346

7.4.1.2 Identifying gaps at the subnational levels in equity of access to necessary health services?

7.4.1.3 Identifying barriers that impede access to necessary health services?

7.4.1.4 Developing strategies to reduce such barriers?

7.4.1.5 Coordinating with complementary programs that promote community outreach activities and equitable access to necessary health services?

EPHF 8: Human Resource Development and Training in Public Health

Definition:

This function includes:

- The development of a public health workforce profile in public health that is adequate for the performance of public health functions and services.
- Educating, training, developing and evaluating the public health workforce to identify the needs of public health services and health care to efficiently address priority public health problems and adequately evaluate public health activities.
- The definition of licensure requirements for health professionals in general and the adoption of ongoing programs that improve the quality of public health services.
- Formation of active partnerships with professional development programs to ensure that all students have relevant public health experience and continuing education in the management of human resources and leadership development in public health.
- The development of skills necessary for interdisciplinary, multicultural work in public health.
- Bioethics training for public health personnel, emphasizing the principles and values of solidarity, equity, and respect for human dignity.

Indicators:

8.1 Description of the Public Health Workforce Profile

Standard:

The NHA:

- Maintains an up-to-date inventory of filled and vacant posts at all levels of the public health system, both governmental and nongovernmental, as well as estimates of the number of volunteer workers who provide services at each level.
- Completes an evaluation at least once every two years of the number, type, geographical distribution, wage structure, minimum education requirements, licensing, recruitment and retention of specialized public health personnel.
- Projects future health manpower needs in terms of quantity and quality.

8.1.1 The NHA identifies current needs with respect to public health workers.

8.1.1.1 Does the NHA have information on the number of workers needed to discharge essential public health functions and deliver public health services:

If so, does this information exist:
8.1.1.1.1 At the national level?
8.1.1.1.2 At the intermediate level?
8.1.1.1.3 At the local level?

8.1.1.2 Does the NHA maintain a profile of workers needed to discharge essential public health functions and deliver public health services:

If so, does the profile exist:
8.1.1.2.1 At the national level?
8.1.1.2.2 At the intermediate level?
8.1.1.2.3 At the local level?

8.1.1.3 Does the NHA define competencies required to discharge the essential public health functions and deliver public health services:

If so, are these competencies defined for:
8.1.1.3.1 The national level?
8.1.1.3.2 The intermediate level?
8.1.1.3.3 The local level?

8.1.2 The NHA identifies gaps in the composition and availability of the public health workforce that must be filled.

8.1.2.1 Does the NHA establish criteria for defining the future needs of the public health workforce?

8.1.2.2 Are current needs for a public health workforce compared with future needs?

8.1.2.3 Does the NHA establish criteria to minimize existing gaps in the public health workforce?

8.1.3 The NHA periodically evaluates the profile of the country's public health workforce.

Does the NHA:

8.1.3.1 Have access to data on the wage structure and other pecuniary benefits?

8.1.3.2 Have access to data on the geographical distribution of the public health workforce?

8.1.3.3 Have access to data on the distribution of the public health workforce categorized according to type of employment (nongovernmental, private, public)?

8.1.3.4 Have access to data on the educational profile required for specific posts?

8.1.3.5 Have access to data on the competencies required for specific posts?

If so,

8.1.3.5.1 Does the NHA evaluate existing competencies to ensure that the existing workforce is capable of performing transcultural tasks?

If so,

8.1.3.5.1.1 Does the NHA develop strategies to achieve a workforce competent to work with communities of diverse cultures and languages?

8.1.3.6 Does the NHA have a management information system capable of monitoring the above data?

8.1.4 The NHA uses a pre-existing profile to maintain an up-to-date inventory of the posts needed to discharge public health functions and deliver services.

Does this inventory include:

8.1.4.1 A preexisting profile of posts?

8.1.4.2 Mechanisms for filling vacancies based on priorities?

8.1.4.3 An in-depth analysis of filled and vacant posts?

8.1.4.4 Information from the national and subnational levels?

8.1.4.5 An estimate of volunteer workers within the public health system?

8.1.4.6 Identification of areas for potential growth?

8.1.5 The NHA's evaluation of the quantity and quality of the workforce takes advantage of input from other institutions.

Does this input come from:

8.1.5.1 Other government agencies?

8.1.5.2 Subnational levels?

8.1.5.3 Academic institutions?

8.1.5.4 Leaders and experts in public health?

8.1.5.5 Nongovernmental organizations?

8.1.5.6 Professional associations?

8.1.5.7 Civil society?

8.1.5.8 International agencies?

8.1.5.9 The Ministry of Education?

8.1.5.10 The Ministry of Labor?

8.2 Improving the Quality of the Workforce

Standard:

The NHA:

- Ensures that public health workers and managers meet the educational level and certification required by law in accordance with pre-established criteria.
- Coordinates training programs and collaborates with educational institutions devoted to public health training, recommending a basic public health curriculum for the training programs offered at the various levels of public health.
- Periodically assesses teaching programs, performance evaluation systems and continuing education courses to ensure that they contribute to developing human resources for public health.
- Offers incentives and implements plans that improve the quality of the country's public health workforce.
- Actively searches for qualified workers to exercise leadership, recruiting and offering incentives for them to remain with the organization.

- Encourages leaders in public health to create effective partnerships for action in all areas of public health and fosters the political and environmental conditions necessary to accomplish this.

8.2.1   The NHA has strategies in place to improve the quality of the workforce.

Does the NHA:

8.2.1.1   Follow guidelines or norms to accredit and certify educational credentials in hiring of public health workers?

If so,

8.2.1.1.1   Does the NHA evaluate compliance with these criteria throughout the country?

8.2.1.2   Have policies in place that ensure the adequate training of public health workers allowing them to exercise their responsibilities?

8.2.1.3   Collaborate and coordinate with academic institutions and scientific professional associations to develop a basic public health curriculum?

8.2.1.4   Encourage participation by the public health workforce in continuing education activities to improve the quality of the workforce?

8.2.1.5   Offer or coordinate training for public health workers needing more experience?

8.2.1.6   Have evaluation activities, at least every three years, that permit an evaluation of the effectiveness of its recruitment policies, the quality of its hiring process and its capacity to retain public health workers?

8.2.1.7   Have strategies that motivate its personnel in their respective career paths?

8.2.1.8   Prepare and implement plans for educating public health workers in bioethics, with emphasis on principles and values such as solidarity, equity and respect for human dignity?

8.2.1.9   Prepare and implement plans to improve the quality of the country's public health workforce?

If so,

8.2.1.9.1   Does the NHA periodically evaluate these plans?

8.2.2   The NHA has strategies to strengthen leadership in public health.

Does the NHA:

8.2.2.1   Provide opportunities for leadership development in the public health workforce?

8.2.2.2   Actively identify potential leaders in the public health workforce?

If so, does the NHA:

8.2.2.2.1   Encourage the retention of the leaders identified?

8.2.2.2.2   Offer incentives to improve leadership capacity?

8.2.2.3   Have mechanisms in place that identify and recruit potential leaders?

8.2.2.4   Establish agreements with academic institutions and other organizations devoted to developing leadership in public health?

8.2.2.5   Have strategies and mechanisms in place to link decision-making with ethical principles and social values in the context of public health leadership?

8.2.3   The NHA has a system to evaluate the performance of public health workers.

Does this system of performance evaluation:

8.2.3.1   Indicate the performance expectations for each worker over a given period?

8.2.3.2   Define measurable work outcomes for each staff member?

8.2.3.3   Communicate to public health workers performance expectations over a given period?

8.2.3.4   Analyze its results and propose improvements to it?

8.2.3.5   Utilize the results of the evaluation to better assign responsibilities and retain workers?

8.3 Continuing Education and Graduate Training in Public Health

Standard:

The NHA:

- Establishes formal ties with academic institutions having graduate programs in public health to facilitate access by the public health workforce to continuing education.
- Evaluates and encourages academic institutions to adapt their programs and teaching strategies to meet the needs of essential public health functions and future challenges.
- Shares the results of the evaluation of its continuing education and graduate training programs and obtains feedback from public health workers on this issue.

8.3.1 The NHA provides orientation and promotes continuing education and graduate training in public health.

Does the NHA:

8.3.1.1 Facilitate formal agreements that permit access to continuing education, with academic institutions having public health programs?

8.3.1.2 Encourage academic institutions to offer programs in public health that meet the needs of the public health workforce?

8.3.1.3 Annually survey public health workers who have participated in continuing education activities?

8.3.1.4 Survey institutions that employ these workers on the knowledge and skills acquired through continuing education and graduate training activities?

If so,

8.3.1.4.1 Does the NHA share the results of these surveys with the academic institutions to encourage quality improvement of the academic programs offered to public health workers?

8.3.1.5 Have strategies and mechanisms in place to ensure the retention of public health workers who have been trained and their reintegration into the workforce commensurate with their acquired skills?

8.4 Improving Workforce to Ensure Culturally-Appropriate Delivery of Services

Standard:

The NHA:

- Trains health workers in the delivery of high quality, culturally-appropriate services to diverse user populations.
- Makes an effort to form public health teams that include workers from the ethnic and cultural groups served.
- Makes an effort to reduce social and cultural barriers by the population in accessing user-oriented health services by the population (e.g., health center admitting offices staffed by multilingual personnel trained as intercultural facilitators).
- Continuously evaluates the ethnic and cultural diversity of public health workers and takes the necessary steps to eliminate ethnic and cultural barriers.

8.4.1 The NHA adapts its human resources to deliver services suited to the different characteristics of its users.

Does the NHA:

8.4.1.1 Factor in gender issues into its workforce training programs?

8.4.1.2 Train its workforce to deliver services to culturally-diverse populations?

8.4.1.3 Utilize the concept of delivering culturally-appropriate services to the community when planning and implementing public health activities?

If so, does the NHA utilize these practices:

8.4.1.3.1 At the national level?

8.4.1.3.2 At the intermediate levels?

8.4.1.3.3 At the local levels?

8.4.1.3.4 Can you cite an example of the use of culturally-appropriate service delivery at any level?

8.4.1.4 Does the NHA identify barriers to attaining the desired diversity in its public health workforce to make it consistent with the characteristics of the population being served?

If so, does the NHA:

8.4.1.4.1 Try to eliminate these barriers preventing the desired diversity in its public health workforce?

8.4.1.5 Does the NHA have policies in place that ensure the recruitment of culturally-appropriate public health workers?

If so, are these policies applied:
8.1.4.5.1 At the national level?
8.1.4.5.2 At the intermediate level?
8.1.4.5.3 At the local level?

8.4.1.6 Does the NHA try to eliminate cultural barriers by employing public health workers capable of improving access to public health services by the country's social and cultural groups (e.g., utilizing intercultural facilitators or bilingual staff)?

8.5 Technical Assistance and Support to the Subnational Levels in Human Resources Development

Standard:
The NHA:

- Collaborates with the subnational levels in conducting a comprehensive inventory and evaluation of human resources.
- Offers guidelines to the subnational levels on ways to reduce gaps in the quality of public health workforce.
- Ensures the availability of continuing education programs for public health workers at all levels, including training in the management of diversity and the improvement of leadership skills.
- Facilitates linkages between public health workers at all levels with national and international academic institutions to ensure access to varied and up-to-date continuing education courses.

8.5.1 The NHA assists the subnational levels in developing their human resources.

Does the NHA:
8.5.1.1 Offer the necessary guidance to the subnational levels to reduce gaps identified in the national public health workforce evaluation?

8.5.1.2 Support the development of culturally- and linguistically-appropriate programs and workforce training at the subnational levels?

If so, does the NHA support those programs at:
8.5.1.2.1 The intermediate level?
8.5.1.2.2 The local level?

8.5.1.3 Have strategies in place that ensure the presence of continuing education programs at the subnational levels?

If so, are they:
8.5.1.3.1 At the intermediate level?
8.5.1.3.2 The local level?

8.5.1.4 Facilitate agreements between the subnational levels and academic institutions that ensure continuing education for the public health workforce at the subnational level?

8.5.1.5 Develop capacity at the subnational level to support decentralized planning and workforce management?

EPHF 9: Ensuring the Quality of Personal and Population-based Health Services

Definition:
This function includes:

- The promotion of systems that evaluate and improve quality.
- The development of standards for quality assurance, quality improvement and oversight of compliance of service providers.
- The definition, explanation and assurance of user rights.
- A system for health technology assessment that supports the decision-making process at all levels and contributes to quality improvement.
- Using evidence-based methodology to evaluate health interventions.
- Systems to evaluate user satisfaction and application of its results to improve the quality of health services.

Indicators:

9.1 Definition of Standards and Evaluation of Quality of Population-based and Personal Health Services

Standard:

The NHA:

- Establishes appropriate standards that permit the evaluation of quality of population-based and personal health services using data from all levels of the health system.
- Uses these standards and scientifically-proven instruments to measure the quality of personal and population-based public health services.
- Adopts results-oriented analytical methods that include scientific identification of the parameters to be evaluated, the data to be collected and the procedures to follow in the collection and analysis of those data.
- Has access to an autonomous entity that accredits and evaluates quality and is independent of health services.

9.1.1 The NHA has a policy that promotes continuous quality improvement in the health services.

Does this policy include:

9.1.1.1 A comparison of national performance goals with standards for population-based and personal health services?

9.1.1.2 The use of varied methodologies to improve quality?

9.1.1.3 Quality improvement processes in all NHA divisions or departments?

9.1.1.4 Measurement of the degree to which defined goals and objectives have been met?

9.1.1.5 Activities that evaluate staff attitudes toward user satisfaction?

9.1.1.6 Activities to develop policies and procedures on quality improvement of population-based and personal health services?

9.1.1.7 Measurement of user satisfaction?

9.1.2 The NHA sets standards and periodically evaluates the quality of population-based health services (public health practice) throughout the country.

To evaluate quality, does the NHA:

9.1.2.1 Promote the definition of standards that evaluate the quality of population-based health services throughout the country?

9.1.2.2 Actively seek input from the subnational levels in developing these standards?

9.1.2.3 Actively seek input from nongovernmental organizations in developing these standards?

9.1.2.4 Have instruments that measure the performance of population-based health services against the defined standards?

If so, do these instruments:

9.1.2.4.1 Measure processes?

9.1.2.4.2 Measure results?

9.1.2.4.3 Identify the performance goals for quality improvement?

9.1.2.4.4 Identify procedures for data collection?

9.1.2.4.5 Identify procedures for data analysis?

9.1.2.5 Disseminate the results of the quality evaluation to the providers of population-based services?

9.1.2.6 Disseminate the results of the quality evaluation to the users of population-based services?

9.1.2.7 Have an autonomous entity that accredits and evaluates quality independently of providers of population-based health services?

9.1.3 The NHA sets standards and periodically evaluates the quality of personal health services throughout the country.

To evaluate quality, does the NHA:

9.1.3.1 Have the authority to accredit and oversee the quality of personal health services?

9.1.3.2 Promote the definition of standards that evaluate the quality of personal health services throughout the country?

9.1.3.3 Actively seek support from the subnational levels to set these standards?

9.1.3.4 Actively seek input from nongovernmental organizations to set these standards?

9.1.3.5 Have instruments that measure the performance of personal health services against the defined standards?

If so, do these instruments:

9.1.3.5.1 Measure processes?

9.1.3.5.2 Measure results?

9.1.3.5.3 Identify the performance goals for quality improvement?

9.1.3.5.4 Identify procedures for data collection?

9.1.3.5.5 Identify procedures for data analysis?

9.1.3.6 Disseminate the results of the quality improvement evaluation to the providers and users of personal health services?

9.1.3.7 Have an autonomous entity that accredits and evaluates quality independently of personal health services providers?

9.2 Improving User Satisfaction with Health Services

<u>Standard:</u>

The NHA:

- Commits to the ongoing measurement and improvement of user satisfaction resulting from continuous quality improvement.
- Focuses on the user in orientating activities to improve staff performance and develop policies and procedures to accomplish this improvement at all levels.
- Clearly defines the rights and responsibilities of users of health services as well as disseminates this information.
- Periodically evaluates improvements in user satisfaction with health services and acts on the results to improve quality of services.
- Provides feedback on user satisfaction with health services to the subnational levels, users and other key actors.

9.2.1 The NHA actively encourages community participation to evaluate public satisfaction with health services in general.

Is input for this evaluation obtained from:

9.2.1.1 Local/community organizations?

9.2.1.2 Community surveys?

9.2.1.3 Focus groups?

9.2.1.4 The Internet?

9.2.1.5 Surveys of users of health services?

9.2.1.6 Surveys of users at point of service?

9.2.1.7 Log of comments, complaints and suggestions?

Are the results of the evaluation:

9.2.1.8 Used for continuous quality improvement of health services?

9.2.1.9 Used to improve the performance of health workers?

9.2.1.10 Communicated to civil society along with any resulting policy changes?

9.2.2 The NHA regularly evaluates user satisfaction with population-based health services.

Does this evaluation include:

9.2.2.1 Collaboration with decisionmakers[11] involved in these population-based services?

9.2.2.2 Input from decisionmakers on those factors to be evaluated?

9.2.2.3 Collaboration with members of civil society affected by these population-based services?

9.2.2.4 Input from members of civil society on the factors to be evaluated?

9.2.2.5 Formal mechanisms for users to provide input to the NHA in a timely and confidential manner?

Does the NHA:

9.2.2.6 Use the results of the evaluations to develop plans for improving the quality of programs and service delivery?

9.2.2.7 Use the results of the evaluation to develop plans that improve access to population-based services?

9.2.2.8 Communicate the results of this evaluation to all participants involved in the evaluation process?

9.2.2.9 Publish a report summarizing the main results of the user satisfaction evaluation?

If so,

9.2.2.9.1 Is this report widely distributed?

9.2.3 The NHA evaluates the degree of user satisfaction with the personal health services available in the country.

---

[11] This involves a broad spectrum that includes providers, industry affected by specific regulations, etc.

Does this evaluation include:

9.2.3.1 Collaboration with decisionmakers involved in personal health services?

9.2.3.2 Input from decisionmakers on the factors to be evaluated?

9.2.3.3 Collaboration with members of civil society affected by personal health services?

9.2.3.4 Input from members of civil society on the factors to be evaluated?

9.2.3.5 Formal mechanisms for users to provide input to the NHA in a timely and confidential fashion?

Does the NHA:

9.2.3.6 Use the evaluation results to develop plans to improve the quality of programs and service delivery?

9.2.3.7 Use the evaluation results to develop plans to improve access to personal health services?

9.2.3.8 Communicate the results of this evaluation to all participants involved in the evaluation process?

9.2.3.9 Publish a report summarizing the main results of the user satisfaction evaluation?

If so,

9.2.3.9.1 Is this report widely distributed?

9.3 Systems for Technology Management and Health Technology Assessment that Support Decision-making in Public Health

Standard:

The NHA:

- Establishes technology management and health technology assessment systems that function as part of an integrated network.
- Uses evidence available on safety, effectiveness and cost-effectiveness of health interventions in order to recommend the adoption and use of health technologies.
- Promotes the use of health technology assessment and evidence-based practices at all levels of the health system including public and private insurers, service providers and consumers.

- Periodically evaluates and improves national and subnational skills and knowledge with regard to the adoption, utilization and assessment of technologies.

9.3.1 The NHA develops and promotes health technology management systems.

9.3.1.1 Has the NHA set up one or more entities for technology management and health technology assessment as part of an integrated network?

If so, do these entities:

9.3.1.1.1. Provide information for decision-making processes that lead to the formulation of health policies?

9.3.1.2 Does the NHA use the above information to formulate better recommendations on available technology to the providers and users of health services?

9.3.2 The NHA ensures the proper functioning of its system for technology management and health technology assessment.

Does the NHA:

9.3.2.1 Define the roles of key individuals responsible for the operations of the technology management and health technology assessment systems?

9.3.2.2 Define the responsibilities and tasks of the above key individuals?

9.3.2.3 Establish channels of communication for the above key individuals?

If so,

9.3.2.3.1 Does the NHA use these channels of communication to also obtain information from the subnational levels?

9.3.3 The NHA utilizes the methodologies available for systematic technology assessment.

Does this evaluation cover:

9.3.3.1 Safety?

9.3.3.2 Effectiveness?

9.3.3.3   Cost-effectiveness?

9.3.3.4   Usefulness?

9.3.3.5   Utility cost (cost utility)?

9.3.3.6   Social acceptance?

9.3.4   The NHA promotes the development of technology management and health technology assessment systems based on the data provided by a national network of decision-making entities.

Does this network include:

9.3.4.1   Public health insurers?

9.3.4.2   Private health insurers?

9.3.4.3   Public health providers?

9.3.4.4   Private health providers?

9.3.4.5   Users?

9.3.4.6   Academic institutions and training centers?

9.3.4.7   Professional associations?

9.3.4.8   Scientific societies?

9.3.5   The NHA regularly evaluates its national capacity for technology management and health technology assessment.

Does the NHA:

9.3.5.1   Issue recommendations to improve this capacity?

9.3.5.2   Periodically evaluate the capacity at the subnational levels for technology management and health technology assessment?

9.3.5.3   Issue recommendations to improve the capacity at the subnational level levels for technology management and health technology assessment?

9.4 Technical Assistance and Support to the Subnational Levels to Ensure Quality Improvement in Personal and Population-based Health Services

Standard:

The NHA:

• Provides assistance to the subnational levels in the collection and analysis of data on quality of health services which includes data on structure, processes and outcomes of services delivered by health providers.

• Provides and trains the subnational levels in the use of technology management and health technology assessment tools, including evidence-based practices, for use in the delivery of personal and population-based health services.

• Supports the subnational levels in evaluating its technology management and health technology assessment systems by using functional criteria supported by available scientific evidence.

• Supports the subnational levels in conducting a formal evaluation of user satisfaction with personal and population-based health services.

9.4.1   The NHA provides technical assistance to the subnational levels for the collection and analysis of data on the quality of population-based public health services.

Does this data on quality cover:

9.4.1.1   Organizational structure and capacity to deliver population-based health services at the subnational levels?

9.4.1.2   Procedures and practices for health services delivery at the subnational levels?

9.4.1.3   Outcomes of services delivered by health providers at the subnational levels?

9.4.1.4   Degree of user satisfaction with population-based health services at the subnational level?

9.4.2   The NHA provides technical assistance to the subnational levels for the collection and analysis of data on the quality of personal health services.

Does the data on quality cover:

9.4.2.1   Organizational structure and capacity to deliver personal health services at the subnational levels?

9.4.2.2   Procedures and practices for health services delivery at the subnational levels?

9.4.2.3   Outcomes of services delivered by health providers at the subnational levels?

9.4.2.4   Degree of user satisfaction with personal health services at the subnational level?

9.4.3   The NHA provides technical assistance at the subnational levels on the use of technology management and assessment instruments.

Does the NHA:

9.4.3.1 Provide technical assistance to the subnational levels to measure management performance at these levels?

If so, is this assistance for:

9.4.3.1.1 Population-based health services?

9.4.3.1.2 Personal health services?

9.4.4 This assistance to the subnational levels covers all areas of health technology assessment.

Does the assistance include health technology assessment terms of:

9.4.4.1 Safety?

9.4.4.2 Effectiveness?

9.4.4.3 Cost-effectiveness?

9.4.4.4 Usefulness?

9.4.4.5 Utility cost (cost utility)?

9.4.4.6 Social acceptance?

EPHF 10: Research in Public Health

Definition:

This function includes:

- Rigorous research aimed at increasing knowledge to support decision-making at the various levels.
- The implementation of innovative solutions in public health whose impact can be measured and assessed.
- Intra- and intersectoral partnerships with research centers and academic institutions to conduct timely studies that support decision-making at all levels of the health system.

Indicators:

10.1 Development of a Public Health Research Agenda

Standard:

The NHA:

- Develops a priority agenda for research in public health based on needs perceived by the population and key actors in public, as well as identifies and mobilizes funding sources to permit this research.

- Encourages schools of public health, universities and other independent research centers to study health problems identified on the public health research agenda.
- Identifies traditional medicine, cultural diversity issues and alternative medicine as being priorities for research.
- Collaborates in implementing the public health research agenda, and collects and disseminates information to interested key actors in the health system.

10.1.1 The NHA has developed a public health research agenda.

Does the agenda:

10.1.1.1 Address the current gaps in knowledge that impede the NHA from meeting national priorities in health?

10.1.1.2 Take into account the need for evidence-based information on which to base policy decisions in public health?

10.1.1.3 Address the need for evidence-based information to improve the management of public health services?

10.1.1.4 Address the need for evidence-based information to ensure feasibility and sustainability of research on the agenda?

10.1.1.5 Identify existing funding sources to conduct research on the agenda?

10.1.1.6 Include input in setting priorities from key actors in public health (in the academic, nongovernmental, private, and community spheres).

Does the NHA:

10.1.1.7 Collaborate with institutions engaged in public health research to put together an agenda and plan its execution?

10.1.1.8 Discuss this research agenda with national and international institutions that fund public health research?

10.1.1.9 Include cultural diversity and a gender approach in the public health research agenda?

10.1.1.10 Have an entity that develops the public health research agenda and conducts the research included in it?

10.1.2 The NHA periodically evaluates progress in terms of adherence to the essential public health research agenda.

Does the NHA:

10.1.2.1 Communicate the results of this progress evaluation to all those involved in implementing the agenda?

    10.1.2.1.1   At the national level?
    10.1.2.1.2   At the subnational levels?

10.1.2.2 Promote the dissemination and use of the findings from the research agenda?

If so, are the findings disseminated and used:

    10.1.2.2.1   At the national level?
    10.1.2.2.2   At the subnational levels?

10.2 Development of Institutional Research Capacity

<u>Standard:</u>

The NHA:

- Assumes a proactive role in collaborating and coordinating with the scientific community working in areas relevant to public health, serving as lead in the interaction with researchers.
- Conducts independent research relevant to public health and has the necessary capacity to prepare timely proposals and research agendas in public health.
- Ensures that procedures exist for the approval of all research involving human subjects.
- Ensures access to adequate analytical tools, including up-to-date databases, computer technology and physical infrastructure.
- Has the capacity to procure funding for research activities.
- Is able to show how recent research findings have been used to improve public health practice.

10.2.1 The NHA is developing institutional capacity in public health research.

Does the NHA:

10.2.1.1 Have technical teams to interact with researchers working on public health priorities?

10.2.1.2 Have the ability to conduct independent research on relevant public health, in the absence external research groups?

If so,

    10.2.1.2.1 Is this research interdisciplinary?

    10.2.1.2.2 Does it take gender and cultural diversity into account?

10.2.1.3 Has NHA established an approval procedure for conducting research in its facilities and on the population?

If so, does this procedure include:

    10.2.1.3.1 A research priority evaluation from the perspective of national priorities and avoiding the duplication of efforts?

    10.2.1.3.2 A formal mechanism that adheres to internationally accepted norms for monitoring of ethical aspects of the research?

    10.2.1.3.3 A formal and transparent mechanism for funding budgets allocated to units responsible for the research?

    10.2.1.3.4 A formal and transparent mechanism for remunerating researchers?

10.2.2. The NHA has adequate qualitative and quantitative analytical tools for conducting research on public health problems.

Does the NHA:

10.2.2.1 Have research databases that are updated with qualitative and quantitative information relevant to public health research?

10.2.2.2 Have statistical software available for analyzing high-volume data[12]?

10.2.2.3 Have experts available who can utilize the above software for analyzing high-volume data?

---

[12] This refers to statistical packages used for the management of population surveys or population databanks; for example, SPSS, SAS, ARIEL, STATA, etc.

10.2.2.4 Have computer support available for analyzing high-volume data?

10.2.2.5 Have capacity for qualitative and quantitative data analysis?

10.2.2.6 Have capacity to communicate research findings to key actors in the health system for use in decision-making?

10.2.2.7 Have regular, internal seminars to present and discuss research findings relevant to decision-making?

10.2.2.8 Have any public health research projects that have been financed during the past 24 months (the research may be conducted by groups external to the NHA)?

10.2.2.9 Can you cite an example, during the past 24 months, in which the findings of research conducted or sponsored by the NHA were used to address a relevant health problem?

10.3 Technical Assistance and Support to the Subnational Levels for Research in Public Health

Standard:

The NHA:

- Establishes a broad network for the dissemination of research findings at all levels, including innovative and new public health practices.
- Encourages the participation of public health workers from the subnational levels in national public health research projects to bolster the subnational capacity for research methodology.
- Facilitates the human resource development in the field of research, particularly that of operations research.

10.3.1 The NHA advises the subnational levels on operations research methodologies in public health.

Does this training include:
10.3.1.1 Research on outbreaks of epidemics?
10.3.1.2 Research on outbreaks of food poisoning?
10.3.1.3 Research on the risk factors for chronic diseases?
10.3.1.4 Evaluation of the effectiveness of public health interventions?

10.3.1.5 Research on health services delivery?
10.3.1.6 Research on community health?

10.3.2 The NHA advises the subnational levels on how to properly interpret research findings.

Does the NHA train the subnational levels to:
10.3.2.1 Critically analyze scientific information?
10.3.2.2 Translate public health research findings into practice?

10.3.3 The NHA has a large network of institutions and individuals who are dedicated to or benefit from public health research findings.

10.3.3.1 Does the network disseminate research findings to members of the scientific community in public health?

Does the network include:
10.3.3.1.1 Decisionmakers?
10.3.3.1.2 Schools of public health?
10.3.3.1.3 Subnational levels of the NHA?
10.3.3.1.4 Medical schools?
10.3.3.1.5 Other institutions involved to public health research?
10.3.3.1.6 Other extrasectoral actors?

10.3.3.2 Does the NHA promote the participation of public health works from the subnational levels in national research projects?

If so, do these public health workers participate in:
10.3.3.2.1 The design of research projects?
10.3.3.2.2 Data collection?
10.3.3.2.3 Analysis of the results?

10.3.3.3 Does the NHA encourage the use of research findings by the subnational levels to improve public health practice?

If so,
10.3.3.3.1 Can you cite an example of such a use in the past two years?

EPHF 11: Reducing the Impact of Emergencies and Disasters on Health[13]

Definition:
This function includes:

- Policy development, planning and execution of activities in the prevention, mitigation, preparedness, early response and rehabilitation programs to reduce the impact of disasters on public health.
- An integrated approach with respect to the damage and etiology of any and all emergencies and disasters that can affect the country.
- Involvement of the entire health system and the broadest possible intersectoral and inter-institutional collaboration to reduce the impact of emergencies and disasters.
- The procurement of intersectoral and international collaboration to respond to health problems resulting from emergencies and disasters.

Indicators:

11.1 Emergency Preparedness and Disaster Management in Health

Standard:
The NHA:

- Promotes an understanding of social and health benefits that reduce the impact of emergencies and disasters in all sectors, including the private sector and the community.
- Facilitates intra- and intersectoral coordination in implementing measures that reduce the impact of disasters and emergencies on the health infrastructure (health services, water and sanitation systems); these include prevention, mitigation, preparedness, early response and rehabilitation as it relates to public health.
- Trains both health and non-health workers alike in the reduction impact of emergencies and disasters on health.
- Protects against various threats to physical and operational infrastructure (e.g. hospitals, health centers, water and sewage systems, etc.)
- Provides public education through mass media campaigns and health education activities.

---

[13] Emergency and disaster reduction in health includes prevention, mitigation, preparedness, early response and rehabilitation.

11.1.1 The NHA has an national institutional plan for reducing the impact of emergencies and disasters on health.

11.1.1.1 Is the emergency component of the national health sector plan part of the national emergency plan?

11.1.1.2 Does the plan include a national map of risks, threats and vulnerability to emergencies and disasters?

11.1.1.3 Does the national plan for the health sector include subnational plans?

11.1.1.4 Is there a unit within the NHA dedicated to emergency preparedness and disaster management in health?

If so,

11.1.1.4.1 Does the NHA have an emergency and disaster unit with its own budget?

11.1.2 The NHA acts as coordinator for the entire health sector in the implementation of emergency and disaster preparedness measures.

Does the NHA:

11.1.2.1 Have a communications network in place that functions in emergencies?

If so,

11.1.2.1.1. Are the operations of this communications network periodically evaluated?

11.1.2.2 Have a transport system in place to function in emergencies and disasters?

If so,

11.1.2.2.1 Are the operations of this transportation system periodically evaluated?

11.1.3 The NHA provides training to its health workers in emergency and disaster preparedness.

Is the NHA's personnel trained:

11.1.3.1 To develop guidelines that deal with emergencies and disasters within the health sector?

11.1.3.2 To coordinate activities within the health sector?

11.1.3.3 To coordinate activities with other sectors?

11.1.3.4 In the prevention and control of communicable and noncommunicable diseases resulting from an emergency or disaster?

11.1.3.5 In the protection against mental illness resulting from an emergency or disaster?

11.1.3.6 To ensure food safety following disasters?

11.1.3.7 In sanitation and environmental health following disasters?

11.1.3.8 To undertake vector control in emergencies?

11.1.3.9 To manage health services in emergencies?

11.1.3.10 To carry out emergency simulation exercises?

11.1.3.11 To conduct rapid risk and needs assessments?

11.1.3.12 To request, obtain and distribute critical equipment/and health supplies for emergencies and disasters?

11.1.3.13 In the operation of communications systems and situation rooms in emergencies?

11.1.3.14 In the operation of emergency transport systems?

11.1.3.15 To disseminate health information through mass media and other means?

11.1.3.16 To ensure transparency and efficiency in the administration of post-disaster aid?

11.1.3.17 In the preparation of emergency rehabilitation projects for the health sector?

11.1.4 The NHA implements strategies to include emergency preparedness and disaster management components in professional education.

Does the NHA:

11.1.4.1 Collaborate with health science schools to include emergency preparedness and disaster management components in the curriculum?

11.1.4.2 Collaborate with the schools of public health to include emergency preparedness and disaster management components in the curriculum?

11.1.4.3 Collaborate with schools related to health to include emergency preparedness and disaster management components in the curriculum?

11.2 Development of Standards and Guidelines that Support Emergency Preparedness and Disaster Management in Health

Standard:

The NHA:

- Prepares standards and guidelines for constructing, updating and maintaining health infrastructure and services, with emphasis on emergency and disaster preparedness and the reduction of physical and organizational vulnerability.
- Develops and maintain norms and standards for health facilities in areas prone to disasters.
- Produces lists of essential drugs and other health supplies necessary in emergencies and disasters.
- Participates in the development of guidelines for the health components of emergency plans.
- Develops and promotes standards and guidelines to support preparedness in emergencies and disasters, particularly outbreaks of communicable disease.

11.2.1 The NHA implements strategies to reduce the impact of emergencies and disasters on health.

Does the NHA:

11.2.1.1. Develop sanitation standards for the national emergency plan?

11.2.1.2. Develop standards and guidelines that help prepare for the consequences of emergencies and disasters?

If so, do these standards and guidelines address:

11.2.1.2.1 Outbreaks of communicable disease?

11.2.1.2.2 Sanitation of lodgings, shelters and camps?

11.2.1.2.3 Norms and regulations for the donating essential drugs and necessary supplies?

11.2.1.2.4 Vector control?

11.2.1.2.5 Equipment, drugs and supplies necessary for emergencies and disasters?

11.2.1.2.6 Basic sanitation?

11.2.1.2.7 Food security and safety?

11.2.1.2.8 Mental health in emergencies?

11.2.1.2.9 Construction and maintenance of health infrastructure and services?

If so, do the standards and guidelines on constructing and maintaining the health infrastructure refer to:

11.2.1.2.9.1 Hospital services?

11.2.1.2.9.2 Outpatient services?

11.2.1.2.9.3 Water services?

11.2.1.2.9.4 Solid waste services?

11.2.1.3 Develop standards and guidelines to deal with the consequences of emergencies and disasters?

If so, do the standards and guidelines take into account:

11.2.1.3.1 The physical infrastructure of the health facilities?

11.2.1.3.2 The management of health facilities and organizations in emergency and disaster situations?

11.2.1.3.3 Health services delivery in emergencies?

If so, does the health service delivery ensure:

11.2.1.3.3.1 The availability and distribution of personnel?

11.2.1.3.3.2 Alternative ways of operating critical care units?

11.2.1.3.3.3 Criteria for setting priorities that meet the demand for emergency care services?

11.3 Coordination and Partnerships with other Agencies and/or Institutions in Emergencies and Disasters

Standard:
The NHA:

- Coordinates and collaborates with the national civil defense agency or other agencies with multisectoral responsibilities.
- Coordinates other key disaster entities, units or commissions.
- Collaborates and coordinates with the existing health sector emergency and disaster programs of other countries in the region.
- Establishes and maintains partnerships with national subnational and international organizations that deal with emergencies.
- Works with other agencies to develop protocols necessary for communication.

11.3.1 The NHA coordinates with other agencies or institutions to reduce the impact of emergencies and disasters.

Do these other agencies/institutions include:

11.3.1.1 National emergency offices?

11.3.1.2 Subnational emergency offices?

11.3.1.3 The transportation sector?

11.3.1.4 The public works sector?

11.3.1.5 The housing sector?

11.3.1.6 The telecommunications sector?

11.3.1.7 The education sector?

11.3.1.8 The Ministry of Foreign Relations?

11.3.1.9 The police and armed forces?

11.3.1.10 Fire departments?

11.3.1.11 The Area Coordinator for the United Nations?

11.3.1.12 UN Children's Fund (UNICEF)?

11.3.1.13 UN High Commissioner for Human Rights (OHCHR)?

11.3.1.14 UN High Commissioner for Refugees (UNHCR)?

11.3.1.15 Food and Agriculture Organization (FAO)?

11.3.1.16 Pan American Health Organization (PAHO)?

11.3.1.17 The National Red Cross? Red Cross Federation (RCF)? Red Cross Committee (RCC)?

11.3.1.18 Professional associations?

11.3.1.19 Other nongovernmental organizations?

11.3.1.20 Other agencies or commissions?

11.3.1.21 Does it coordinate with the national civil defense or other agencies with multisectoral responsibilities?

If so,

11.3.1.21.1 Do the agencies and institutions work together to develop the necessary protocols to disseminate information through the mass media?

11.3.1.22 Does the NHA establish and maintain international partnerships to deal with emergencies?

If so, does the NHA:

11.3.1.22.1 Collaborate and coordinate with existing health sector emergency and disaster programs of other neighboring countries?

11.3.1.22.2 Collaborate and coordinate with national, subnational and international organizations and institutions that deal with emergency and disaster preparedness?

11.4 Technical Assistance and Support to the Subnational Level to Reduce the Impact of Emergencies and Disasters on Health

Standard
The NHA:

- Promotes, provides and facilitates technical assistance to the subnational levels to build local capacity for mobilizing and coordinating efforts that reduce the impact of emergencies and disasters on health.
- Provides support to the subnational levels to build capacity for intersectoral collaboration in emergencies and establishes links with emergency service providers.
- Helps to identify leaders who will promote efforts that reduce the impact of emergencies at the local level.
- Establishes standards and guidelines to reduce the impact of emergencies and disasters at the subnational levels.
- Provides technical assistance to the subnational levels to conduct a needs assessment with respect to reducing the impact of emergencies and disasters on health, as well as contributes resources necessary to strengthen areas of weakness in the capacity to respond to them in a timely manner.

11.4.1 The NHA helps the subnational levels to reduce the health impact of emergencies and disasters.

Does the NHA:

11.4.1.1 Facilitate technical assistance to the local levels to strengthen local capacity to mobilize activities in emergencies or disasters?

11.4.1.2 Support the subnational levels in strengthening local capacity to collaborate with other sectors in emergencies or disasters?

11.4.1.3 Help the subnational level establish links with other local emergency service providers?

If so, are these emergency services in:
11.4.1.3.1 Health?
11.4.1.3.2 Other sectors?

11.4.2 The NHA collaborates with the subnational levels to build capacity for reducing the impact of emergencies and disasters on health.

Does this collaboration include:

11.4.2.1 Assistance to the subnational levels in identifying local leaders to promote efforts aimed at reducing the impact of emergencies or disasters on health?

11.4.2.2 Design of standards and guidelines at the subnational levels for emergency preparedness and disaster management?

11.4.2.3 Definition of the responsibilities for each level in emergencies or disasters?

11.4.2.4 Analysis of the vulnerability of the health infrastructure for which these levels are responsible in emergencies and disasters?

11.4.2.5 Preparation of emergency and disaster risk maps for these levels?

11.4.2.6 Needs assessment at the subnational levels?

Does the NHA provide:
11.4.2.6.1 The necessary assistance to correct any deficiencies identified by such an assessment?

11.4.2.6.2 The necessary resources to correct deficiencies identified by such an assessment?

APPENDIX B

Sample National Measurement Report

Executive Report

Background

The Directing Council of the Pan American Health Organization (PAHO) approved an initiative aimed at strengthening public health in the Americas and improving the practice of public health, as well as strengthening the steering role of health authorities at all levels of the State by defining and measuring the performance of essential public health functions (EPHF). This has improved the dialogue between the actors in the field of health and those of related disciplines at various levels in the Region.[1]

The national authorities measured performance of the EPHF using the instrument designed for this purpose and held a workshop to discuss the experi-

ences and opinions of the participating professionals from relevant public areas of health in Country X.[2]

For its application in Country X, the process and measurement instrument were submitted for the consideration of a group of decisionmakers at the NHA in order conduct an exercise to measure the performance of EPHF.[3] This exercise took place between X and X and involved the participation of a large group of professionals from various areas of public health in the country.

The event was organized by the Ministry of Health of X, with the collaboration of the PAHO/WHO Representative Office in that country and of the Division of Health Systems and Services Development of PAHO. It was strongly backed by the Minister of Health, who pledged his support for this initiative, which seeks to strengthen

the public health services infrastructure in the country and the Region.

Description of the Process

The Ministry of Health of Country X, in collaboration with the local PAHO/WHO Representative Office, held a workshop to coordinate and organize the preparatory phases of the EPHF measurement exercise.

The PAHO/WHO Representative Office in Country X, with the cooperation of authorities from the Ministry of Health, coordinated and organized the workshop on application of the instrument to measure the EPHF. The Ministry of Health and PAHO likewise decided to hold a training workshop for national facilitators who would be those responsible for the definitive application of the EPHF performance measurement instrument.

X representatives from the National Health Authority participated in the

---

[1] Resolution CD42.R14. Essential Public Health Functions. 42nd Directing Council of PAHO. Washington, DC, 25 to 29 September 2000.

[2] The list of participants in the event is presented as an Annex.
[3] Id.

training workshop for facilitators, which resulted in the formation of a local team that was prepared to continue the process and support the exercise.

Application of the Instrument

X professionals (including health personnel, academicians, and other specialists) were selected and convened by the Ministry of Health, worked throughout the X days of the exercise. X groups were formed, distributing the professionals in accordance with their profiles and experience in specific operations.

Each group was supported by a local facilitator (who helped build consensus for a group response), a secretary (who kept track of the responses and confirmed the degree of consensus in the group), and a technical assistant (who recorded the responses). At the same time, an external facilitator from PAHO contributed to the effort by obtaining the comments and suggestions of the participants to refine the terminology or make editorial improvements to the instrument.

The mechanics of the exercise involved having each facilitator read out loud the definition, standards, measures, and submeasures of each function the group was to discuss. The external facilitator, supported by the local facilitator from the Ministry, ensured that the result of the voting reflected a consensus by the participating group.

Results of the Measurement

Description of the Scoring and Measurement Mechanism

The score for each indicator that was part of the measurement for each func-

tion is based on the score obtained by the variable being measured.

The questions for the measures and submeasures allow for only a "Yes" or "No" response. It is therefore important to understand how the collective response to each measure and submeasure was obtained. For the purposes of this exercise, it was determined that if a response could not be agreed on in a group discussion, or if a second round of voting yielded another tie, then the response would automatically be "No" due to the existing uncertainty.

In order to record and process the results of the responses, a computer program was used to tally the final score of each question directly and instantaneously, as a function of the responses to its measures and submeasures. This calculation of the final score of every variable is essentially the average of the affirmative responses to the measures and submeasures, except in the case of the exceptions mentioned in the instrument.

The score assigned to the indicator is the weighted average of the results obtained for each of the respective measures, and the simple weighted average of the results of all the indicators determines the score for the performance of that particular essential public health function.

Since this was the first time the EPHF were measured in the Region, a uniform scoring method was used, in which all the essential functions, indicators, and measures have the same relative weight. Lending the same degree of consideration to all the measurements facilitates the analysis and subsequent decisions by the country.

As a convention, the following scale is proposed as a guide for the overall interpretation:

76 – 100%   (0.76 to 1.0)
Quartile of optimal performance

51 – 75%   (0.51 to 0.75)
Quartile of above average performance

26 – 50%   (0.26 to 0.50)
Quartile of below average performance

0 – 25%   (0.0 to 0.25)
Quartile of minimum performance

In the final plenary session of the workshop, the results of the EPHF performance measurement were shared with the participants in order to identify areas of intervention, focusing on processes and results, and decentralized capacities, infrastructure, and competencies.

This was considered to be the most useful and important part of the measurement process, because it gave the participants an opportunity to express their opinions and revealed strengths and weaknesses. Thus, it was possible for the NHA to design an institutional development plan to improve the EPHF in its immediate sphere of influence.

Overall Analysis of Results

The results of the exercise were analyzed by the competent authorities of Country X, taking into account the unique characteristics and circumstances of the exercise of the essential public health functions established by the health authorities. It should also be noted that in interpreting the results, it might be necessary to compensate for possible biases in the groups analyzing each function.

Figure 1   Results of the Measurement by Function[4]

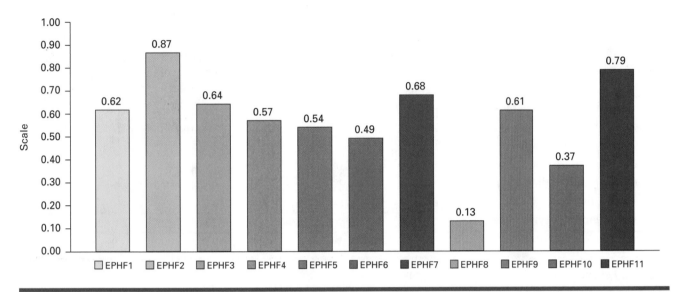

The figure 1 provides an overview of the performance of each of the 11 EPHF in Country X.

This overview of the performance of the 11 essential public health functions measured by the instrument shows high levels for EPHF 2 (Public Health Surveillance, Research, and Control of Risks and Threats to Public Health), for EPHF 7 (Evaluation and Promotion of Equitable Access to Necessary Health Services), and for EPHF 11 (Reducing the Impact of Emergencies and Disasters on Health). Medium performance levels were seen for EPHF 1 (Monitoring, Evaluation and Analysis of Health Status), for EPHF 3 (Health Promotion), for EPHF 5 (Development of Policies and Institutional Capacity for Planning and Management in Public Health) and for EPHF 4 (Social Participation in Health). The lowest levels were observed for EPHF 6 (Strengthening of Institutional Capacity for Regulation and Enforcement of Public

Health), for EPHF 8 (Human Resources Development and Training in Public Health), and for EPHF 10 (Research in Public Health). The internal structure of each of these functions will be analyzed in greater detail further on.

It is important to note in this report that both the highest and lowest scores described in the overall analysis should be studied with extreme care, avoiding the drawing of conclusions about the degree of importance of each score when the NHA makes health decisions. Actually, a high-scoring function could show that what remains to be done to achieve a score of 100% is extremely important in high-level decision-making.

Moreover, low scores could reflect a low degree of performance in certain key areas of the measurement instrument that may not necessarily coincide with priorities in the health policy of Country X.

In the overall performance analysis of the 11 EPHF (figure 1), the results for EPHF 2 (Public Health Surveillance,

Research, and Control of Risks and Threats to Public Health) were the highest. This could be interpreted as the result of the importance the country has placed on surveillance, in terms of both training and operations.

The function with the second highest score was Function 11 (Reducing the Impact of Emergencies and Disasters on Health). The group that analyzed it had little knowledge of the subject, and the issue of evacuating the population directly involved in these situations dominated the discussion. This is an example of possible biases that, as noted above, make it necessary to exercise caution in interpreting the results.

At the other end of the spectrum, the very low score in Function 8 (Human Resources Development and Training in Public Health) may reflect the manifest dissatisfaction by the group with the conditions for staff development.

Function 10 (Research in Public Health) also received a score that places it in the below-average performance quartile,

[4] The list of the essential public health functions is presented as an Appendix.

which might reflect concerns over the apparently little attention devoted to research.

The low score assigned to each of these EPHF 8 and 10 might reflect neglect of investments in human capital and the scientific apparatus to sustain the development of public health in the country. This hypothesis would warrant a more exhaustive analysis within the context of a process aimed at improving public health, given the medium- and long-term implications of investment in this area.

Likewise, Function 6 (Strengthening of Institutional Capacity for Regulation and Enforcement in Public Health) scored in the below-average performance quartile. This explains the concern manifested even before the beginning of the exercise about including additional aspects of regulation, specifically with regard to insurance companies.

What can be deduced from the scores obtained in these three Functions (6, 8, and 10) is that they can be used to identify certain gaps or weaknesses that might warrant priority attention from the health authority.

In general, the remaining functions obtained scores that place them in the quartile of above-average performance, not the optimum described as the final objective of the process.

In order to delve further into the analysis of the results, the figures on the profile of indicators for each function are provided below, accompanied by comments. It should be noted that the remarks on these results were made during the workshop and were a first attempt at analysis. They reflect the

EPHF 1 Monitoring, Analysis and Evaluation of the Health Situation of the Population

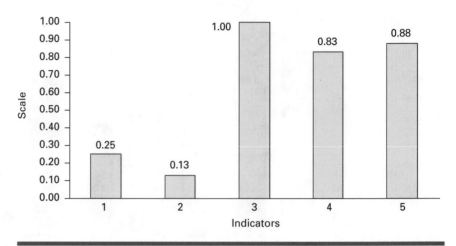

Indicators:
1. Guidelines and processes for monitoring health status
2. Evaluation of the quality of information.
3. Expert support and resources for monitoring health status.
4. Technical support for monitoring and evaluating health status.
5. Technical assistance and support to the subnational levels of public health.

conclusions reached by the different groups during the exercise.

What is striking in this profile are the low scores of the first two indicators, which describe the process and outcome of the monitoring, analysis, and evaluation of the health situation, notwithstanding the fact that the institutional capacity to exercise this function well is considered to be optimal (indicators 3, 4 and 5). This could be interpreted as an institutional management problem, rather than one of resources and infrastructure.

As noted in the overall analysis, the score for this function indicated virtually optimal performance, a result of the high scores for each indicator. It is worth asking whether some degree of bias might have been present in the group that did the analysis it. In any

case, there is a marked consistency in the positive results.

Contrary to what was seen in Function 1, here it seems that the analysis was favorable to one of the processes involved: the process carried out within the organization of the health services, notwithstanding the recognition that there is little development of decentralized capacity for the exercise of this function (Indicator 5).

It should be noted that the processes involving the work of the health authority outside the sector (Indicators 2 and 3) obtained a moderately unsatisfactory score. This may pose a challenge to the health authority in terms of strengthening its leadership in the extrasectoral dynamic affecting the quality of life; to some extent it explains the interest expressed prior to

EPHF 2 Public Health Surveillance, Research, and Control of Risks and Harm to Public Health

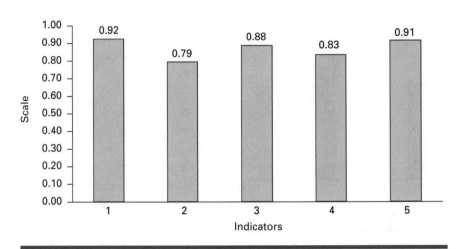

Indicators:
1. Surveillance system to identify threats and harm to public health.
2. Capacities and expertise in public health surveillance.
3. Capacity of public health laboratories.
4. Capacity for timely and effective response to control public health problems.
5. Technical assistance and technical support for the subnational levels of public health.

EPHF 3 Health Promotion

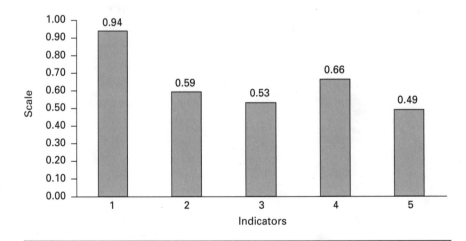

Indicators:
1. Support for health promotion activities, the development of norms, and interventions to promote healthy behaviors and environments.
2. Building of sectoral and extrasectoral partnerships for health promotion.
3. National planning and coordination of information, education, and social communication strategies for health promotion.
4. Reorientation of the health services toward health promotion.
5. Technical assistance and support to the subnational levels to strengthen health promotion activities.

the meeting to further promote the determinants of the quality of life, which was proposed as a potential area for expansion in the instrument.

As with the first function, the exercise reveals a remarkably high degree of dissatisfaction with performance, in contrast to the recognition of the effort to improve the decentralized capacity to carry out the two processes implied in this function.

Despite the unsatisfactory performance in both processes, it might be interesting to delve further into the considerable difference in the scores for citizen empowerment and social participation.

The profile for this function reveals weaknesses in the development of the institutional capacity for management, in contrast to the moderately satisfactory performance in defining objectives and public health policies; it also reveals a low score with regard to strengthening the subnational levels for decentralized planning and management.

If these deficiencies actually do exist, they might explain the performance gap between some processes and the available installed capacity, as noted in Functions 1, 4, 7, and 10.

The deficiencies in this Function refer to the health authority's capacities and the exercise of its inspection and enforcement roles, in tandem with its regulatory role.

The little effort recognized for strengthening regulatory and enforcement capacities at the subnational levels is noteworthy; this could warrant in-depth analysis, given its implications for the exercise of the steering role of health

EPHF 4   Citizen Participation in Health

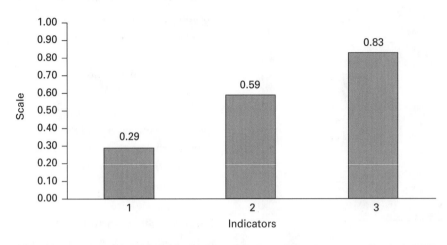

Indicators:
1. Empowering citizens for decision-making in public health.
2. Strengthening of social participation in health.
3. Technical assistance and support to the subnational levels to strengthen social participation in health.

EPHF 5   Development of Policies and Institutional Capacity for Planning and Management in Public Health

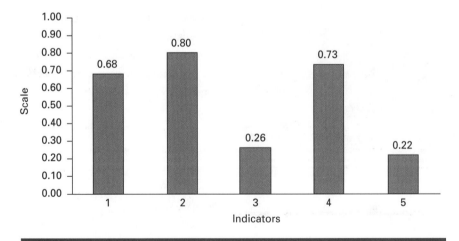

Indicators:
1. Definition of national and subnational health objectives.
2. Development, monitoring, and evaluation of public health policies.
3. Development of institutional capacity for the management of public health systems.
4. Negotiation of international cooperation in public health.
5. Technical assistance and support to the subnational levels for policy development, planning, and management in public health.

and the territorial expanse and demographic diversity of the country.

The profile of this function reflects, yet again, the aforementioned gap between the exercise of processes and the abilities to perform them.

Also evident is the remarkable difference between satisfaction with advocacy for improving access and dissatisfaction with knowledge of the conditions of access and possible interventions to improve access. It would be advisable to analyze these in depth. Furthermore, it is evident that the efforts to strengthen decentralized capabilities to address problems of access are regarded as optimal.

The profile of this function reflects the national evaluation group's strong dissatisfaction with the performance of the health authority in human resource development. There is a remarkably low score for continuing education efforts and for support to the subnational levels.

It would be necessary to provide a context and perform an in-depth analysis of the results in these five indicators in order to validate their objectivity and understand the underlying factors if a pertinent intervention strategy is to be developed.

Once more, there is a clear asymmetry between the normative processes (Indicator 1) and the executive processes (Indicators 2 and 3), with the latter lagging behind. Also evident is the occasional disjunction between the quality-assurance capacity at the decentralized levels and the action taken to improve user satisfaction.

These are clear examples indicating that the analysis of the exercise of these

FESP 6 Strengthening of Institutional Capacity for Regulation and Enforcement in Public Health

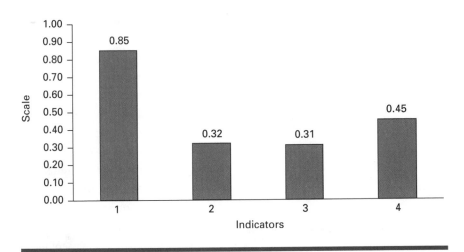

Indicators:
1. Periodic monitoring, evaluation, and modification of the regulatory framework.
2. Enforcement of laws and regulations.
3. Knowledge, skills, and mechanisms for reviewing, improving, and enforcing the regulations.
4. Technical assistance and support to the subnational levels of public health in developing and enforcing laws and regulations.

EPHF 7 Evaluation and Promotion of Equitable Access to Necessary Health Services

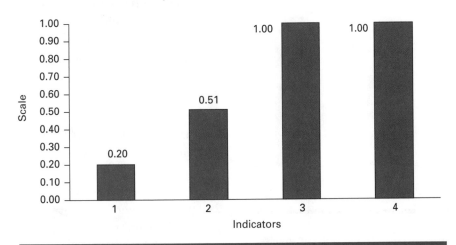

Indicadores:
1. Monitoring and evaluation of access to necessary health services.
2. Knowledge, skills, and mechanisms for improving access by the population to necessary health services.
3. Advocacy and action to improve access to necessary health services.
4. Technical assistance and support to the subnational levels to promote equitable access to health services.

functions should rely on in-depth knowledge of the national situation and be geared to identifying determinants for the preparation of pertinent intervention strategies.

As noted above, this function yet again reflects the gap between installed capacity and its utilization in research.

The low score for the indicators of this function may reflect limited efforts by the health authority to support the process of generating knowledge, implementing a national research agenda, or making use of the research findings of other actors.

More in-depth analysis may be called for with regard to possible relationships between the low results obtained in Function 8 (human resources development) and this research function.

The profile of this function reflects yet again the gap between the normative (Indicator 2) and executive (Indicator 1) capacities, and between developed capacity and its utilization in work processes. Given the characteristics of the group that analyzed it and the knowledge available to it, a review of the results obtained in previous iterations of the instrument is recommended.

Identification of Priority Intervention Areas for the Institutional Development Plan

In preparing a plan to develop the institutional capacity of the health authorities to improve the exercise of the EFPH pertaining to them (the immediate objective of this exercise in perform-

EPHF 8 Human Resources Development and Training in Public Health

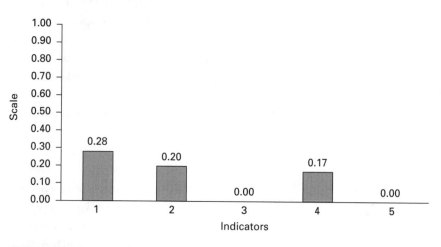

Indicators:
1. Description of the public health workforce.
2. Improving the quality of the workforce.
3. Continuing education and graduate training in public health.
4. Upgrading human resources to ensure culturally appropriate delivery of services.
5. Technical assistance and support to the subnational levels in human resources development.

EPHF 9 Ensuring the Quality of Personal and Population-based Health Services

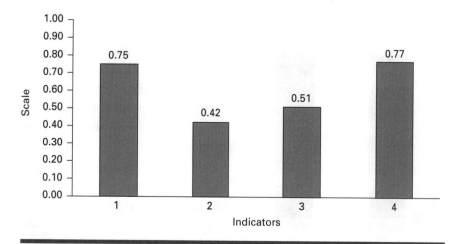

Indicators:
1. Definition of standards and evaluation to improve the quality of population-based and personal health services.
2. Improving user satisfaction with the health services.
3. Systems for technological management and health technology assessment to support decision-making in public health.
4. Technical assistance and support to the subnational levels to ensure quality improvement in the services.

ance measurement), two basic premises have been observed:

1) Development efforts should be institutional in nature. This implies a comprehensive approach, rather than isolated interventions targeting the actors and areas of each function. To this end, all the functions have been merged into three strategic intervention areas:

- **Final achievement of outcomes and key processes**, the substantive component of the work of the health authority in public health, and thus, the primary goal of interventions to improve performance.

- **Development of capacities and infrastructure**, understood as the human, technology, knowledge, and resources situation necessary for the optimal exercise of the public health functions appertaining to the health authority.

- **Development of decentralized competences**, in terms of faculties and capacities directed to supporting the subnational levels or to transferring responsibilities to them, so as to strengthen the decentralized exercise of the health authority with regard to public health, consistent with the requirements of State modernization and sectoral reform.

2) Interventions for institutional development must seek to overcome *weaknesses* by taking advantage of *strengths*. In order to rate performance in the different indicators as strengths or weaknesses, a *reference value* is needed; this needs to be

EPHF 10   Research in Public Health

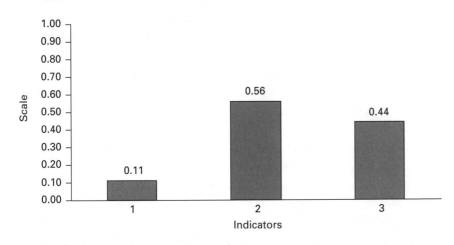

Indicators:
1. Development of a public health research agenda.
2. Development of institutional research capacity.
3. Technical assistance and support for research in public health at the subnational levels.

EPHF 11   Reducing the Impact of Emergencies and Disasters on Health

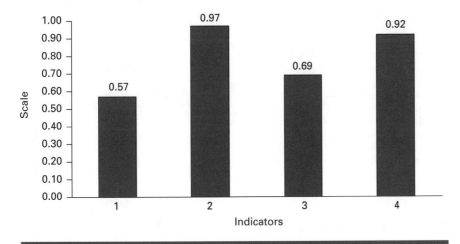

Indicators:
1. Reducing the impact of emergencies and disasters.
2. Development of standards and guidelines that support emergency preparedness and disaster management in health.
3. Coordination and partnerships with other agencies and/or institutions.
4. Technical assistance and support to the subnational levels to reduce the impact of emergencies and disasters on health.

identified for each country at different points in the process, as a function of the level of performance and development goals. The basic criteria for establishing the reference values are: a) that the weaknesses diagnosed not be accepted or consolidated and, b) that they represent an achievable challenge and a reasonable incentive for continuing efforts at improvement.

Nevertheless, for the purposes of these pioneering applications of the instrument, and in order to facilitate consolidation of the results of all the evaluations in the countries of the Region (with a view to formulating a regional plan of action), as a convention, the reference value has been set as the average of the overall results in the 11 functions. The majority of deficiencies thus remain qualified as weaknesses to be overcome.

The workshop discussed whether the reference value for X should be 50% or more. The view was that on this occasion the country's track record and national public health resources warranted raising the value closer to 70%. In any case, this presentation of results uses the reference value adopted for the regional exercise, without prejudice to the future ability of the national authorities to change it when preparing their development plan.

What follows is the classification of the indicators as strengths or weaknesses resulting from the application of the aforementioned reference value, along with comments, for example, on possible areas for priority intervention in the three components of institutional development that have been identified.

The main weaknesses that the priority interventions should probably focus on in order to improve the processes and results of the exercise of the essential public health functions corresponding to the health authority would be, first, those related to developing human resources and the research agenda and improving the quality of information used in monitoring and evaluating the health situation and access. These were indicated as being in the range of minimum performance. Second would be those involving empowerment of the citizens, communication for health promotion and the improvement of user satisfaction, inspection activities to enforce existing regulations, and management to reduce the impact of emergencies and disasters.

The interventions to improve processes and outcomes are generally of a managerial type. They involve adopting measures for installed capacity to be used more efficiently and to improve operations and results. Such actions can be based on the identified strengths in areas related to these weaknesses, such as: operation of the surveillance and response system for the control of public health problems (this can serve as a reference to improve monitoring and evaluation of the health situation). For example, the development of standards and promotional interventions should serve as the basis for improving communication strategies for promotion; social participation actions could be used to empower citizens in decision-making. Obviously, implementation of the regulations must be the starting point for actions aimed at improving regulatory enforcement.

The main weaknesses that the priority interventions to develop human, technical and infrastructure capacities

---

Area of Intervention   Final Achievement of Results and Key processes

EPHF		Indicators	Classification	
1	1.1	Guidelines and processes for monitoring health status	0.25	D
1	1.2	Evaluation of the quality of information	0.13	D
2	2.1	Surveillance system to identify threats and harm to public health.	0.92	F
2	2.4	Capacity for timely and effective response to control public health problems	0.83	F
3	3.1	Support for health promotion activities, the development of norms, and interventions to promote healthy behaviors and environments	0.94	F
3	3.2	Building of sectoral and extrasectoral partnerships for health promotion	0.59	F
3	3.3	National planning and coordination of information, education, and social communication strategies for health promotion	0.53	D
3	3.4	Reorientation of the health services toward health promotion	0.66	F
4	4.1	Empowering citizens for decision-making in public health	0.29	D
4	4.2	Strengthening of social participation in health	0.59	F
5	5.1	Definition of national and subnational health objectives	0.68	F
5	5.2	Development, monitoring, and evaluation of public health policies	0.80	F
6	6.1	Periodic monitoring, evaluation, and modification of the regulatory framework	0.85	F
6	6.2	Enforcement of laws and regulations	0.35	D
7	7.1	Monitoring and evaluation of access to necessary health services	0.20	D
7	7.3	Advocacy and action to improve access to necessary health services	1.00	F
8	8.1	Description of the public health workforce	0.28	D
8	8.2	Improving the quality of the work force	0.20	D
8	8.3	Continuing education and graduate training in public health	0.00	D
8	8.4	Upgrading of human resources to ensure culturally appropriate delivery of services	0.17	D
9	9.1	Definition of standards and evaluation to improve the quality of population-based and personal health services	0.75	F
9	9.2	Improving user satisfaction with the health services	0.42	D
10	10.1	Development of a public health research agenda	0.11	D
11	11.1	Reducing the impact of emergencies and disasters	0.57	D
11	11.2	Development of standards and guidelines that support emergency preparedness and disaster management in health	0.97	F
11	11.3	Coordination and partnerships with other agencies and/or institutions	0.69	F

Final Achievement of Results and Key Processes

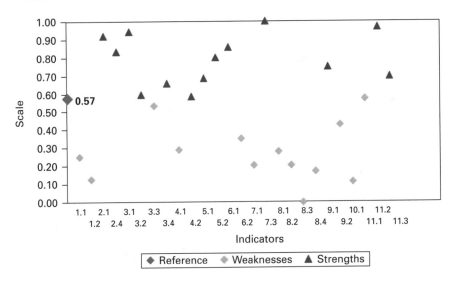

Indicators

◆ Reference   ◆ Weaknesses   ▲ Strengths

Area of Intervention   Capacity and Infrastructure Development

EPHF		Indicators	Classification	
1	1.3	Expert support and resources for monitoring health status	1.00	F
1	1.4	Technological support for the monitoring and evaluation of health status	0.83	F
2	2.2	Capacities and expertise in public health surveillance	0.79	F
2	2.3	Capacity of public health laboratories	0.88	F
5	5.3	Development of institutional capacity for the management of public health systems	0.26	D
5	5.4	Negotiation of international cooperation in public health	0.73	F
6	6.3	Knowledge, skills, and mechanisms for reviewing, improving, and enforcing the regulations	0.31	D
7	7.2	Knowledge, skills, and mechanisms for improving access by the population to programs and services	0.51	D
9	9.3	Systems for technology management and health technology assessment to support decision-making in public health	0.51	D
10	10.2	Development of institutional research capacity	0.56	D

---

should target in order to improve the processes and results of the exercise of the essential public health functions corresponding to the health authority would be, first, those related to increasing the institutional capacity of management, regulation and control, and, second, those related to improving access to the services, technology management, and research. The interventions to increase institutional capacity are more likely to involve investment in training, acquisition of expertise, and procure-

ment of technology resources to improve performance in functions where capacities are deficient.

The main weaknesses that the priority interventions related to the development of human resources and the capacity for planning and management at the subnational levels should focus on in order to improve the processes and results of the exercise of the essential public health functions corresponding to the health authority would probably

be, first, those which are in the range of minimum performance; and second, those related to technical support to the subnational levels in health promotion, research, and decentralized oversight.

Interventions in this area of institutional development generally have to do with the delegation of functions, along with the strengthening of the capacity to exercise them, and technical support from the central levels for optimal performance by the subnational levels.

Development of Capacities and Infrastructure

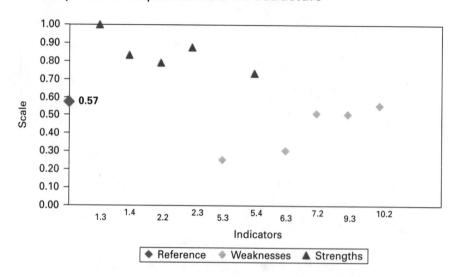

Area of Intervention   Development of Decentralized Competencies

EPHF		Indicators	Classification	
1	1.5	Technical assistance and support to the subnational levels of public health	0.88	F
2	2.5	Technical assistance and support to the subnational levels of public health	0.91	F
3	3.5	Technical assistance and support to the subnational levels to strengthen health promotion activities.	0.49	D
4	4.3	Technical assistance and support to the subnational levels to strengthen social participation in health	0.83	F
5	5.5	Technical assistance and support to the subnational levels in policy development, planning, and management in public health	0.22	D
6	6.4	Technical assistance and support to the subnational levels of public health in developing and enforcing laws and regulations	0.45	D
7	7.4	Technical assistance and support to the subnational levels of public health to promote equitable access to health services	1.00	F
8	8.5	Technical assistance and support to the subnational levels in human resources development	0.00	D
9	9.4	Technical assistance and support to the subnational levels of health to ensure quality improvement in the services	0.77	F
10	10.3	Technical assistance and support for research in public health at the subnational levels	0.44	D
11	11.4	Technical assistance and support to the subnational levels to reduce the impact of emergencies and disasters on health	0.92	F

Conclusion

The test application in X was a success, as reflected in the strong interest and motivation of the participants and their contributions to improve the instrument, based on their professional expertise and the shared experience in issues pertaining to the EFPH.

This experience will be of assistance in adapting the measurement instrument and improving the methodology for applying it, pursuant to the resolution of the Directing Council of PAHO. It is furthermore assumed that it will serve the country as a baseline for future implementation and evaluation activities.

Development of Decentralized Competencies

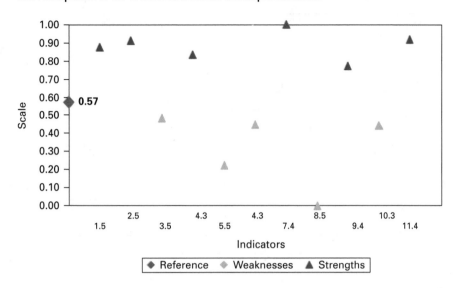

Annex 1   List of Essential Public Health Functions

Essential Public Health Functions

EPHF 1   Monitoring, Evaluation, and Analysis of the Health Situation of the Population

EPHF 2   Public Health Surveillance, Research, and Control of Risks and Harm to Public Health

EPHF 3   Health Promotion

EPHF 4   Citizen Participation in Health

EPHF 5   Development of Policies and Institutional Capacity for Planning and Management in Public Health

EPHF 6   Strengthening of Institutional Capacity for Regulation and Enforcement in Public Health

EPHF 7   Evaluation and Promotion of Equitable Access to Necessary Health Services

EPHF 8   Human Resources Development and Training in Public Health

EPHF 9   Quality Assurance in Personal and Population-based Health Services

EPHF 10   Research in Public Health

EPHF 11   Reducing the Impact of Emergencies and Disasters on Health[1]

[1] Reducing emergencies and disasters in health includes prevention, mitigation, preparedness, response, and rehabilitation.

Annex II   List of Participants in the Workshop

No.	Name	Position and Institution
1		
2		
3		
4		
5		
6		
7		
8		
9		
10		
11		
12		
13		
14		
15		
16		
17		
18		
19		
20		
21		
22		
23		
24		
25		
26		
27		
28		
29		
30		
31		
32		
33		
34		
35		
36		
37		
38		
39		
40		
41		
42		
43		
44		
45		

Essential Function No. 1: Monitoring, Evaluation and Analysis of Health Status

	FINAL SCORE EPHF No. 1	0.00

1.1 Guidelines and Processes for Monitoring Health Status		**0.00**

1.1.1	*Has the NHA developed guidelines for measuring and evaluating the population's health status?*	*0.00*
	Have the guidelines or other instruments for monitoring health status:	
1.1.1.1	Been developed for use by the health system at the national level?	0
1.1.1.2	Been developed for use by the health system at intermediate levels?	0
1.1.1.3	Been developed for use by the health system at local levels?	0
1.1.1.4	Described suitable methods for collecting data and selecting appropriate sources of information which provide that data?	0
1.1.1.5	Described the roles of the national and subnational levels in collecting data?	0
1.1.1.6	Provided access to information by civil society and organized community groups in a manner that protects the individual's privacy?	0
1.1.1.7	Included a process that continuously improves information systems to better meet user needs at both national and subnational levels (decision-makers, program directors, etc.)?	0
	If so, does the process:	
1.1.1.7.1	Include uniform standards at all levels (national and subnational) of the information system?	0
1.1.1.7.2	Include procedures that provide information to national and international agencies that form part of the health system?	0
1.1.1.7.3	Include a periodic review of standards and procedures that evaluate their relevance in view of the technological advances and changes in health policy?	0
1.1.1.8	Described procedures for communicating information to the mass media and general public?	0
1.1.1.9	Protected the confidentiality of information through the use of specific protocols for accessing data?	0
1.1.1.10	Described the procedures to organize a health status profile that contains information on national health objectives?	0

1.1.2	*Does the NHA identify and annually update the data collected in a country health status profile?*	*0.00*
	Does this profile include:	
1.1.2.1	Social and demographic variables?	0
1.1.2.2	Mortality data?	0
1.1.2.3	Morbidity data?	0
1.1.2.4	Data on risk factors?	0
1.1.2.5	Information on lifestyles?	0
1.1.2.6	Data on environmental risks?	0
1.1.2.7	Data on access to personal health services?	0
1.1.2.8	Data on contact with population-based health services?	0
1.1.2.9	Data on utilization of population-based and personal health services?	0
1.1.2.10	Data on cultural barriers in accessing health care?	0

1.1.3	*Does the NHA use the health status profile:*	*0.00*
1.1.3.1	To monitor the health needs of the population?	0
1.1.3.2	To evaluate inequities in health conditions?	0
1.1.3.3	To monitor trends in health status?	0
1.1.3.4	To monitor changes in the prevalence of risk factors?	0
1.1.3.5	To monitor changes in utilization of health services?	0
1.1.3.6	To determine the adequacy and significance of reported data?	0
1.1.3.7	To identify the population's priorities and needs in terms of access to services, participation in health promotion activities, resource allocation, focusing on the elimination of inequities in access and improving health services?	0
1.1.3.8	To define national health objectives and goals?	0
1.1.3.9	To evaluate compliance with national health objectives and goals?	0
1.1.3.10	To improve the efficiency and quality of the health system in discharging the essential public health functions by the NHA?	0
1.1.3.11	Can you cite an example where this profile has been used?	0

1.1.4	*Does the NHA disseminate information on the health status of the population?*	*0.00*
	Does the NHA:	
1.1.4.1	Produce an annual report?	0
1.1.4.2	Disseminate this report and its information to interested parties?	0
1.1.4.3	Present this report to groups of key decision-makers in the country?	0

(continued)

1.1.4.4	Regularly organize seminars or other activities that explain and raise awareness of key decision-makers about the implications of the information on the health status of the population contained in the annual report?	0
1.1.4.5	Provide data on trends in health outcomes, comparing them with standards and goals specifically mentioned in the profile?	0
1.1.4.6	Provide communities with a common set of measures that help them make comparisons, prioritize community health problems and determine allocation of resources?	0
1.1.4.7	Periodically solicit and evaluate suggestions that improve the content, presentation and dissemination of the health profile?	0
1.1.4.8	Regularly evaluate how the recipients of the health profile report use the information?	0

1.2 Evaluation of the Quality of Information   0.00

1.2.1	*Is there a unit that evaluates the quality of the information generated by the health system?*	*0.00*
1.2.1.1	Is the unit outside the direct control of the NHA?	0
1.2.1.2	Does the unit conduct periodic audits of the information system that assesses the country's health status?	0
1.2.1.3	Does the unit suggest modifications to the system in areas recognized as being weak or in need of improvement?	0
1.2.1.4	Does the NHA take into consideration the suggestions made by the evaluation unit for improving the measurement of health status?	0

1.2.2	*Is there a national organization for statistics of which the NHA is a part?*	*0.00*

Do the NHA and the national organization for statistics:

1.2.2.1	Meet at least once a year to propose modifications to the information systems to make these systems more compatible?	0
1.2.2.2	Take the proposed modifications into account to improve the NHK's information systems?	0
1.2.2.3	Propose specific measures to improve the quality and usefulness of information from the NHA?	0
1.2.2.4	Know the percentage of medically certified deaths known? If so,	0
1.2.2.4.1	Does the NHA consider that this percentage makes the mortality data reliable?	0

1.3 Expert Support and Resources for Monitoring Health Status   0.00

1.3.1	*Does the NHA use or have access at the national level to personnel with expertise in epidemiology and statistics?*	*0.00*

Does this personnel have expertise in the following areas:

1.3.1.1	Was this personnel trained in epidemiology at the Doctoral level?	0
1.3.1.2	Sampling methodologies for collecting qualitative and quantitative data?	0
1.3.1.3	Consolidating data from various sources?	0
1.3.1.4	Data analysis?	0
1.3.1.5	Interpreting results and formulating scientifically valid conclusions based on the data analyzed?	0
1.3.1.6	Translating data into clear and useful information to produce comprehensible and well-designed documents for different audiences?	0
1.3.1.7	Design and maintenance of disease registries (e.g. cancer registries)?	0
1.3.1.8	Communicating health information to decision-makers and members of community organizations?	0
1.3.1.9	Research and quantitative analysis?	0

1.3.2	*Does the NHA use or have access to personnel with expertise in epidemiology and statistics at the intermediate levels?*	*0.00*

Does this personnel have training and expertise in the following areas:

1.3.2.1	Sampling schemes for data collection?	0
1.3.2.2	Consolidating data from various sources?	0
1.3.2.3	Data analysis?	0
1.3.2.4	Interpreting results and formulating scientifically valid conclusions based on data analyzed?	0
1.3.2.5	Translating data into clear and useful information?	0
1.3.2.6	Design and maintenance of disease registries (e.g., cancer registries)?	0
1.3.2.7	Communicating health information to the population?	0
1.3.2.8	Communicating health information to decision-makers?	0
1.3.2.9	Was this personnel trained in public health at the Master's degree level?	0

1.4 Technical Support for Monitoring and Evaluating Health Status   0.00

1.4.1	*Does the NHA utilize computer resources to monitor the population's health status?*	*0.00*

Does the NHA:

1.4.1.1	Utilize computer resources to monitor the health status of the country's population at the intermediate levels?	0
1.4.1.2	Utilize computer resources to monitor the health status of the population at the local level?	0
1.4.1.3	Have personnel trained in the use and basic maintenance of these computer resources?	0
1.4.1.4	Use a system that includes one or more computers with high-speed processors?	0

1.4.1.5	Have programs with commonly used utilities (word processors, spreadsheets, graphic design and presentation software)?	0
1.4.1.6	Have the capacity to convert data from various sources to standard formats?	0
1.4.1.7	Have a dedicated line and high-speed access to the Internet?	0
1.4.1.8	Have electronic communication with the subnational levels that generate and utilize information?	0
1.4.1.9	Have sufficient storage capacity to maintain the databases on the country's health profile?	0
1.4.1.10	Meet the design requirements for compiling vital statistics?	0
1.4.1.11	Have rapid access to specialized maintenance of the computer system?	0
1.4.1.12	Annually assess its need for upgrading its computer resources?	0
1.4.1.13	Can you give an example in which computer resources were used to monitor health status?	0

1.5	**Technical Assistance and Support to the Subnational Levels of Public Health in Monitoring, Evaluating and Analysis of Health Status**	**0.00**
1.5.1	*During the past 12 months, has the NHA advised one or more subnational levels on data collection and analysis?*	*0.00*
1.5.1.1	Has the NHA advised the subnational levels on the design of instruments for collecting relevant health data?	0
1.5.1.2	Have all subnational levels been informed of the NHK's availability to advise them on data collection methodology?	0
1.5.1.3	Have the subnational levels been informed of the NHK's availability to advise them on methodology for the analysis of data collected locally?	0
1.5.1.4	During the past 12 months, has the NHA actually advised one or more subnational levels on the methodology to analyze data collected locally?	0
1.5.2	*During the past 12 months, has the NHA constantly disseminated information periodically to users at the subnational levels?*	*0.00*
1.5.2.1	Has feedback been sought from these users of this information?	0
1.5.2.2	Have these users been advised on how to interpret these analyses?	0
1.5.2.3	During the past 12 months, has the NHA advised those responsible for producing the community health profile at the subnational levels?	0
1.5.2.3.1	Have those responsible for publishing the community health profile been informed that provisions exist to advise them on this?	0

COLOPHON

This book has been produced by the
Pan American Health Organization.
Two-thousand copies have been printed in the English language
in September 2002, in Washington, D.C., USA.